DIABETES MANAGEMENT

CLINICAL PATHWAYS, GUIDELINES, AND PATIENT EDUCATION

HEALTH & ADMINISTRATION DEVELOPMENT GROUP

Jo Gulledge
Executive Director

Shawn Beard
Research Editor

AN ASPEN PUBLICATION®
Aspen Publishers, Inc.
Gaithersburg, Maryland
1999

Library of Congress Cataloging-in-Publication Data

Diabetes management : clinical pathways, guidelines, and patient
education / Health & Administration Development Group;
Jo Gulledge, executive director; Shawn Beard, research editor.
p. cm. — (Aspen chronic disease management series)
Includes index.
ISBN: 0-8342-1703-1
1. Diabetes Handbooks, manuals, etc. 2. Medical protocols
Handbooks, manuals, etc. 3. Patient education Handbooks,
manuals, etc. I. Gulledge, Jo. II. Beard, Shawn. III. Health and
Administration Development Group (Aspen Publishers) IV. Series.
[DNLM: 1. Diabetes Mellitus—therapy. 2. Critical Pathways.
3. Patient Education. 4. Self Care.
WK 815 D5356 1999]

RC660.D4516   1999
616.4'62—dc21
DNLM/DLC
for Library of Congress
99-31853 CIP

Editorial Services: Marsha Davies

Copyright © 1999 by Aspen Publishers, Inc.

Orders: (800) 638-8437
Customer Service: (800) 234-1660

About Aspen Publishers • For more than 35 years, Aspen has been a leading professional
publisher in a variety of disciplines. Aspen's vast information resources are available in both
print and electronic formats. We are committed to providing the highest quality information
available in the most appropriate format for our customers. Visit Aspen's Internet site for more
information resources, directories, articles, and a searchable version of Aspen's full catalog,
including the most recent publications: **http://www.aspenpublishers.com**
Aspen Publishers, Inc. • The hallmark of quality in publishing
Member of the worldwide Wolters Kluwer group

Library of Congress Catalog Card Number: 99-31853
ISBN: 0-8342-1703-1

Printed in the United States of America

1 2 3 4 5

Table of Contents

Editorial Board

Claire B. Rossé, RN, BS, MBA
Founder and CEO
FutureHealth Corporation
Timonium, Maryland

Rachel Stipe, RN, BS, CPHQ
Quality Improvement/Reimbursement Specialist
Spectracare, Inc.
Louisville, Kentucky

Maura J. Sughrue, MD
Medical Director
Fairfax Family Practice Centers
Fairfax, Virginia

Warren E. Todd, MBA
Vice President, Business Development
Hastings Healthcare Group
Pennington, New Jersey

Marcus D. Wilson, PharmD
President
Health Core, Inc.
Newark, Delaware

Introduction

Disease management is based on the understanding that a small proportion of the population—individuals with chronic conditions—consumes the vast majority of health care resources. Focusing on chronic illnesses, disease management programs strive to reduce costly hospitalizations through continual, rather than episodic, care. The logic is straightforward: providing a continuum of care dramatically reduces the incidence of acute episodes requiring inpatient treatment.

Because of disease management's emphasis on continual care, effective education of patients, families, and other informal caregivers is a vital component. Providers form partnerships with patients and families, teaching them to take daily responsibility for managing disease.

Diabetes is one of several chronic disease states affecting millions of Americans. Without proper management, diabetes can lead to blindness, amputations, kidney disease, or renal failure. Because of its prevalence and gravity, it is imperative to create a disease-management program that aids clinicians in diagnosing and effectively treating the disease.

Diabetes Management provides comprehensive, detailed guidelines on all aspects of managing diabetes from the initial diagnosis in the clinical examination to the treatment strategy which may include drug therapy, lifestyle modification, and nutrition intervention. *Diabetes Management* couples these clinical guidelines with patient education handouts, which teach patients to comply with interventions, while also learning the principles of demand management: recognizing and prioritizing their health care needs. Through education, patients know when professional interventions are required, and use resources accordingly.

To ensure quick access to the information clinicians need most, *Diabetes Management* is divided into two parts.

Part I, "Managing Diabetes: Clinical Pathways and Guidelines," addresses the essentials of administering diabetes management programs, with information on developing and implementing clinical guidelines/pathways, measuring and managing outcomes, and monitoring and improving patient satisfaction. While the guidelines originate from nationally recognized sources, their purpose is to serve as a starting point for providers and payers pursuing disease management. They are meant to be adapted to meet the needs of specific populations and to be further refined for individual patients.

Part II, "Self-Management of Diabetes: Patient Education," recognizes the patient education component of disease management. Consisting entirely of large-print patient handouts, including Spanish-language patient information sheets, this section is designed for clinicians across the care continuum to distribute freely to patients. The educational materials encourage patients and their families to become active partners in managing chronic conditions.

Diabetes Management is not intended to add new information to the abundant literature relevant to disease management, but rather to extract from hundreds of publications the most sound and useful information available. The goal is to provide this information in such a manner that is concise, practical, and pertinent. To that end, *Diabetes Management* distills the traditional narrative text and presents it in a quick-read format.

Shawn K. Beard
Research Editor
Health & Administration Development Group

Acknowledgments

Creating a reference volume such as *Diabetes Management* demands tremendous effort during the development period—shaping the manual's focus, collecting and evaluating materials, and ensuring that the format is practical and easy to use.

Foremost among the people who help us fulfill these responsibilities are the editorial board members. By answering queries, providing contacts, and reviewing materials, they play an instrumental role in the development of a high quality resource.

I am grateful to all the health care facilities, organizations, individual professionals, and others who generously shared their clinical guidelines, pathways, and patient education materials with us—special thanks to Jose Arevalo, MD, Diabetes Coalition of California, Sacramento, California; Midwest Regional Medical Center, Midwest City, Oklahoma; Linda Snetselaar, Associate Professor, University of Iowa, Iowa City, Iowa; Anna M. Sousa, MS, RD, Nutrition Consultant, Howell, New Jersey; and Janet Yozura, RD, Clinical Nutrition Manager, Youville Hospital and Rehabilitation Manager, Cambridge, Massachusetts; Harvard Pilgrim Health Care, Brookline, Massachusetts; Janet Schwarz, Publisher, American Association of Diabetes Educators, Chicago, Illinois; and American Diabetes Association, Inc., Alexandria, Virginia.

In addition, this project never could have progressed from a bare-bones idea to a comprehensive resource without the untiring support of Rosemarie Cooper, Administrative Assistant; the skill of Marsha Davies, Editorial Services; and the guidance of Jo Gulledge, Executive Director, Health & Administration Development Group.

Shawn Beard
Research Editor
Health & Administration Development Group

Tracking Form

POLICY

Patient education documentation

PURPOSE

To provide interdisciplinary documentation of patient/family education

PROCEDURE

1. On admission, stamp the Tracking Form with patient's Addressograph plate and place in front of chart.
2. Within first three days of admission, have licensed nursing/therapy staff identify patient/family educational needs.
3. Read and follow directions 1–3 on the Tracking Form.
4. Fill out specific sections of the Tracking Form.

- **Document:** List of materials from manual by chapter.
- **Initial/Date Given:** As material is given, initial and date in the space provided.
- **Primary Caregiver:** Indicate who is receiving education information (the caregiver or the patient).
- **Comments:** Write comments regarding when material was reviewed (provide date/initials), with whom, and any required special needs.
- **Demonstrates Understanding of Activity:** Initial and date when primary caregiver has demonstrated understanding of activity (must be completed before discharge).
- **Other Classes Attended:** List other education opportunities (classes attended and additional handouts) not already listed.

5. Sign full name, with initials and title, on back of form.

Place Facility Logo Here

Diabetes Management

DIRECTIONS:
1. Highlight APPROPRIATE patient education materials.
2. Initial and date when material was given/reviewed/completed.
3. Use comments column for:
   a. Charting dates reviewed.
   b. Special patient/family needs.
   c. Receiver of education.

ADDRESSOGRAPH

DOCUMENT	Init/Date Given	Primary Caregiver	COMMENTS Init/Dates Material Reviewed • Special Needs • Who Received Education	Init/Date States &/or Demonstrates Understanding of Activity
4. Overview of Diabetes				
About Diabetes				
What Is Diabetes?				
Diabetes Mellitus				
Symptoms of Diabetes				
What Causes Noninsulin-Dependent Diabetes?				
Who Develops Noninsulin-Dependent Diabetes?				
Diagnosing Diabetes				
5. Managing Diabetes				
Treating Diabetes				
Diabetes Diet				
Why Is Diet Important?				
Alcoholic Beverages and Diabetes				
Exercise and Diabetes				
Why Is Exercise Important?				
Checking Blood Glucose Levels				
Keep Daily Records				
Diabetes To Do List				
Sample Record for Each Physician Evaluation				
Record for Each Physician Evaluation				
Things To Do At Least Once a Year				
Sample Record for Annual Test Results				
Record for Annual Test Results				
Questions To Ask Your Doctor about Blood Sugar Control				

DOCUMENT	Init/Date Given	Primary Caregiver	COMMENTS Init/Dates Material Reviewed • Special Needs • Who Received Education	Init/Date States &/or Demonstrates Understanding of Activity
Managing Hypoglycemia				
How Is Hypoglycemia Treated?				
Guidelines for Sick Days				
Diabetic Emergencies				
Surgery and Diabetes				
Pregnancy and Diabetes				
Pregnancy, Diabetes, and Women's Health				
Stress and Illness and Diabetes				
Dealing with Diabetes				
Traveling with Diabetes				
6. Medications for Diabetes				
Oral Medications for Diabetes				
Oral Hypoglycemic Agents				
What Are Diabetes Pills?				
Insulin				
What Is Insulin?				
How To Give an Insulin Shot				
Where Is Insulin Injected?				
How To Draw Up and Inject Insulin				
How To Care for Insulin				
Alternative Therapies for Diabetes				
7. Nutrition for Diabetes				
Diabetes Mellitus Nutritional Goals				
Noninsulin-Dependent Diabetes Mellitus and Diet				
Insulin-Dependent Diabetes Mellitus and Diet				
How Can I Find Out How Much To Eat Each Day?				
Make Your Own Food Pyramid				
Simplified Diabetic Diet				
No Concentrated Sweets				
How To Calculate Total Available Glucose				
Examples of Foods To Add for Exercise				
Carbohydrate Content of Foods Appropriate for Sick-Day Use				
Diabetic Toddler Feeding Guidelines				

DOCUMENT	Init/Date Given	Primary Caregiver	COMMENTS Init/Dates Material Reviewed • Special Needs • Who Received Education	Init/Date States &/or Demonstrates Understanding of Activity
Exchange Lists for Meal Planning for Vegetarian Diabetics				
Sample Diet Plan Handout for Low Literacy Client with Diabetes				
8. Complications of Diabetes				
Diabetes Complications				
What Are Possible Complications of Diabetes?				
Managing Complications				
Heart Disease and Diabetes				
Women with Diabetes: Risk Factor for Heart Disease				
Kidney Disease and Diabetes				
Diabetes and Your Kidneys				
Kidney Disease: Options for Prevention and Treatment				
End-Stage Renal Disease and Hemodialysis				
Hemodialysis—Know Your Number				
End-Stage Renal Disease and Peritoneal Dialysis				
End-Stage Renal Disease and Kidney Transplantation				
Eye Problems and Diabetes				
Diabetes and Your Eyes				
Diabetic Retinopathy				
Leg and Foot Problems and Diabetes				
For People with Diabetes—How To Care for Your Feet				
How To Take Care of Your Feet				
Skin and Mouth Infections				
Diabetes and Periodontal Disease				
Enfermedad periodontal en los diabéticos (Spanish-language information on diabetes and periodontal disease)				
Constipation and Diabetes				
Diabetic Neuropathy: The Nerve Damage of Diabetes				
Diabetic Ketoacidosis				
Ketoacidosis and Hyperosomolar Nonketotic Coma				

DOCUMENT	Init/Date Given	Primary Caregiver	COMMENTS Init/Dates Material Reviewed • Special Needs • Who Received Education	Init/Date States &/or Demonstrates Understanding of Activity
9. Patient Pathways				
Diabetes, Type I, Adult				
Diabetes, Type I, Pediatric— Sample 1				
Diabetes, Type I, Pediatric— Sample 2				
Diabetes, Type II—Sample 1				
Diabetes, Type II—Sample 2				
Diabetes, Type II—Sample 3				

OTHER CLASSES ATTENDED/HANDOUTS GIVEN	INIT	SIGNATURE

PART I
Managing Diabetes: Clinical Pathways and Guidelines

1. Diabetes Mellitus and Disease Management*

IMPORTANCE

Approximately seven million Americans have been diagnosed with diabetes mellitus and an additional five million may have the disease and be unaware of it. Diabetes is an underlying cause of death for 37,000 persons and a contributing factor in another 100,000 deaths. Complications related to diabetes are quite high, with an estimated 5,800 cases of blindness, 40,000 amputations, and 4,000 cases of renal failure annually.

There are two types of diabetes mellitus. Type I (insulin-dependent or IDDM) and Type II (noninsulin-dependent or NIDDM) are quite different in their epidemiology and risk of complications. Type I most often afflicts children and young adults whereas Type II (accounting for 92% of all diabetes cases) tends to afflict older adults. Type II diabetes is more likely to be mild and asymptomatic and may frequently be undetected and untreated. Type I is more serious and generally requires ongoing insulin therapy.

IDDM is one of the more common chronic conditions among children. The prevalence is estimated to be 1.2 to 1.9 cases per 1,000 children and the peak age at onset is between 10 and 14 years of age; the peak age of onset for girls is earlier (10–12 years old) than for boys, probably due to earlier onset of puberty. There is both seasonal and geographic variation in the incidence of cases with more cases being diagnosed in cooler months and more cases being identified in cooler climates. There is no significant difference in the prevalence of IDDM between males and females. There are racial differences in the incidence of IDDM with whites being considerably more likely to develop IDDM than nonwhites.

EFFICACY OR EFFECTIVENESS OF INTERVENTIONS

Primary prevention of either Type I or Type II diabetes is currently considered infeasible. Secondary and tertiary prevention of acute and long-term complications of the disease is the principal focus of treatment strategies.

Annually, more than 67,000 cases of acute metabolic complications (ketoacidosis or nonketotic hyperosmolar coma) occur. Although there is evidence that some acute complications of diabetes can be reduced or prevented through improved management, many may not be preventable and some management strategies may actually increase the likelihood of complications. However, both ketoacidosis and hyperosmolar coma can be effectively treated in the hospital, implying that death from these conditions is preventable and high rates of deaths due to acute complications may signal possible problems of quality.

The long-term management of IDDM presents a challenge for the health professional, child, and family. The major goals of treatment are: (1) normal physical and emotional development; (2) reduction in symptoms associated with excessive glycemic excursion; and (3) lessening of the long-term complications. Children who are undertreated are likely to experience growth retardation and delays in sexual maturation. Children with IDDM are at risk for hypoglycemia, which can cause an altered level of consciousness, seizures, and brain damage. Long-term problems include significant retinal, renal, and nerve damage. Management of the disease is important and requires education of the family and the child so that they can participate in independent decision making around daily decisions related to diet, activities, and insulin dose adjustment to reduce hyperglycemia and hypoglycemia. Avoiding metabolic abnormalities requires monitoring blood glucose multiple times daily as well as intermittent urinary ketone checks. Frequent health care visits are recommended to monitor HbA_{1c} levels, blood lipids, and blood pressure, although no specific guidelines exist that specify the exact number of recommended visits.

The Diabetes Control and Complications Trial (DCCT) established that intensive insulin therapy was superior to conventional therapy in delaying the onset and slowing the progression of retinopathy, nephropathy, and neuropathy in patients with IDDM. In the primary prevent cohort, the adjusted mean risk of developing retinopathy was reduced by 76% in the intensive insulin therapy group as compared to the conventional therapy group. In the secondary prevention group, the progression of retinopathy was slowed by 54% in the intensive, as compared to the conventional, therapy group. Intensive therapy also resulted in significant reductions in the occurrence of microalbuminuria, albuminuria, and clinical neuropathy. The major adverse event was a two- to threefold increase in severe hypoglycemia.

Prevention of long-term complications may be feasible using strategies other than tight glycemic control. For example, patient education programs may improve outcomes among persons with diabetes. Annual eye examinations have been recommended to identify and treat proliferative retinopathy and diabetic macular edema, cataracts, and glaucoma at an early stage. The incidence of foot infections may be reduced by patient education about foot care and encouraging smoking cessation; among those who develop foot infections, medical and surgical management may reduce morbidity. Persons with diabetes are at increased risk of developing hypertension and hypercholesterolemia. Atten-

*Source: Elizabeth A. McGlynn, "Choosing Chronic Disease Measures for HEDIS: Conceptual Framework and Review of Seven Clinical Areas," *Managed Care Quarterly*, Vol. 4:3, Aspen Publishers, Inc., © 1996.

tion to the prevention and treatment of these risk factors may reduce the incidence of cardiovascular complications. Decline in renal function may be mitigated for patients with diabetic nephropathy through aggressive treatment of hypertension or microalbuminuria.

POTENTIAL FOR IMPROVING QUALITY

The evidence suggests that substantial shortcomings exist in the care of diabetics. One study found that only one third of diabetics seen by university internists were under adequate control; among diabetics with hypertension, 40% were found to have poorly controlled blood pressures. Foot examinations are infrequently done in physician visits. The recent HEDIS Pilot Project found that overall annual funduscopic examinations were performed for 47% of persons in the 21 participating health plans, with a range from 12% to 58%. These exams may need to be done by ophthalmologists because primary care physicians may not be able to perform an adequate funduscopic examination.

Because the DCCT results are only recently available, there may be considerable variation in the use of intensive insulin therapy versus conventional therapeutic approaches. This may represent one area of potential improvement in the quality of care for persons with IDDM.

COST-EFFECTIVENESS OF INTERVENTIONS

Probably because there are not many alternatives in diabetes treatment, few studies examining cost effectiveness have been conducted. One study examining classroom versus individual education found that classroom education was more cost effective, and more conducive to learning than individual instruction. Failure to adequately treat individuals who have diabetes is likely to result in complications, hospitalization, and death; these are likely to be extremely expensive relative to the cost of high-quality care.

HEALTH PLAN ROLE IN PROVIDING INTERVENTION

The health plan role in providing treatment of diabetes, both Type I and Type II, is consistent with a traditional role. Perhaps the greatest challenge is the provision of educational interventions designed to facilitate self-management of the disease. This may be best accomplished by special clinics. For example, the DCCT treatment team included diabetologists, nurses, dietitians, and behavioral specialists. During the first month of the trial, the treatment team was in daily phone contact with study participants. Such team management may be beyond the coverage of many insurance policies, but may be more feasible to accomplish in the managed care setting than in a solo practice.

AREAS FOR OUTCOMES MEASUREMENT

1. Proportion of persons with diabetes mellitus whose most recent HbA_{1c} levels are within the normal range.
2. Proportion of persons with diabetes mellitus who have an annual retinal examination (existing HEDIS measure).
3. Proportion of persons with diabetes mellitus and hypertension whose blood pressure is within the normal range.
4. Proportion of persons with diabetes mellitus who have a competent annual foot examination.

TIPS FOR DESIGNING DIABETES MANAGEMENT PROGRAMS

The tips provided here draw on the experiences of Lifeguard Health Care in San Jose, California, in developing a diabetes management program.

1. Seek out members with diabetes and encourage them to enroll.

Lifeguard used a database from its drug management company that listed all members who are dependent on insulin or oral medication. A letter with a response card was sent out. About 400 replies were received.

Members on the list who did not respond to the original mailing were called and asked if they would be willing to participate.

The program was also announced in a newsletter to health plan physicians and members.

Future plans include targeting letters to physicians who are most likely to treat patients with diabetes.

2. Contract with a local group of experts.

The Diabetes Society of Santa Clara Valley, a well-known group in the region, has been contracted to work on the Lifeguard project.

Diabetes educators from the society assess program enrollees, determining where the patient needs the most assistance. They find out what area of diabetes control the member is most confident in. From that point, the diabetic educators at the society brainstorm different strategies to get the patient moving to the next stage of controlling diabetes.

3. Use of a multifaceted approach.

Lifeguard is building a network between its physicians, the Diabetes Society, the members, and the health care plan to take a united front in dealing with diabetes.

Take a multifront approach to dealing with the problem.

Instead of focusing efforts only on the individual with diabetes or better educating physicians, target all aspects.

Encourage the members to be their own best health advocates. To work with members to better control this condition, be sure the provider and member approach the problem from the same perspective.

4. Assess members' readiness to change.

Lifeguard's health behavior questionnaire asks the members to rate their behaviors according to a continuum that measures them against the ideal behavior.

For example, members are asked if they follow their diets in the way they were instructed. Members can state whether they have been complying for more than six months or less than six months.

Members who are not following the diet have the option of stating they are considering complying in the next month or the next six months, or that they have no intention of complying.

Other questions examine the amount of exercise the member gets, how often the member complies with instructions for medication, how frequently the member tests blood sugar level, and how frequently the member receives various preventive exams.

5. Promote change in a way that works for the individual.

Try to develop an intervention for an individual who is at a specific stage of readiness. For example, if the individual is not thinking about dealing with exercise and doesn't intend to exercise in the next six months, deal with that member differently than someone who is planning on making a change within the next month.

6. Assist members in planning for change.

Counselors should help members set dates to start a physical activity or an improved diet. They should also develop strategies to overcome potential barriers to change.

7. Recognize that change takes time.

If a member is unable to change behavior, that should not be considered a failure.

Just moving people toward the more optimal behavior can be a goal.

Don't expect everybody to be compliant with the ideal behaviors right away. It takes time.

8. Keep physicians informed.

Enter information from patient questionnaires into a database, track changes, and distribute that information to physicians so they can understand how well their patients are doing in changing their behaviors.

Let physicians know what areas the member has committed to working on.

Physicians must be kept well informed because they play a key role in delivering potent health messages.

9. Track utilization of resources.

Lifeguard asks program enrollees to report how many times in the last six months they have visited the hospital, the emergency department, and urgent care clinics.

This information is analyzed before the member begins the program and at specific times during member enrollment.

Take a look at how these trends may change as a result of the program being in place and how assertive people are in taking care of themselves.

10. Monitor effectiveness of the program.

Lifeguard asks members to complete surveys, such as the SF-36 health status form, before enrollment and during the program. Look at change scores for all those completing surveys.

Source: Peter Sepsis, "Diabetes," *Inside Preventive Care,* Vol. 2:5, Aspen Publishers, Inc., © 1996.

DIABETES STATISTICS

PREVALENCE OF DIABETES IN THE UNITED STATES

Total (diagnosed and undiagnosed): 16 million (1995 estimate)

- **Diagnosed:** 8 million
- **Undiagnosed:** 8 million
- **Insulin-dependent diabetes (IDDM):** Estimates range up to 800,000 (No national registry for diabetes exist. These estimates are extrapolated from several regional registries.) IDDM is a chronic condition in which the pancreas makes little or no insulin because the insulin-producing beta cells have been destroyed by the body's immune system. To treat the disease, the person must inject insulin. IDDM usually begins before age 30.
- **Non–insulin-dependent diabetes (NIDDM):** About 7 to 7.5 million diagnosed cases (1993 estimate) NIDDM is a chronic condition in which the pancreas produces insulin, but the insulin is ineffective in lowering blood sugar. In contrast to IDDM, NIDDM patients may be treated with diet, exercise, pills, or insulin injections, although about 40% require insulin to control blood sugar. NIDDM usually develops in people who are over age 40; most are overweight. NIDDM accounts for 90% to 95% of diabetes.

COST

Total (direct and indirect): $92 billion (United States, 1992).

- **Direct medical costs:** $45 billion (The figure for direct medical costs includes only those costs directly attributable to diabetes. This is in contrast to figures cited elsewhere that estimate all health care costs incurred by people with diabetes, including costs not related to diabetes.)
- **Indirect costs:** $47 billion (disability, work loss, premature mortality)

DEATHS

- In 1993 about 400,000 deaths from all causes are estimated to have occurred in people with diabetes. This figure represents 5% of all persons known to have diabetes and 18% of all deaths in the United States in persons age 25 years and older.
- Based on death certificate data, diabetes contributed to the deaths of more than 169,000 persons in 1992. It is well known that death certificate data underrepresent diabetes deaths.
- Diabetes was the seventh leading cause of death listed on US death certificates in 1993, according to the National Center for Health Statistics. It is the fourth leading cause of death by disease.

INCIDENCE

Total New Cases Diagnosed Every Day: About 1800 (1990–1992 averaged)
Total New Cases Diagnosed Each Year: 625,000 (1990–1992 averaged)

- **NIDDM:** About 595,000 new cases per year
- **IDDM:** About 30,000 news cases per year

Who Has Been Diagnosed with Diabetes? (1993 estimates)

- **Women:** 4.2 million
- **Men:** 3.6 million
- **Children age 19 years or younger:** About 100,000
- **Adults age 65 years or older:** 3.2 million

PERCENT OF ADULTS WITH DIABETES, BOTH DIAGNOSED AND UNDIAGNOSED, BY RACE AND ETHNICITY

- **African-Americans:** 9.6%
- **Mexican-Americans:** 9.6%
- **Cuban-Americans:** 9.1%
- **Puerto Rican–Americans:** 10.9%
- **White Americans:** 6.2%
- **Native Americans:** Ranges from 5% to 50%
- **Japanese-Americans:** Among second-generation Japanese-Americans 45 to 74 years of age residing in King County, Washington, 20% of the men and 16% of the women had diabetes.

TREATMENT FOR DIABETES

Treatment for diabetes may include physical activity, meal planning, education, attention to relevant medical and psychosocial factors, blood glucose monitoring, and, if needed, oral medications or insulin.

- **IDDM:** By definition, people with IDDM require insulin injections.
- **NIDDM:** About 40% use insulin, 49% use oral agents, 10% use combination of insulin and oral medications.

LONG-TERM COMPLICATIONS

Heart disease

- Cardiovascular disease is two to four times more common in people with diabetes.
- Cardiovascular disease is present in 75% of diabetes-related deaths.

continues

Diabetes Statistics continued

- Middle-aged people with diabetes have death rates twice as high and heart disease death rates about 2 to 4 times as high as middle-aged people without diabetes.

Stroke

- The risk of stroke is 2.5 times higher in people with diabetes.

High blood pressure

- Affects 60% to 65% of people with diabetes.

Blindness

- Diabetes is the leading cause of new cases of blindness among adults 20 to 74 years of age.
- From 12,000 to 24,000 new cases of blindness per year are caused by diabetic retinopathy.

Kidney disease (treatment by dialysis or transplantation)

- Diabetes is the leading cause of end-stage renal disease, accounting for 36% of new cases.
- 19,800 new cases occurred in 1992 in people with diabetes.
- 56,000 people with diabetes were undergoing dialysis or transplantation treatment in 1992.

Nerve disease

- About 60% to 70% of people with diabetes have mild to severe forms of diabetic nerve damage (with such manifestations as impaired sensation in the feet or hands, delayed stomach emptying, carpal tunnel syndrome, peripheral neuropathy).
- Severe forms of diabetic nerve disease are a major contributing cause of lower-extremity amputations.

Amputations

- More than half of lower-limb amputations in the United States occur among people with diabetes; from 1989 to 1992, the average number of amputations performed each year among people with diabetes was 54,000.

Dental disease

- Studies show that periodontal disease, which can lead to tooth loss, occurs with greater frequency and severity in people with diabetes. In one study, 30% of IDDM patients age 19 years or older had periodontal disease.
- The rate of tooth loss is 15 times higher in Pima Indians with NIDDM, compared to those without diabetes, and the incidence of periodontal disease is 2.6 times higher.

Pregnancy

- The rate of major congenital malformations in babies born to women with preexisting diabetes varies from 0% to 5% in women who receive preconception care to 10% in women who do not receive preconception care.
- 3% to 5% of pregnancies in women with diabetes result in death of the newborn; this compares to a rate of 1.5% in women who do not have diabetes.

GESTATIONAL DIABETES

Gestational diabetes is a type of diabetes that develops in some pregnant women; the condition disappears when the pregnancy is over. A history of gestational diabetes, however, is a risk factor for eventual development of NIDDM.

- Occurs in 2% to 5% of pregnancies, with higher rates in African-Americans, Hispanics/Latino Americans, and Native Americans (rates in Native Americans range from 1% to 14%).

IMPAIRED GLUCOSE TOLERANCE (IGT)

IGT refers to a condition in which blood sugar levels are higher than normal but not high enough to be classified as diabetes (between 140 to 199 mg/dL in a 2-hour oral glucose tolerance test). IGT is a major risk factor for NIDDM.

- Present in about 11% of adults
- About 40% to 45% of persons age 65 years or older have either NIDDM or IGT.

Source: "Diabetes Statistics," National Diabetes Information Clearinghouse, National Institute of Diabetes and Digestive and Kidney Diseases, NIH Publication No. 96-3926, October 1995.

2. Managing Diabetes

BASIC GUIDELINES FOR DIABETES CARE

PHYSICAL ASSESSMENT

Blood Pressure, Weight (for children, add height; plot on growth chart)
Every visit. Blood Pressure target goal <130/85 mm Hg (children: <90th pctl age standard).
Children: normal weight for height (see standard growth charts)

Foot Exam (for adults)
Thorough visual inspection every "diabetes visit"; pedal pulses, neurological exam annually.

Dilated eye exams
Type 1 (Insulin-Dependent Diabetes Mellitus): 5 years post diagnosis, then every year by a trained expert.
Type 2 (Noninsulin-Dependent Diabetes Mellitus): shortly after diagnosis, then every year by a trained expert.

LABORATORY EXAM

HbA1c
Quarterly, if treatment changes or is not meeting goals; 1–2 times/year if stable. Target goal <7.0% or <1% above lab norms; children, modify if necessary to prevent significant hypoglycemia.

Microalbuminuria
Type 1: 5 years post diagnosis, then every year.
Type 2: begin at diagnosis, then every year.

Blood Lipids (for adults)
On initial visit, then annually for adults. Target goals: Cholesterol, Triglycerides (mg/dL) <200; LDL <130 unless CHD, then <100; HDL >35.

SELF-MANAGEMENT TRAINING

Management Principles and Complications
Understanding diabetes, medications, glucose self-monitoring, hypo/hyperglycemia, chronic complications, psychosocial assessment (special attention needed for adolescents) initially and in follow-up visits. Children: appropriate for developmental stage.

Self Glucose Monitoring
Type 1: typically test 4 times a day; Type 2 and others: as needed to meet treatment goals.

Medical Nutrition Therapy
Initial: assess needs/condition, assist patient in setting nutrition goals. Follow-up: assess progress toward goals; identify problem areas by a trained expert.

Physical Activity
Assess patient initially; prescribe physical activity based on patient's needs/condition initially and in follow-up visits.

Weight Management
Must be individualized for patient initially and in follow-up visits.

INTERVENTIONS

Preconception Counseling and Management
Consult with high-risk perinatal programs where available (e.g., "Sweet Success" Regional Perinatal Programs of California). Adolescents: special counseling advisable, beginning with puberty.

Pregnancy Management
Consult with high-risk perinatal programs where available.

Aspirin Therapy
(81–325 mg/day) in adults as primary and secondary prevention of CHD, unless contraindicated

Smoking Cessation
Screen, advise, and assist initially, then annually.

Vaccinations
Influenza and Pneumococcal, per CDC recommendations.

EXPLANATORY NOTES TO BASIC GUIDELINES FOR DIABETES CARE

1. These guidelines are intended for use by primary care professionals.
2. The guidelines are meant to be basic **guidelines,** not enforceable standards.
   (Where an internal quality assurance program has demonstrated that less frequent testing does not jeopardize patient care, less frequent testing may be acceptable; e.g., dilated eye exams every two years vs. every year.)
3. One or more of the following criteria were used for inclusion of an item in the guidelines.
   a. Published evidence demonstrated either the **efficacy** or the **effectiveness** of the item.
   b. Published studies on **cost-identification, cost-effectiveness,** or **cost-benefit** analysis of the item demonstrated favorable economic results.
   c. A preponderance of **expert opinion** held that the item is considered to be essential to the care of persons with diabetes.
4. It is assumed that the following are routinely occurring in the medical setting:
   a. A history and physical appropriate for a person with diabetes are performed. Visits are sufficiently frequent to meet the patient's needs and treatment goals.
   b. **Abnormal physical or laboratory findings result in appropriate interventions which are individualized for each patient.**

continues

Basic Guidelines for Diabetes Care continued

c. Self-Management Training is provided by allied health professionals who are experts in the provision of this training. For children/adolescents and their families, training from a diabetes team or team member with experience in child and adolescent diabetes is strongly recommended to begin at diagnosis.

d. Physicians consult current references for normal values and for appropriate treatment goal values, both for children and adults.

e. Specialists should be consulted when patients are unable to achieve treatment goals in a reasonable time frame, when complications arise, or whenever the primary care physician deems it appropriate. Under similar circumstances, children/adolescents should be referred to specialists who have expertise in managing children and adolescents with diabetes.

5. Additional comments on specific items included in the guidelines:

HcA1c/Self Blood Glucose Monitoring—HcA1c target goals should be achieved gradually over time. Target goals should be less stringent for children, the elderly, and other fragile patients. Clinicians have found that making the patient aware of his/her HcA1c values and their significance help motivate the patient toward improved glucose management. This principle also applies to self blood glucose monitoring. **Target goals should be individualized for each patient.**

Blood Lipids—Abnormal blood lipids are often undertreated. An active, progressive treatment and monitoring plan should be instituted.

Microalbuminuria—Need not test for microalbuminuria if albumin has previously been found in the urine.

Note: **These materials have been produced through the collaborative efforts of the Diabetes Coalition of California and the California Diabetes Control Program** © 1998. These guidelines should be used in conjunction with the Explanatory Notes attached. These guidelines are consistent with ADA Clinical Practice Recommendations.

Source: Copyright © 1995 Diabetes Coalition of California, Sacramento, California.

ALGORITHM FOR THERAPY FOR GLYCEMIC CONTROL OF
TYPE II DIABETES MELLITUS IN ADULTS

- The terms "Asymptomatic Hyperglycemia," "Symptomatic Hyperglycemia," and "Very Symptomatic Hyperglycemia" are not formal classifications or stages of type 2 diabetes. They are used to indicate degrees of metabolic decompensation. "Asymptomatic" refers to abnormal blood sugars diagnostic of diabetes without signs or symptoms. "Symptomatic" might include blurred vision, itching, recurrent infections such as skin infections, vaginal yeast infections and urinary tract infections, leg cramping, and mild increased thirst and urination. "Very symptomatic" would include marked increase in thirst and urination, dehydration and ketosis.
- This algorithm emphasized the need to evaluate regularly the patient's response to therapy and identify the therapy which achieve and maintain glycemic control with the least pharmacologic intervention possible.
- Generic and trade names for classes of medications named in the algorithm.

Class	Generic	Trade	Manufacturer
Alpha Glucosidase Inhibitor	Acarbose	Precose	Bayer
Biguanide	Metfarmin	Glucophage	Bristol-Myers Squibb
Insulin Secretagogues			
Benzoic Acid Analogue (Meglitinides)	Repaglinide	Prandin	Novo-Nordisk
Sulfonylurea	Chlorpropamide	Diabinese	Pfizer
	Glimepiride	Amaryl	Hoechst-Roussel
	Glipizide	Glucotrol	Pfizer
	Glyburide	DiaBeta	Hoechst-Roussel
	Tolazamide	Micronase	Upjohn
	Tolbutamide	Glynase	Upjohn
			Mylan
			Mylan
Thiazolidnedione	Troglitazone	Rezulin	Parke-Davis

Class	Generic	Trade	Manufacturer

Insulin

Class	Generic	Trade	Manufacturer
Rapid Acting	Lispro	Humalog	Lilly
Short Acting	Regular (R)		
	Purified Pork	Regular Iletin II	Lilly
	Pork	Regular Purified Pork insulin	Novo Nordisk
	Human	Humulin R	Lilly
		Novolin R	Novo Nordisk
		Velosulin BR	Novo Nordisk
Intermediate Acting	NPH (N)		
	Purified Pork	Pork NPH Iletin II	Lilly
	Pork	NPH Purified N	Novo Nordisk
	Human	Humulin N	Lilly
		Novolin N	Novo Nordisk
	Lente (L)		
	Purified Pork	Lente Iletin II (Pork)	Lilly
	Pork	NPH Purified N	Novo Nordisk
	Human	Humulin L	Lilly
		Novolin L	Novo Nordisk
Long Acting	Ultralente		
	Human	Humulin U	Lilly
Pre-Mixed	NPH/Regular (70/30)	Humulin 70/30	Lilly
	Human	Novolin 70/30	Novo Nordisk
	NPH/Regular (50/50)		
	Human	Humulin 50/50	Lilly

DIABETES CONTROL AND COMPLICATIONS TRIAL (DCCT)*

What Is the DCCT?

The DCCT is a clinical study conducted from 1983 to 1993 by the National Institute of Diabetes and Digestive and Kidney Diseases (NIDDK). The study showed that keeping blood sugar levels as close to normal as possible slows the onset and progression of eye, kidney, and nerve diseases caused by diabetes. In fact, it demonstrated that *any* sustained lowering of blood sugar helps, even if the person has a history of poor control.

The largest, most comprehensive diabetes study ever conducted, the DCCT involved 1,441 volunteers with insulin-dependent diabetes mellitus and 29 medical centers in the United States and Canada. Volunteers had diabetes for at least 1 year but no longer than 15 years. They also were required to have no, or only early signs of, diabetic eye disease.

The study compared the effects of two treatment regimens—standard therapy and intensive control—on the complications of diabetes. Volunteers were randomly assigned to each treatment group.

How Did Intensive Treatment Affect Diabetic Eye Disease?

All DCCT participants were monitored for diabetic retinopathy, an eye disease that affects the retina. Study results showed that intensive therapy reduced the risk for developing retinopathy by 76%. In participants with some eye damage at the beginning of the study, intensive management slowed the progression of the disease by 54%.

The retina is the light-sensing tissue at the back of the eye. According to the National Eye Institute, one of the National Institutes of Health, as many as 24,000 persons with diabetes lose their sight each year. In the United States, diabetic retinopathy is the leading cause of blindness in adults under age 65.

How Did Intensive Treatment Affect Diabetic Kidney Disease?

Participants in the DCCT were tested to assess the development of diabetic kidney disease (nephropathy). Findings showed that intensive treatment prevented the development and slowed the progression of diabetic kidney disease by 50%.

Diabetic kidney disease is the most common cause of kidney failure in the United States and the greatest threat to life in adults with IDDM. After having diabetes for 15 years, one third of people with IDDM develop kidney disease. Diabetes damages the small blood vessels in the kidneys, impairing their ability to filter impurities from blood for excretion in the urine. Persons with kidney damage must have a kidney transplant or rely on dialysis to cleanse their blood.

How Did Intensive Treatment Affect Diabetic Nerve Disease?

Participants in the DCCT were examined to detect the development of nerve damage (diabetic neuropathy). Study results showed the risk of nerve damage was reduced by 60 percent in persons on intensive treatment.

Diabetic nerve disease can cause pain and loss of feeling in the feet, legs, and fingertips. It can also affect the parts of the nervous system that control blood pressure, heart rate, digestion, and sexual function. Neuropathy is a major contributing factor in foot and leg amputations among people with diabetes.

How Did Intensive Treatment Affect Diabetes-Related Cardiovascular Disease?

DCCT participants were not expected to have many heart-related problems because their average age was only 27 when the study began. Nevertheless, they underwent cardiograms, blood pressure tests, and laboratory tests of blood fat levels to look for signs of cardiovascular disease. The study proved that volunteers on intensive treatment had significantly lower risks of developing high blood cholesterol, a cause of heart disease. The risk was 35% lower in these volunteers, suggesting that intensive treatment can help prevent heart disease.

DCCT Study Findings

Lowering blood sugar reduces risk:

- eye disease, 76% reduced risk
- kidney disease, 50% reduced risk
- nerve disease, 60% reduced risk
- cardiovascular disease, 35% reduced risk

---

*Source: "Diabetes Control and Complications Trial," National Diabetes Information Clearinghouse, National Institute of Diabetes and Digestive and Kidney Diseases, NIH Publication No. 95-3874, September 1994.

Elements of Intensive Management in the DCCT

- Testing blood sugar levels 4 or more times a day.
- Four daily insulin injections or use of an insulin pump.
- Adjustment of insulin doses according to food intake and exercise.
- A diet and exercise plan.
- Monthly visits to a health care team composed of a physician, nurse educator, dietitian, and behavioral therapist.

What Are the Risks of Intensive Treatment?

In the DCCT, the most significant side effect of intensive treatment was an increase in the risk for low blood sugar episodes severe enough to require assistance from another person. This is called severe hypoglycemia. Because of this risk, DCCT researchers do not recommend intensive therapy for children under age 13, people with heart disease or advanced complications, older adults, and people with a history of frequent severe hypoglycemia. Persons in the intensive management group also gained a modest amount of weight, suggesting that intensive treatment may not be appropriate for people with diabetes who are overweight.

DCCT researchers estimate that intensive management doubles the cost of managing diabetes because of increased visits to health care professionals and the need for more frequent blood testing at home. However, this cost is offset by the reduction in medical expenses related to long-term complications and by the improved quality of life of people with diabetes.

BENEFITS OF BLOOD GLUCOSE CONTROL CONFIRMED— INCORPORATING THE DCCT RESULTS INTO PRACTICE*

The DCCT, a 10-year study conducted by the National Institutes of Health, provides convincing scientific evidence about the benefits of near-normal blood glucose control. The

---

*Source: *The Prevention and Treatment of Complications of Diabetes Mellitus: A Guide for Primary Care Practitioners*, Department of Health and Human Services, Public Health Service, Centers for Disease Control, National Center for Chronic Disease Prevention and Health Promotion, Division of Diabetes Translation, January 1, 1991.

Centers for Disease Control and Prevention (CDC) believes that the DCCT results have therapeutic implications for persons with diabetes and clinical practice implications for health care providers.

The DCCT, which involved 1,441 persons with IDDM at 29 medical centers in the United States and Canada, showed that intensive therapy can prevent the development and slow the progression of microvascular and neurologic complications among persons with IDDM. The volunteers, who were aged 13–39 years at baseline and did not have advanced complications, were randomly assigned to an intensive treatment group or a conventional treatment group. Those in the intensive treatment group received care from an experienced multidisciplinary team that included a nurse, a dietitian, a diabetologist, and a behavioral counselor. Participants tested their blood sugar four or more times a day, injected insulin three or more times a day or used an insulin pump, performed insulin self-adjustment, received intensive diabetes education and nutritional instruction, and visited a clinic monthly. In addition, they were in telephone contact with their diabetes treatment team at least weekly. Volunteers in the conventional treatment group used the type of regimen followed by the majority of persons with IDDM treated in university medical centers: one or two insulin injections a day, daily self-monitoring of blood glucose, a program of diabetes education that included nutritional instruction, and a clinic visit every three months.

The cumulative risks for the onset and progression of three complications of diabetes—diabetic retinopathy, nephropathy, and neuropathy—were approximately 40%–75% less for persons in the intensive treatment group than for those in the conventional treatment group.

The intensive treatment group achieved mean glucose values of 155 mg/dL (normal 110 mg/dL) and hemoglobin A1c levels of about 7.2% (normal). A goal of achieving glucose levels and hemoglobin A1cs similar to those achieved by the DCCT's intensive treatment group is reasonable for most persons with IDDM, with the expectation that their long-term outcome will be measurably improved. The complex nature of diabetes requires that the recommendations from the DCCT be individualized. Further, it should be noted that the intensive treatment volunteers received sustained, comprehensive, multidisciplinary diabetes treatment, education, and counseling. Optimal glucose control requires (1) an individual with diabetes who makes an informed decision to attempt optimal control and is intellectually, emotionally, physically, and financially prepared to adopt an intensified regimen, and (2) a health care team that provides resources, guidance, and support.

There are several contraindications for intensive therapy among persons with IDDM. Intensive therapy is contraindicated for the following persons:

- those who are unable or unwilling to participate actively in their glucose management
- children under the age of two

Extreme caution should be used with children aged two to seven because the benefits are unproven, risk of hypoglycemia may be greater, and hypoglycemia occurrence may impair normal brain development. (The danger of hypoglycemia in young children is greater because food intake, activity, and adherence to schedules may be less predictable than in adults.)

Other relative contraindications may include:

- persons with other diabetes-related problems (eg, autonomic neuropathy resulting in hypoglycemic unawareness and severe hypoglycemia; end-stage renal disease)
- older adults with significant coronary artery disease or cerebrovascular disease who may be more vulnerable to injury from hypoglycemia

Intensive treatment requires more attention and skilled services than may be routinely available in clinical practice. Broad implementation of intensive therapy will require expanded health care teams (diabetes educators, dietitians, physicians, and behavioral counselors), major professional and public educational efforts, and enhanced partnerships between primary care providers and specialists.

The core message of the DCCT—"Metabolic Control Matters"—is relevant to all persons with diabetes. If near-normal control is not feasible, improved control should be the goal. Persons with non–insulin-dependent diabetes mellitus, who make up over 90% of persons with diabetes, were not studied. The CDC feels it is reasonable to anticipate that better glucose control would also benefit persons with NIDDM. The role of diet and exercise in improving glycemic control should be evaluated for persons with NIDDM before additional treatment (ie, oral hypoglycemic agents or insulin) is recommended. The recommendations contained in *The Prevention and Treatment of Complications of Diabetes: A Guide for Primary Care Practitioners* remain extremely important in the prevention, detection, and treatment of major complications of diabetes.

Comprehensive training in self-management is essential. Persons with diabetes should learn how to

- monitor their blood glucose
- negotiate a meal plan with a dietitian
- achieve and maintain recommended exercise/activity levels
- adjust their insulin as needed (if applicable)

- prevent and treat hypoglycemia
- track hemoglobin A1c or glycosylated hemoglobin tests, with the help of their diabetes team, approximately every three months

Persons with diabetes should be encouraged to record hemoglobin A1c values on tracking sheets, such as those contained in the CDC publication *Take Charge of Your Diabetes: A Guide for Care*. Single copies of this publication may be obtained by writing to the address below:

Centers for Disease Control and Prevention
Technical Information Services Branch
Mailstop K-13
4770 Buford Highway, NE
Atlanta, GA 30341-3724
(404) 488-5080

For reprints and more information about the DCCT, contact:

The National Diabetes Information Clearinghouse
Box NDIC
Bethesda, MD 20892
(301) 654-3327

MANAGING AND PREVENTING PSYCHOSOCIAL PROBLEMS WITH DIABETES*

Background

Description. Like other chronic illnesses, diabetes mellitus poses a wide range of problems for patients and their family members. These problems include pain, hospitalization, changes in lifestyle and vocation, physical disabilities, and threatened survival. Direct psychological consequences can arise from any one of these factors, making it harder for patients to treat their diabetes and live productive, enjoyable lives.

Populations at Risk

Diabetes itself does not cause changes in personality or psychiatric illness, but particular subgroups of the diabetic

*Source: *The Prevention and Treatment of Complications of Diabetes Mellitus: A Guide for Primary Care Practitioners*, Department of Health and Human Services, Public Health Service, Centers for Disease Control, National Center for Chronic Disease Prevention and Health Promotion, Division of Diabetes Translation, January 1, 1991.

population appear to be at risk for developing psychosocial problems. Young people with insulin-dependent diabetes mellitus may have a higher prevalence of eating disorders, such as anorexia nervosa and bulimia, and adults with long-standing diabetes and major medical complications have a higher prevalence of symptoms of depression and anxiety. Elderly persons who have non–insulin-dependent diabetes mellitus and other symptomatic medical conditions may also have a higher risk of developing psychological problems.

Patients with IDDM diagnosed before age five and older patients with NIDDM may have associated alterations in cognitive or intellectual functioning. The pathophysiology of these cognitive changes is not well understood. In the young patients, these cognitive changes may be linked to recurring episodes of severe hypoglycemia. In the older patients, both microvascular and artherosclerotic disease are possible factors.

Barriers to Self-Care

Research has indicated that psychological and social factors can profoundly influence a patient's success at adhering to a prescribed regimen of self-care. Patients may fail to care for themselves if they have certain attitudes or beliefs, including the following:

- anticipating an early cure
- believing that their self-care regimen is too difficult
- believing that treatment is unlikely to improve or control their health problems

Several other psychosocial factors can influence how well patients care for themselves:

- stressful events in the patient's life
- development of a new complication
- the availability and quality of social support for the patient
- psychiatric problems unrelated to the patient's diabetes
- the health care provider's approach to medical care

Prevention

To help anticipate or identify psychosocial problems that could interfere with a patient's self-care regimen, the practitioner should strive to establish an ongoing therapeutic alliance with the patient. The stronger the alliance, the more likely the patient is to share inner concerns and psychosocial issues. This leads to improved detection and permits more rapid institution of treatment.

This therapeutic alliance will take shape through discussions identifying the patient's expectations of, and feelings about, treatment. Although the patient should not be forced to set particular goals, the practitioner may be able to broaden or refine existing objectives to include improving the patient's adjustment to having diabetes.

Over time, this alliance may lead to better glycemic control by helping the patient address such self-care barriers as low motivation, preconceived judgments about treatment, and fears about diabetes.

Detection

The practitioner should be sensitive to possible psychosocial issues when diabetes is first diagnosed and when complications, however minor, first develop.

Some psychosocial barriers stem from personal, family, and cultural beliefs that may conflict with suggested treatment. A patient may resist following a prescribed diet, for instance, because of certain cultural beliefs about weight. Such beliefs should be given their due respect; patients respond best to advice that does not seem to prejudge their beliefs.

Certain medical conditions can be reliable indicators of psychosocial barriers. Recurrent hypoglycemia, frequent episodes of diabetic ketoacidosis, and very high glycosylated hemoglobin levels should each be recognized as a possible sign of personal or family problems. Although brittle, or unstable, diabetes can sometimes have a metabolic basis, interrupted or erratic self-care is by far a more common cause—and psychosocial problems may underlie this cause.

To help uncover problem areas, the practitioner may want to conduct discussions along the following lines:

- Ask patients to describe how they feel about the following issues of self-care:
  - the importance of glycemic control
  - the feasibility of adhering to a prescribed diet
  - the importance of self-monitoring of blood glucose
  - the patient's susceptibility to developing complications
  - the efficacy of treating complications
  - the reasonableness of the practitioner's recommendations and expectations
- Ask patients to describe any stressful events or situations, such as changes in job, school, place of residence, and immediate family (for example, death or divorce). Ask whether any other events could be creating barriers to a self-care program.
- Determine whether patients have adequate social and family support. Specifically, ask patients to whom they can turn for help in caring for themselves.

- Ask about problems concerning mood, anxiety, and sense of well-being.
- Ask young women who might be at risk for eating disorders whether they have skipped insulin doses, dieted excessively, eaten in binges, or vomited.
- Ask specific questions about topics that patients may hesitate to talk about, such as sexual problems.
- Determine how effectively patients use available information about diabetes. Ask whether they find it difficult to retain or add to such knowledge.

The practitioner may then be able to counsel patients and provide useful solutions.

Treatment

Try to actively engage the patient in determining as well as pursuing a course of treatment. Ask the patient both specific and open-ended questions. Open-ended questions may elicit information that can help detect problems as well as tailor the course of treatment. Such discussions may identify individual strengths and problem-solving strategies that have helped the patient successfully face previous challenges.

The practitioner will need to identify, for possible referral, mental health professionals who are knowledgeable about diabetes and who can serve as collaborators in treating the patient. If these individuals are not familiar with diabetes, they can be given materials (such as this guide) that provide basic information.

Refer the following persons:

- Parents of children or adolescents in whom diabetes has recently been diagnosed. A single psychosocial evaluation of the family unit may be important to the overall educational process of raising a child who has diabetes.
- Patients who in one year have had two or more episodes of severe hypoglycemia or diabetic ketoacidosis without obvious causes
- Patients whom you—the health care professional—find frustrating. The mental health professional may prove a valuable consultant for treating these patients.

Remember that diabetes is a chronic illness. Even if treatment activities fail to bring change within a short time, remaining involved with the patient and the patient's family and providing an accepting atmosphere may lead to increased motivation for change.

Encourage patients and their families to attend group sessions. Medical and psychosocial information can be given at these sessions, which can also provide a forum for discussion of personal concerns. These sessions can be led by health care professionals, including physicians, nurses, and dietitians, and may meet several times a year. Local diabetes organizations may sponsor or know of such groups.

Patient Education Principles

- Inform patients about the typical personal concerns that come with diabetes, about the problems faced in accepting the disease and adapting to it, and about the impact diabetes has on emotional and social functioning.
- Involve families in treatment and education sessions.
- Encourage parents to help their young children and adolescents who are having problems controlling their diabetes.
- Encourage parents to give adolescents increasing responsibility for their diabetes—but not to force them to take these steps.
- Encourage families to provide help for their older relatives, who may find insulin difficult or frightening to use or who may have trouble changing lifelong dietary habits.
- Encourage families to ensure that school nurses and teachers are educated about the needs of children with diabetes and that nursing homes provide proper treatment to elderly patients with diabetes.

MANAGING AND PREVENTING ACUTE GLYCEMIC COMPLICATIONS*

Introduction

In diabetes mellitus, severe hyperglycemia may result from absolute or relative insulin deficiency. In some patients, the condition may culminate in diabetic ketoacidosis or hyperglycemic hyperosmolar nonketotic coma. Profound hypoglycemia may result from a relative excess of insulin. Symptoms associated with acute hyperglycemia generally develop more slowly (over hours or days) than do symptoms associated with an acute fall in the level of blood glucose (over minutes).

Diabetic Ketoacidosis

Definition. Diabetic ketoacidosis (DKA) develops when absolute insulin deficiency and excess contrainsulin hor-

*Source: *The Prevention and Treatment of Complications of Diabetes Mellitus: A Guide for Primary Care Practitioners*, Department of Health and Human Services, Public Health Service, Centers for Disease Control, National Center for Chronic Disease Prevention and Health Promotion, Division of Diabetes Translation, January 1, 1991.

mones increase hepatic glucose production, decrease peripheral glucose utilization, and stimulate release of fatty acids from fat cells and production of ketones by the liver. These changes cause hyperglycemia, osmotic diuresis, volume depletion, and acidosis.

Occurrence. The annual incidence of DKA ranges from three to eight episodes per 1,000 persons with diabetes. It is much more common among persons with insulin-dependent diabetes mellitus than among those with non–insulin-dependent diabetes mellitus.

DKA may be the initial manifestation of previously unrecognized IDDM. More often, DKA develops in persons known to have diabetes. Patients with IDDM who fail to take insulin or who do not receive extra insulin during flulike illness, pneumonia, or myocardial infarction may develop DKA. Patients with NIDDM who experience severe stress may secrete more contrainsulin hormones; these further compromise limited insulin secretion, which may in turn lead to DKA.

Morbidity and mortality. Before insulin was available, patients with diabetes often died of DKA; now, the mortality rate associated with DKA is less than 5%. However, persons who develop DKA experience pain and suffering, lose time from school or work, have increased hospitalization rates, and have high medical costs. Serious medical sequelae include cerebral edema (in young people), aspiration pneumonia, and adult respiratory distress syndrome.

Prevention

Why DKA occurs. Ultimately, DKA results from lack of insulin. Early recognition of metabolic disarray, by monitoring glucose and ketones and by properly using exogenous insulin and fluids, can prevent further decompensation. Thus, DKA should be considered preventable. When DKA occurs, a breakdown in care has occurred that should have been prevented.

Three general circumstances may allow DKA to develop:

1. low index of suspicion
2. inappropriate cessation of insulin therapy
3. mismanagement of intercurrent illness, often due to inadequate education

Index of suspicion. Many people may not know the signs and symptoms of diabetes. At times, even when a person seeks medical help, a health care provider may fail to recognize the warning signs of hyperglycemia—particularly when the patient is very young (an infant), is very old (such as an octogenarian), or has unusual symptoms (such as mental deterioration without nausea or vomiting).

Therefore, to prevent DKA or to minimize its extent, the health care provider must have a high index of suspicion for DKA. In emergency rooms, clinics, and physicians' offices, routine use of a glucose/ketone urine dipstick may allow for early identification of decompensating diabetes.

Inappropriate cessation of insulin therapy. Under circumstances such as those described below, insulin therapy may be inappropriately discontinued.

- Adolescents with diabetes may not adhere to a prescribed program, and their parents may not provide appropriate supervision.
- Patients with major emotional or psychosocial problems may fail to adhere to their usual medical program.

Intercurrent illness. Both patients and health care providers may incorrectly assume that when no food or fluid is consumed, no insulin should be taken. However, when ill or stressed, the patient with diabetes should promptly test the glucose level in blood and/or urine and test the urine for ketones. The patient should follow a sick-day protocol and consult with the health care provider. Both patients and providers must understand the proper management of diabetes during intercurrent illness.

Analysis and referral. For the patient who has experienced DKA, the health care provider should do the following:

- determine why DKA occurred
- assess the patient's self-care practices
- modify individual guidelines (as appropriate)
- implement preventive measures to prevent subsequent episodes

When recurrent episodes of DKA occur, the practitioner should determine the medical and psychosocial components of the episodes. Patients with difficult-to-manage IDDM should be referred to a diabetologist. Patients with underlying psychosocial problems should be referred to a mental health professional.

Detection

Symptoms. Suspect diabetes and DKA in any person at any age who has symptoms compatible with hyperglycemia and ketosis, including:

- altered mental status
- fatigue
- weight loss
- blurred vision

- thirst
- excessive urination
- enuresis
- abdominal pain
- nausea and vomiting

Results of a simple glucose/ketone urine dipstick may give guiding information about the presence of diabetes or DKA. If glucose or ketones are present in the urine, the blood glucose level must be measured.

Monitoring. All patients with IDDM should be taught to prevent DKA. Encourage patients to monitor their blood glucose level and advise them to monitor the urine for ketones when the blood glucose level is 240 mg/dL or more and/or acute illness develops.

Insist that patients contact you promptly when the blood glucose level remains at 240 mg/dL or more, ketonuria develops, or acute illness persists.

Periodically assess how proficient patients are with self-monitoring and reassess their understanding of self-care during acute illness.

Treatment

Identify the causes of DKA by taking a thorough history, performing a physical examination, and requesting appropriate laboratory tests. In adult patients, an electrocardiogram should be performed to rule out a silent acute myocardial infarction. Treatment should be initiated while this information is being collected.

If DKA is mild and the patient is quickly responding to therapy, replacement of fluids, electrolytes, and insulin may occur in the emergency department. If DKA is more severe, hospitalize the patient at once to ensure adequate treatment and monitoring of the clinical state until recovery ensues. An intensive care unit is the preferred site for the treatment of severe DKA.

Health care providers whose experience with DKA is episodic and infrequent should not hesitate to arrange for the patient's prompt referral to a specialist experienced in the care of patients with DKA. A detailed summary of the treatment of DKA is available in the American Diabetes Association's Physician's Guide to Insulin-Dependent (Type I) Diabetes.

MANAGING HYPERGLYCEMIC HYPEROSMOLAR NONKETOTIC COMA*

Background

Definition. Hyperglycemic hyperosmolar nonketotic coma (HHNKC) is characterized by severe hyperglycemia (glucose level typically greater than 600 to 800 mg/dL), dehydration, and altered mental status—in the absence of ketosis. In HHNKC, hyperglycemia causes glycosuria. Osmotic diuresis results in volume contraction and a reduction in both the glomerular filtration rate and glucose excretion. Worsening hyperglycemia causes further extracellular hypertonicity and intracellular dehydration.

Central nervous system dysfunction in persons with HHNKC is probably due to hyperosmolarity. The absence of ketosis has not been entirely explained but may be due to the secretion of insulin in amounts sufficient to suppress ketogenesis.

Occurrence. HHNKC occurs most often among persons over 60 years of age. Most persons with HHNKC have a history of NIDDM, but in a sizable minority, NIDDM is undiagnosed or untreated. When persons who are chronically ill, debilitated, or institutionalized have mild renal insufficiency and lack normal thirst mechanisms or access to water, they are at risk of developing HHNKC. Acute illnesses (stroke, myocardial infarction, or pneumonia), drugs (diuretics or glucocorticoids), surgery, and, occasionally, large glucose loads (through enteral or parenteral nutrition or peritoneal dialysis) may precipitate HHNKC.

Severity. The mortality rate for HHNKC has been reported to be as high as 50%, primarily because of the age of the population most at risk and the acute precipitating causes.

---

*Source: *The Prevention and Treatment of Complications of Diabetes Mellitus: A Guide for Primary Care Practitioners*, Department of Health and Human Services, Public Health Service, Centers for Disease Control, National Center for Chronic Disease Prevention and Health Promotion, Division of Diabetes Translation, January 1, 1991.

Prevention

Be alert to the elderly patient who:

- has a history of NIDDM
- has an altered level of consciousness
- takes diuretics or glucocorticoids
- lacks free access to drinking water
- has a poor support system at home or lives in a nursing home
- is receiving enteral or parenteral nutrition

For persons with several of these characteristics, periodically monitor the glucose level in the urine or blood. (Monitoring blood glucose is preferred.) If the fasting blood glucose level is above 200 mg/dL, monitor the glucose level more frequently and initiate or adjust hypoglycemic medications as necessary.

Early diagnosis of diabetes or early identification of worsening hyperglycemia will permit appropriate therapy that will prevent the development of HHNKC.

Detection

The patient with HHNKC has severe hyperglycemia and azotemia without ketoacidosis. The intravascular volume is contracted, and the patient shows signs and symptoms of hypovolemia and severe dehydration. Both diffuse and focal central nervous system deficits may occur. These may include hallucinations, aphasia, nystagmus, hemianopsia, hemiplegia, hemisensory deficits, and focal or grand mal seizures. Coma may ensue.

Treatment

Therapy is primarily directed at replacement of fluid and electrolytes while supportive care is given. Insulin therapy is designed to slowly—over 24 to 48 hours—return the blood glucose level to a near normal range.

When therapy is successful, the patient may be significantly sensitive to further insulin. Ultimately, the patient may achieve metabolic control through diet and/or oral agents.

MANAGING HYPOGLYCEMIA*

Background

Occurrence. Any person with diabetes who takes an oral hypoglycemic agent or insulin may experience low blood glucose. Severe hypoglycemia occurs more often in patients who are following an intensified insulin therapy protocol (with the target glucose level near the normal range), whose diet and activity vary widely, who have a long duration of diabetes, and/or who have autonomic neuropathy. Patients with a history of severe hypoglycemia are at increased risk for future episodes. Often the cause is multifactorial. A delay or decrease in food intake, vigorous physical activity, and alcohol consumption all may contribute.

Prevention

Patient education and self-monitoring of blood glucose are the best approaches to preventing hypoglycemia.

By emphasizing the relation between hypoglycemia and delayed or decreased food intake or increased physical activity, you may help patients anticipate and avoid the condition. If patients regularly and correctly monitor their blood glucose levels, impending hypoglycemia may be avoided. Patients who know how to treat hypoglycemia can reduce its impact and severity.

To minimize the risk of hypoglycemia, cooperation is required between the patient, family members, other persons close to the patient (including friends, teachers, and colleagues), and health care providers. Stress the importance of such persons knowing the signs and symptoms of hypoglycemia and how to treat it.

Detection

Clinical hypoglycemia (blood glucose level below approximately 60 mg/dL) is associated with adrenergic symptoms (apprehension, tremors, sweating, or palpitations) and

---

*Source: *The Prevention and Treatment of Complications of Diabetes Mellitus: A Guide for Primary Care Practitioners*, Department of Health and Human Services, Public Health Service, Centers for Disease Control, National Center for Chronic Disease Prevention and Health Promotion, Division of Diabetes Translation, January 1, 1991.

neuroglycopenic symptoms (fatigue, headache, confusion, coma, or seizure). Usually, the symptoms of low blood glucose are mild, related to catecholamine release, and easily treated by the patient.

Severe hypoglycemia occurs when the patient ignores, inappropriately treats, lacks, or does not recognize the early warning signs or when glucose counterregulation fails to return the blood glucose level to normal.

Treatment

Guidelines for treating hypoglycemia are as follows:

Person	Action
Patient	Eat 10 to 15 grams of rapidly absorbable carbohydrate (3 to 5 pieces of hard candy, 2 to 3 packets of sugar, or 4 ounces of fruit juice) to abort the episode. Repeat in 15 minutes, as necessary.
Friend or family member	If the patient is unable to treat himself or herself, administer oral carbohydrate. If the patient is unable to swallow, administer glucagon subcutaneously or intramuscularly. For children younger than 3 years of age, give 0.5 mg glucagon; for children 3 years of age and older and for adults, give 1.0 mg.
Practitioner	If the patient shows signs and symptoms of severe hypoglycemia, administer glucagon or inject 25 grams of sterile 50% glucose intravenously.
	Analyze the cause of the episode. Often, a modest reduction in the insulin dosage should be advised. Reeducate the patient about preventing hypoglycemia by discussing the timing of meals and physical activity, the use of alcohol, and the frequency of self-monitoring of blood glucose.
	Those patients who develop hypoglycemia while taking oral hypoglycemic agents should be closely monitored for at least 48 to 72 hours to prevent a possible recurrence.

Teaching Patients To Avoid Acute Glycemic Complications

Thorough and repetitive patient education is essential to prevent the development of acute glycemic complications. In particular, teach patients how to care for themselves when they are ill and how to monitor themselves.

Patient Education Principles

For patients with diabetic ketoacidosis:

- Be sure your patients with diabetes know the following:
  - whether they are at risk for DKA
  - when they are most susceptible to DKA
  - what they can do to prevent DKA
  - when they should contact you

For patients with hyperglycemic hyperosmolar nonketotic coma:

- Remind persons responsible for the elderly, the infirm, or the chronically ill to look for the signs and symptoms of diabetes when their patients do not thrive. Recommend that a blood glucose screening test be performed at the bedside.

For patients with hypoglycemia:

- Ensure that patients who use oral hypoglycemic agents or insulin understand the signs and symptoms, causes, and treatment of hypoglycemia.
- Instruct patients who use oral hypoglycemic agents or insulin to wear a bracelet or necklace that identifies them as having diabetes and to carry sugar or some other source of simple carbohydrate that can be used to promptly treat hypoglycemia.
- Advise persons with diabetes to tell close friends, teachers, or colleagues about their diabetes, how to recognize hypoglycemia, and what to do if an emergency occurs.
- Ensure that patients particularly prone to hypoglycemia who are treated with insulin have glucagon available and that family members and friends know how to administer it.
- Instruct patients with diminished awareness of the signs and symptoms of hypoglycemia to monitor their blood glucose levels at frequent intervals so that unexpected episodes can be recognized early and more severe hypoglycemia forestalled.
- Consider changing the level of diabetes control in the following patients:
  - those who do not or cannot recognize the early warning signs of hypoglycemia
  - those who do not understand the educational details of avoiding or treating hypoglycemia
  - those whose lifestyle makes them vulnerable to life-threatening episodes of hypoglycemia

MANAGING ADVERSE OUTCOMES OF PREGNANCY WITH DIABETES*

Introduction

When a woman who is known to have diabetes becomes pregnant, she is said to have pregestational diabetes. When a woman develops diabetes during pregnancy or is first recognized as having this condition during pregnancy, she is said to have gestational diabetes. Each year, approximately 10,000 infants are born to women with pregestational diabetes, and 60,000 to 90,000 infants are born to women with gestational diabetes.

The factor most important to the outcome of pregnancy is how well the mother's glucose level is controlled before and during pregnancy. When women with diabetes receive optimal care, the perinatal mortality rate for their offspring approaches the corresponding rate for the general population. However, when pregnant women with diabetes do not receive expert treatment, the perinatal mortality rate for their offspring more than doubles.

Pregestational and Gestational Diabetes

Metabolic changes. Normal pregnancy is characterized by increasing insulin resistance, which is probably due to human placental lactogen, a growth hormone–like protein secreted by the placenta. Although pregnant women develop compensatory hyperinsulinemia, postprandial glucose levels increase significantly throughout pregnancy. During late pregnancy, fasting glucose levels fall because of increased glucose consumption by the placenta and the fetus.

Human placental lactogen reaches its peak late in pregnancy; during the third trimester, insulin requirements rise. Gestational diabetes most often appears during this period of maximum insulin resistance, and ketoacidosis may be seen, particularly in patients with insulin-dependent diabetes mellitus who do not increase their insulin dose appropriately.

Effect on the fetus. Because glucose crosses the placenta by facilitated diffusion, maternal hyperglycemia produces fetal hyperglycemia. Fetal hyperinsulinemia occurs in response to this abnormal metabolic environment. Hyperinsulinemia, combined with hyperglycemia, leads to excessive fetal growth. It may also contribute to intrauterine fetal death, delayed fetal pulmonary maturation, and neonatal hypoglycemia.

Source: The Prevention and Treatment of Complications of Diabetes Mellitus: A Guide for Primary Care Practitioners, Department of Health and Human Services, Public Health Service, Centers for Disease Control, National Center for Chronic Disease Prevention and Health Promotion, Division of Diabetes Translation, January 1, 1991.

The incidence of major congenital malformations is increased approximately fourfold among infants of women with pregestational diabetes. Approximately 9% of pregnancies complicated by pregestational diabetes result in the birth of infants with central nervous system, cardiac, renal, skeletal, and other malformations. Major malformations may occur in 20% to 25% of infants born to women with very poor glycemic control during organogenesis, as evidenced by markedly elevated glycosylated hemoglobin levels during the first trimester.

Other factors that may increase the risk for fetal anomalies include early age at onset of maternal diabetes and microvascular disease in the mother. The earlier the age at onset of pregestational diabetes, the worse the prognosis is for successful pregnancy.

Effect on the mother. Pregnancy may be associated with exacerbation of diabetic eye disease, especially in women with unrecognized or untreated proliferative diabetic retinopathy. Diabetic women with nephropathy and hypertension are at greater risk for preeclampsia and fetal growth retardation than are women without nephropathy. Death has been reported among pregnant women with diabetes and coronary artery disease.

Caring for the Patient with Pregestational Diabetes

Prevention

The outcome of pregnancy complicated by pregestational diabetes is improved when care begins before conception. Each visit with a woman of childbearing age who has diabetes should be considered a preconceptional visit. Discuss family planning and ask the patient her thoughts about a future pregnancy.

Results of a glycosylated hemoglobin test provide overall assessment of glycemic control. Pregnancy should be deferred until excellent glycemic control is achieved, as indicated by a normal or near normal glycosylated hemoglobin level. Counsel patients about nutrition and teach them how to monitor their blood glucose levels and how to adjust their insulin treatment.

For patients who are planning to become pregnant, establish baseline data that can be used to assess maternal and perinatal risk, including the following:

- history of diabetic ketoacidosis and severe hypoglycemia
- blood pressure measurement
- eye examination
- quantitative assessment of renal function and urinary protein or albumin excretion
- electrocardiogram (if indicated)

Patients whose pregnancy is complicated by diabetes often experience significant emotional and financial stresses. Assess the patient's emotional or psychosocial support and financial resources through discussion with the patient, her partner, and her family.

Emphasize the dangers of smoking and of consuming alcohol when pregnant.

Treatment

Health care team. An experienced health care team is required to care for a patient with pregestational diabetes. The team should include the following persons:

- obstetrician or a specialist in maternal-fetal medicine
- internist or diabetologist
- pediatrician or neonatologist
- diabetes educator
- dietitian
- social worker

Every effort should be made to refer patients to medical centers that can provide comprehensive support. If such referral is not possible, members of the health care team should frequently consult with each other by telephone.

Glucose level. Excellent control of maternal diabetes is a critical objective both before and during pregnancy. During normal pregnancy, mean maternal plasma glucose levels rarely exceed 120 mg/dL and range from fasting levels of 60 mg/dL to 2-hour postprandial levels of 120 mg/dL. Use these values as the therapeutic objective for patients whose pregnancies are complicated by pregestational diabetes.

Diet. During the latter half of pregnancy, the patient with pregestational diabetes needs to eat approximately 35 kilocalories per kilogram of her ideal prepregnancy body weight each day, or approximately 2200 to 2400 calories per day. A weight gain of 24 to 28 pounds is recommended for most patients; however, for obese patients with non–insulin-dependent diabetes mellitus, the preferred daily intake is 25 kilocalories per kilogram of ideal prepregnancy body weight, or approximately 1600 to 1800 calories per day.

The calories should be derived as follows: approximately 50% from complex carbohydrates, 30% from fats, and 20% from proteins. Patients will require three meals and up to three snacks each day. A bedtime snack is particularly important to decrease the risk of nocturnal hypoglycemia.

Monitoring. Patients with insulin-treated diabetes should monitor their blood glucose levels at least four times a day—either before or two hours after each meal and at bedtime. Before breakfast, patients should test for ketones in their urine. Ask patients to record results in a logbook and to note any changes in diet and exercise and any problems with hypoglycemia.

Measure the glycosylated hemoglobin level at least once each trimester to assess overall glycemic control.

Insulin therapy. Patients treated with oral hypoglycemic agents should be switched to insulin before they become pregnant. Human insulin should generally be used. Patients with insulin-treated diabetes require an individualized insulin regimen based on their exercise plan and blood glucose levels.

Most patients will require at least two injections a day of a mixture of intermediate-acting (NPH or Lente) and short-acting (regular) insulin. Selected patients may be treated with multiple daily injections (that is, regular insulin before each meal and an injection of intermediate- or long-acting Ultralente insulin at bedtime). For some patients, continuous subcutaneous insulin infusion is an option, but it appears to offer no significant advantage over multiple daily injections. Patients who prefer the flexibility offered by the pump may be started on such therapy, and those who have used a pump before pregnancy may continue to do so.

Fetal assessment. Maintain a program of fetal assessment throughout pregnancy. Measure the maternal serum alpha-fetoprotein level at 16 weeks of gestation to screen for neural tube defects and other fetal anomalies. Perform a detailed ultrasonographic examination at 16 to 18 weeks of gestation. If indicated, assess the fetal cardiac structure by echocardiography at 20 weeks of gestation. When performed by experienced professionals, such tests allow detection of most major fetal malformations. If an anomaly is found, skilled counseling must be provided for the patient.

During the third trimester, assessment of fetal growth and well-being becomes most important. Fetal growth may be evaluated by serial ultrasonographic examination every four to six weeks. Fetal well-being may be determined by a variety of techniques, including the following:

- maternal monitoring of fetal activity
- antepartum heart rate testing by using the nonstress or contraction stress test
- biophysical profile that includes an ultrasonographic evaluation of fetal activity, fetal breathing movements, fetal tone, and amniotic fluid volume

Although these tests may be initiated at 28 weeks of gestation, they are most often begun at 32 weeks and performed once or twice a week until delivery.

Delivery. If the patient maintains excellent glucose control, if her blood pressure is normal, and if antepartum fetal testing shows no evidence of fetal compromise, delivery may occur at term. If delivery is planned before term, assess fetal pulmonary maturation by measuring the ratio of amniotic fluid lecithin to sphingomyelin (L/S) and the level of acidic phospholipid phosphatidyglycerol. If ultrasound suggests excessive fetal size, delivery by cesarean section may be elected.

Delivery must take place where expert maternal and neonatal care is available. Breastfeeding should be encouraged.

Postpartum care. In the immediate postpartum period, reassess the patient's meal plan and adjust her treatment program. Maternal insulin requirements fall significantly, usually to, or even below, prepregnancy levels.

During the patient's postpartum follow-up visit, encourage her to diet, if necessary, to achieve her ideal body weight. Contraception should be discussed. Low-dose oral contraceptives or a progestin-only pill may be offered to patients who have no evidence of hypertension or vascular disease. For patients with hypertension or vascular disease, a barrier method of contraception, such as a diaphragm, is preferred. If the patient has completed her family or if she has serious vascular disease, sterilization should be discussed.

Caring for the Patient with Gestational Diabetes

Detection

Screening. All pregnant women should be screened for gestational diabetes. If only those patients with recognized historical or clinical risk factors are screened, a significant number of cases of gestational diabetes will be missed.

Timing. Screen for gestational diabetes at approximately 24 to 28 weeks of gestation. Screening may be indicated before 24 weeks if the patient has a history of any of the following:

- polydipsia or polyuria
- recurrent vaginal and/or urinary tract infections
- glycosuria of 1+ or greater on two or more occasions or 2+ or greater on one occasion
- hydramnios
- having given birth to an infant who was large for gestational age
- gestational diabetes

Method for screening. Patients need not be fasting when the screening test is performed. Use a 50-gram oral glucose load and measure the patient's glucose level after one hour. If the venous plasma glucose is 140 mg/dL or higher, schedule a 100-gram oral glucose tolerance test (see next paragraph).

Method for diagnosis. In pregnancy, the oral glucose tolerance test should be performed as follows:

- Perform the test in the morning, after at least three days of unrestricted diet (more than 150 grams of carbohydrate per day) and unrestricted physical activity and after an overnight fast of at least 8 hours but not more than 14 hours.
- Ask the patient to remain seated. If she smokes, ask her not to do so during the test.
- Administer a 100-gram oral glucose load.
- Measure venous plasma glucose when the patient is fasting and at one, two, and three hours after administering the glucose load.
- Diagnose gestational diabetes when two or more of the following concentrations are met or exceeded:

Time of Test	Glucose Concentration
Fasting	105 mg/dL
After glucose	
1 hour	190 mg/dL
2 hours	165 mg/dL
3 hours	145 mg/dL

- If the initial glucose tolerance test is normal but the patient is thought to be at high risk for gestational diabetes, or if one concentration is met or exceeded, consider repeating the glucose tolerance test at 32 weeks of gestation.

Although blood glucose measurements using glucose-oxidase–impregnated test strips are useful for monitoring treatment, they are not sufficiently precise for diagnostic purposes. Glycosuria and glycosylated hemoglobin tests are also not sensitive enough to be used to diagnose gestational diabetes.

Treatment

Most women with gestational diabetes can be cared for as outpatients. The patient should be seen at one- to two-week intervals to assess glucose control, weight gain, and blood pressure. The patient may need to be hospitalized if she does not maintain acceptable glucose control or if she develops hypertension or an infectious complication such as pyelonephritis.

Diet. Dietary therapy is the mainstay of treatment for patients with gestational diabetes. The daily dietary plan should contain approximately 2000 to 2400 calories distributed among three meals and a bedtime snack.

Monitoring. Ideally, the efficacy of the diet is assessed by daily self-monitoring of blood glucose. Weekly measurements of fasting and postprandial glucose levels are also an acceptable method of monitoring.

Pharmacologic therapy. If the fasting plasma glucose level exceeds 105 mg/dL and/or the two-hour postprandial value exceeds 120 mg/dL, treatment with human insulin should be initiated. Patients who require insulin should be instructed in glucose self-monitoring.

Oral hypoglycemic agents should not be used during pregnancy.

Fetal assessment. Patients with insulin-treated gestational diabetes require a program of fetal surveillance identical to that recommended for patients with pregestational diabetes. Begin fetal surveillance by 34 weeks of gestation for patients with non–insulin-treated gestational diabetes who develop preeclampsia or have a history of intrauterine death. Begin fetal surveillance at 40 weeks of gestation for patients with uncomplicated non–insulin-treated gestational diabetes who have not delivered.

Postpartum care. All patients with gestational diabetes should undergo a 75-gram oral glucose tolerance test at six to eight weeks postpartum to determine whether abnormal carbohydrate metabolism has persisted.

The glucose tolerance test should be performed as follows:

- Perform the test in the morning, after at least three days of unrestricted diet (more than 150 grams of carbohydrate per day) and unrestricted physical activity and after an overnight fast of between 8 and 14 hours.
- Ask the patient to remain seated. If she smokes, ask her not to do so during the test.
- Administer a 75-gram oral glucose load.
- Measure the venous plasma glucose when the patient is fasting and 30, 60, 90, and 120 minutes after administering the glucose load.
- Diagnose abnormal glucose tolerance according to the following criteria:

Glucose Concentration

Time of Test	Normal Glucose Tolerance
Fasting	<115 mg/dL and
After glucose (30, 60, and 90 minutes)	<200 mg/dL and
120 minutes	<140 mg/dL

Time of Test	Impaired Glucose Tolerance
Fasting	<140 mg/dL and
After glucose (30, 60, and 90 minutes)	1 value >200 mg/dL and
120 minutes	>140 mg/dL but <200 mg/dL

Time of Test	Diabetes Mellitus
Fasting	>140 mg/dL and
After glucose (30, 60, and 90 minutes)	1 value >200 mg/dL and
120 minutes	>200 mg/dL

Encourage patients to achieve their ideal body weight to decrease their likelihood of developing non–insulin-dependent diabetes mellitus. Patients with a history of gestational diabetes should be annually evaluated for onset of diabetes.

For contraception, patients may use low-dose oral contraceptive pills, progestin-only pills, or barrier methods.

Patient Education Principles

For patients with pregestational diabetes:

- Emphasize the importance of prepregnancy care.
- Work with the patient, her partner, her family, and other health care providers to improve the patient's nutrition, exercise program, and glucose control.
- Recommend that conception be delayed until the patient's blood glucose control is excellent and the glycosylated hemoglobin level is normal or near normal.
- Explain the risks of birth defects and adverse perinatal outcomes and the need for fetal surveillance.
- Recommend that the patient's vascular condition be thoroughly evaluated before she becomes pregnant. Explain that pregnancy may exacerbate advanced diabetic retinopathy but generally does not permanently worsen diabetic nephropathy.
- Explain that, overall, pregnancy does not shorten the life expectancy of a woman with diabetes but does increase her risk for hypoglycemia and ketoacidosis and for associated mortality.
- Inform patients with coronary atherosclerosis that their risks for morbidity or mortality may be greater during pregnancy.

- Discuss the emotional and financial demands of pregnancy with the patient, her partner, and her family.
- Inform patients about lifestyle elements—such as drinking alcoholic beverages and smoking—that increase the risk for a poor outcome of pregnancy. Emphasize that patients will need to modify such behaviors before becoming pregnant.

For patients with gestational diabetes:

- Work with the patient, her partner, her family, and other health care providers to improve the patient's nutrition, exercise program, and glucose control.
- Explain the risks of adverse perinatal outcomes and the need for fetal surveillance.
- Inform patients that they are at increased risk both for developing gestational diabetes during future pregnancies and for developing overt diabetes later in life.
- Encourage physical activity and postpartum weight loss to decrease the likelihood of developing diabetes later in life.
- Recommend an evaluation at six to eight weeks postpartum, and annually thereafter, for detecting the development of diabetes.

For patients with a history of gestational diabetes:

- Recommend screening for overt diabetes before subsequent pregnancies.
- Recommend early screening for the onset of carbohydrate intolerance during subsequent pregnancies.

MANAGING THE CHILD WITH DIABETES*

IDDM and Non-IDDM

The word diabetes is derived from the Greek language and means "to run through," referring to the excessive urination (polyuria) that is a classic symptom of the condition. Mellitus is derived from the Latin language and means "sweetened" or "honeyed" because urine from an untreated patient is sweet due to the presence of sugar. As described above, high blood sugar can be caused by an autoimmune reaction that destroys the source of insulin (IDDM) or may be due to an interference with the action of insulin (insulin resistance), as in the case of non-IDDM (NIDDM). While the vast majority of diabetes is NIDDM (90%), most children with diabetes have IDDM. Families need to be taught that in IDDM the insulin-producing beta cells have been destroyed and the function of these cells does not return. Therefore insulin injections will be necessary for the lifetime of the child. Alternatively, NIDDM patients continue to produce insulin but cannot use this insulin properly; these patients (NIDDM) do not rely on exogenous insulin but may need it during periods of stress or illness or to achieve optimal glycemic control.

Many families initially believe that insulin will be needed until the child is fully grown or until blood glucose levels stabilize or improve. These misunderstandings need to be quickly and accurately clarified; specifically they must realize that children do not "outgrow" their need for exogenous insulin and that IDDM does not "change to" NIDDM as blood glucose levels stabilize.

Additionally, many parents feel tremendous guilt about the diagnosis, especially if they or another family member have diabetes. Many young children believe that they somehow caused diabetes by eating too much sugar. They frequently worry that IDDM is contagious and express concern about giving diabetes to siblings or friends. Families and children need to be reassured about the etiology of IDDM and that nothing that the child or family did or did not do could have prevented the diagnosis. Children, siblings, and friends need to be reassured in developmentally appropriate language that IDDM is not contagious and that there is a minimally increased risk to family members and no increased risk to friends.

Education

Children with newly diagnosed diabetes should be hospitalized and generally stay an average of 3 to 5 days, with some families being ready for discharge in 2 days while others may need up to 1 week. For every family, parents or primary caregivers as well as the child need to commit themselves full time to the educational process. Families come from various ethnic backgrounds, have different levels of education, and various lifestyles and eating habits; some families have more effective support systems than others. All these factors have to be evaluated and taken into consideration when developing a diabetes management and educational plan for each child and family.

An initial interaction with a family is to ensure the parents that even though this experience seems impossible, they will

*Source: Joanne D. Moore, Christine Kaiser, and Javier E. Aisenberg, "Care and Management of the Child with Diabetes," *Home Health Care Management & Practice,* Vol 9:3, Aspen Publishers, Inc., © April 1997.

be able to once again take care of their child at home. Families need to understand that the educational program during the hospital stay will provide them with basic information (survival skills) about insulin, food, exercise, stress, blood glucose monitoring, urine ketones, hypoglycemia, and hyperglycemia, to care for the child. The ultimate goal for diabetes education is to teach families how to be independent and learn self-management, but families should not expect to become "diabetes experts" prior to discharge. Comprehensive information needs to be provided during follow-up care when families have had some time to adjust to the diagnosis and begin to assimilate diabetes into the daily routine. Acute complications of diabetes are emphasized, but chronic complications are mentioned only briefly. Detailing information on chronic complications at this early stage is not particularly helpful and may interfere with the educational process at hand, especially in light of the Diabetes Control and Complications Trial (DCCT), which proved that better metabolic control of diabetes can reduce the complications associated with diabetes. Families need to be instructed on how and when to contact the DMT for problems, questions, or need of assistance. Most DMTs have 24-hour-a-day coverage for families to use. In other words, families learn a "new language" that will allow them to communicate with their DMT and help them take control again.

There is no place like home (ie, usual food, activity, routine). Once the family is at home, a home care professional can be very valuable in reassessing the family level of knowledge and in establishing a bridge between the DMT and the family. Ideally the home care professional should be part of the DMT to share and reinforce the same philosophic points of view about caring for a child with diabetes, but that is not always possible. Therefore home care professionals, themselves, need to have adequate knowledge and technical skills for caring for children with diabetes.

Technical Skills

The acquisition of diabetes skills and knowledge is essential in ensuring that families of a child with diabetes are prepared to safely and effectively care for that child at home. Additionally opportunities to practice procedures repetitively is paramount. Periodic reassessment of diabetes skills should be planned into educational programs and carried out on an ongoing basis.

Blood Glucose Monitoring

Blood glucose monitoring (BGM) is a necessary and integral component in the diabetes management of children with diabetes. It is a means of achieving the goal of optimal glycemic control. Many children with diabetes and their families rely on BGM for day-to-day, moment-to-moment decision making. BGM is a means of assessing therapeutic regimens and for making adjustments in the regimen. Terms such as "good" and "bad" in reference to specific BGM values should be actively avoided, since this can lead to feeling "good" and "bad" about the child with diabetes. Rather, using words such as "in range," "high," or "low" has less emotional impact for the child and parents. Therefore target ranges for BGM should be established cooperatively between the family and the DMT. Families should also be educated on the percentage of BGM in the target range that represents adequate or optimal glycemic control. Sample target ranges for BGM for various ages during childhood are outlined in Table 1.

Numerous methods for BGM are commercially available. These include visually read strips, reflectance meters that detect color differences in reagent strips to determine a blood glucose value, and biosensor technology in which a chemical reaction creates an electrical impulse to determine blood glucose value. Most systems measure whole blood glucose, but some measure plasma glucose; whole blood glucose produces a lower value than does plasma glucose. To evaluate meter accuracy, meters should only be compared with a laboratory measurement done simultaneously; ideally, a result yielded within 10% is deemed acceptable. Most individuals who have been trained on BGM are able to obtain results within 20%. A meter-to-meter comparison, while simpler, is not an adequate determination of accuracy. The decision for BGM systems should be made in consultation with the child, family, and DMT. Consideration of what insurance covers and does not cover may be a limiting factor in BGM system selection and the family's ability/willingness to continue with this component in the child's care. Several other factors to consider are accuracy, cost to family, ease of use, portability, and blood sample size. Whatever system for BGM is selected, children and families need to be instructed on use and care of the equipment and supplies. A return demonstration by any person who will use the equipment and supplies is highly recommended. Manufacturer instruction

Table 1. Sample BGM target ranges by child's age

< 2 years of age	120–200 mg/dl
2–5 years of age	100–200 mg/dl
6–8 years of age	100–180 mg/dl
9–12 years of age	90–150 mg/dl
≥ 13 years of age	80–120 mg/dl

These target ranges are generalizations. Individual consideration must be given to each child and family. These target ranges are the opinion of the authors and may not be representatives of other DMTs.

for use and care of the equipment and supplies should be read and followed explicitly to ensure accurate BGM results. While individual systems vary, several steps in the procedures are universal:

- Obtaining a capillary blood sample: Most children use a finger-lancing device. There are a multitude of these devices available; most are springloaded. Proper attention should be given to the assembly of the device, selection of lancet (most are universally sized), and insertion of lancet into device.
- Cleaning the finger: Either soap and water or alcohol may be used to clean the finger prior to lancing. When alcohol is used, the alcohol should be allowed to dry completely before lancing. This will minimize stinging caused by alcohol in the puncture site as well as reduce the possibility of interfering with accurate BGM results.
- Puncture depth: Many lancing devices include several caps or a dial system to provide for varying degrees of penetration. Care should be taken to obtain an adequate capillary sample to cover the test strip area while minimizing discomfort associated with the puncture.
- Site selection: The sides of the finger should be the site used for finger lancing. Avoid the fingertips, which may increase pain, and the pads of the fingers, which may interfere with obtaining an adequate sample. Rotation of the site is important in reducing callous formation.
- Sample size: This is dependent upon the methodology chosen. A sample sufficient to cover the entire test strip area is necessary to avoid erroneous results. Some methods require that a "hanging drop of blood" be dropped onto the test strip while others allow for contact by the finger to test strip pad. Refer to manufacturer's recommendations or contact the manufacturer directly for further information on specific devices.
- Procedure: Testing procedures are too variable to discuss in depth. However, manufacturer instructions are available for all products and should be followed exactly. Many manufacturers offer written literature and videotapes to facilitate learning as well as technical assistance phone lines. Some questions to keep in mind for meter selection and use are: Does the meter need to be turned on or does it have an automatic start? Does the meter need to be kept on a flat surface or can it be lifted during the procedure? How are strips to be stored? When do the strips expire? How and when does the test strip get inserted into the meter? Does the test strip have a code number that needs to be matched with the meter code number? How does the meter get coded—code chip, calibration strip, button on meter? Does the strip need to be blotted or wiped and, if so, with what material and at what point in the procedure? What is the range of results available—the highest and lowest results measurable?

What energy source (battery) is used? How often will the battery need to be replaced? Does the family have a backup battery available at home or an alternate way to perform BGM? Does the family have control solutions, check strip/paddle? When are these to be done? Does the meter need to be cleaned? For example, a meter that requires a large drop of blood applied to a strip held in place by a platform and a stable surface on which to rest the meter may not be appropriate for a toddler who is struggling during BGM. A better choice may be a meter that can be moved during the test or one during which the sample is applied to a strip and then is inserted into a strip guide.

- Disposal of sharps and prevention of transmission of blood-borne disease: Lancets should be properly disposed of either in a medical waste container or other puncture-resistant container. Disposal of sharps varies by locality. Families should check with local sanitation departments or township offices for restrictions to avoid problems. These containers should be kept out of the reach of children. Finger-lancing devices should be used by one person only in an effort to prevent possible transmission of blood-borne disease. Replacement caps may be available through individual manufacturers or may be purchased at local pharmacies. Some meters that require placement of a blood drop onto a test strip which rests in a test strip guide or platform require individual guides or platforms for each person using the meter.
- Recording results: Families need to record diabetes information in a logbook, on a record sheet, or on a computer printout to identify patterns in glycemic control and as a record to communicate with the DMT. While many meters have memories of 1 to 250 test results, it is generally recommended that alternate records described above be maintained in the event of meter malfunction or battery depletion resulting in the loss of the meter memory.
- Reportable information: Families should know at what point they are responsible to contact the DMT. Some DMTs give specific BGM values that should be reported immediately as well as intervals of time during which families are expected to contact the DMT for routine review of records.

Children at various ages can participate in the process of BGM. Very young children can be encouraged to participate in their own care by holding still or selecting the finger to be used or by pressing a button to turn the meter on. Most school-aged children can perform the lancing and testing procedures with minimal adult assistance but should always be supervised. Adolescents can perform procedures independently but may require adult supervision of task completion and may need intermittent supervision that technique is correct. They may need "breaks" or "vacation" from these tasks as well. Parents should avoid "nagging" but should be available to their children to ensure accuracy of testing and recording and to facilitate completion of diabetes tasks.

BGM is ideally done before breakfast, lunch, dinner, and bedtime snack. However, DMTs, children, and parents need to be willing to negotiate what realistically can be expected from individual children. Frequently a compromise can be found, for example, daily BGM before breakfast and dinner (before insulin injections), 2 days/week before bedtime snack, and 2 days/week before lunch. Unreasonable expectations or rigidity in recommendations for BGM may increase the likelihood that the results are unreliable or fabricated, since it is easier to record what is expected than to cope with the consequences of not testing or reporting abnormal results.

Noninvasive BGM systems are currently being developed or are in US Food and Drug Administration (FDA) review. While no system is commercially available for patient use at present, the advent of these systems is greatly anticipated by families, children, and DMTs. These systems are expected to use near infrared light, skin patches, or to be surgically implanted to produce a reproducible BGM result. There will be no pain associated with these systems, which may make BGM more feasible and advantageous for children with diabetes. Initially the cost of these devices is expected to be quite high, and the issue of insurance reimbursement remains to be addressed.

Urine Ketone Testing

Urine ketone testing is another important component to diabetes control and is essential in preventing or identifying diabetes ketoacidosis (DKA), a life-threatening, medical emergency caused by insulin deficiency and characterized mainly by hyperglycemia and acidosis. Ketone bodies are formed when fat is broken down and used for energy. This occurs during insulin deficiency and during periods of starvation. During insulin deficiency, there is an insufficient amount of insulin to open the body cells and to drive glucose inside the cells for use as energy. The cells begin to starve, and eventually fat utilization for energy begins. This fat breakdown produces an acidic byproduct, ketones, which are excreted and measured in the urine. If the process goes unchecked, DKA is likely to occur.

During periods of starvation, such as fasting or bouts of gastrointestinal (GI) upset where nutritional intake is disturbed, ketone production can occur even with sufficient amounts of insulin. This process is due to insufficient amounts of glucose available for cellular metabolism, resulting in the production of ketones as an alternative energy source.

Several methods for urine ketone testing are commercially available: Ketostix® or Ketodiastix® (includes urine glucose measurement), Chemstrip® K or Chemstrip® uGK (includes urine glucose measurement), and Acetest® tablets. Each product contains specific directions for the product use, such as timing, and these instructions must be followed exactly.

The schedule for urine ketone testing may vary from DMT to DMT. Specific recommendations for each child should be obtained from the DMT. Generally accepted recommendations for urine ketone testing as outlined by the American Diabetes Association (ADA) available in the October 1990 Position Statement include "periods of:

- acute illness or stress;
- blood glucose levels consistently >240 mg/dL;
- any symptoms of DKA (eg, nausea, vomiting, abdominal pain)"

Some DMT will additionally recommend testing the first morning urine to assess for undetected nocturnal hypoglycemia (positive ketones with normal or low blood glucose) or insulin waning (positive ketones with elevated blood glucose) or both.

Appropriate and immediate treatment of ketones is essential in preventing DKA. This includes:

- notification of the DMT,
- rest since exercise may aggravate and/or increase fat mobilization and utilization,
- increased caloric-free fluids to prevent dehydration caused by hyperglycemia and increased urine output,
- additional insulin if insulin deficiency is the cause, and
- continued urine ketone testing until negative.

Insulin Therapy

Insulin acts by allowing glucose to enter the cell (no insulin > glucose remain in the blood > high blood glucose). Once inside the cell, glucose is used for energy, but when enough glucose is available it is also stored in the liver as glycogen. Insulin facilitates this process, and if there is sufficient insulin, glycogen will remain in the liver ready to be slowly released when food is not available, for example, at night. When insulin is unavailable or deficient, those stores never form, and glucose again remains in the blood, causing high blood glucose. Another function of insulin is to maintain fat deposits, again to be used as energy when glucose is not available. In insulin deficiency, for example, undiagnosed diabetes or missed insulin, glucose cannot be used for energy, fat cannot be stored, and fat begins to break down. When fat breakdown occurs, ketone bodies are formed and acidosis can occur.

While it is true that children with IDDM do not outgrow the need for insulin, a short honeymoon period may occur. The honeymoon period occurs because once blood glucose is controlled, that per se allows better function of the remaining beta cells. Consequently insulin requirements may decrease significantly. Since treatment with insulin will not alter the underlying autoimmune reaction, those remaining cells will continue to be destroyed. The honeymoon period, when it occurs, may last from weeks to months; it is very rare for the honeymoon period to last longer than 1 year. At that point the need for exogenous insulin replacement is the rule.

Manufacturers

Two companies manufacture insulins used in the United States—Eli Lilly and NovoNordisk. While neither Lilly nor NovoNordisk insulin appears to be better for individual patients, families should use only one brand at a time and should change brands only after discussion with their DMT. Neither company recommends mixing brands.

Types

Several types of insulin are commercially available.

- Rapid-acting insulins, called Regular and Semilente®. Onset of these insulins is one half to 1 hour, peak effect is 2 to 4 hours, and duration of action is 4 to 8 hours.
- Intermediate-acting insulins, called neutral protamine hagedorn (NPH) and Lente®. Onset of these insulins is 1 to 4 hours, peak effect is 6 to 10 hours, and duration of action is 10 to 16 hours. The protamine in NPH, and higher levels of zinc in Lente®, prolong the actions of these insulins.
- Long-acting insulin, called Ultralente® insulin. Onset of this insulin is 4 to 6 hours, a peak effect is not expected, and duration of action is 18 to 24 hours.
- Premixed insulins are also available as 70/30 and 50/50, with NPH and Regular in these percentages respectively. These premixed insulins are less commonly used in pediatric populations than in the adult population, since they do not allow as much flexibility in dosing as do self-mixing doses.

Species

Human, purified pork, and beef-pork insulins are commercially available throughout the United States. While human insulin is chemically identical to endogenous insulin and the most commonly used insulin, some DMTs prefer to use purified pork insulin in children with diabetes. Human insulins are absorbed more rapidly and have a shorter duration; purified pork insulins allow young patients to take two injections per day instead of three or more. For families who have religious or personal preference for human insulin, many DMTs will use Lente® instead of NPH insulin, since the former insulin has a longer duration of action than does the latter. Families need to be educated on the species of their insulin and should be instructed on the importance of using only the species prescribed by their DMT. Changes in the species of insulin should be done only after consulting with the DMT, since the action of insulins may differ between species. Families should always check supplies obtained from their pharmacies or mail order services. It should be noted that religions allow use of pork products for medicinal purposes, but families may still feel uneasy about the use of such products.

Concentration

The concentrations of insulin commercially available in the United States are U-100 (100 U insulin/1 mL volume) and U-500 (500 U insulin/1 mL volume). U-500 is available by prescription only and used in cases of insulin resistance, more commonly found in NIDDM, and therefore is beyond the scope of this article. U-100 is the insulin used by most children with diabetes. Some children and families do, however, use diluted insulin, such as U-10 (10 U insulin/1 mL volume) or U-50 (50 U insulin/1 mL volume) as prescribed by their DMT. Only Regular insulin can be diluted. Using diluted insulin allows for more accurate dosing of small doses of regular insulin, particularly in infants and very young children. Diluted insulin is mixed by a pharmacist using the manufacturer's diluent. It can be used for up to 30 days, and any unused insulin should be discarded. Caution should be used whenever diluted insulin is used. Careful documentation by families on the dosage of insulin given rather than the volume drawn into the syringe is essential. See Table 2 for conversion information for diluted insulin.

Storage

Insulin that is currently in use can be stored at room temperature (36° to 86°) and used within 30 days. Insulin that is unopened or will not be used within 30 days should be stored in the refrigerator. Insulin being used and stored in the refrigerator may degrade over time and should be discarded within 90 days whenever possible. Insulin that is stored in the refrigerator should be allowed to warm up to room temperature before drawing up and injecting to reduce discomfort. Insulin bottles can be set out ahead of time or gently rolled between the palms to warm up.

Table 2. Using U-10 and U-50 insulins

U-10 regular insulin dose to be given (units)	Dose to be drawn into U-100 syringe* (units)	U-50 regular insulin dose to be given† (units)	Dose to be drawn into U-100 syringe (units)
0.1	1	0.5	1
0.2	2	1.0	2
0.3	3	1.4	3
0.4	4	2.0	4
0.5	5	2.5	5
0.6	6	3.0	6
0.7	7	3.5	7
0.8	8	4.0	8
0.9	9	4.5	9
1.0	10	5.0	10

*Dose to be given multiplied by 10.
†Dose to be given multiplied by 2.

Timing

Insulin is generally given before breakfast and dinner and approximately 30 minutes prior to the meal when Regular insulin is used, since the onset of action of Regular is 30 minutes after injecting. Some DMTs have timing schedules based on the blood glucose value obtained before the meal, for example, longer waiting period for higher blood glucose reading, shorter waiting period for blood glucose readings that are normal or low. When intermediate or long-acting insulins are used exclusively, the insulin can be given along with the meal. Children on more intensive regimens (multiple injections of 3 or more/day) should follow similar guidelines. For infants and toddlers who have erratic eating patterns, some DMTs will instruct families to inject insulin after the food is eaten and the amount of foods can be assessed. This is done to lessen the risk of hypoglycemia for these young children. This practice may be controversial, since no studies have been conducted to assess the potential negative effect of performing painful procedures following eating and its impact on feeding behaviors. Evaluation of the child's individual regimen, including onset, peak, and duration of action(s) is necessary in determining timing/frequency of insulin injection. Home health care professionals should be aware that many children with diabetes do not wait between insulin and food as prescribed. This is an important area to assess because studies have demonstrated improved glycemic control when timing schedules between insulin and food are observed.

MANAGING THE GERIATRIC PATIENT WITH DIABETES*

Type II or noninsulin-dependent diabetes mellitus (NIDDM) is commonly seen in the geriatric age group (older than 65 years of age). Twenty percent of this population has been diagnosed with NIDDM, although, due to underdiagnosis, the frequency has been estimated at 30 to 50 percent. More than half of these cases are in females, and those who have undergone multiple childbirths have a greater statistical chance of developing diabetes. The hyperglycemia associated with NIDDM occurs because of a combination of factors: impaired glucose uptake into skeletal muscle cells due to insulin resistance; increased hepatic glucose production; and initially, impaired second phase pancreatic insulin secretion, followed, later in the course of the disease, by impaired first phase secretion. If left untreated, NIDDM is associated with the development of retinopathy, nephropathy, neuropathy, and atherosclerotic disease, which cause a 10 percent decrease in the 10-year survival rate of geriatric patients. The evaluation and treatment of NIDDM in the older patient must consider factors that may differ from those seen in younger patients, including risk factors, complica-

*Source: Gordon A. Ireland, PharmD, "Issues in Treating the Geriatric Patient with Diabetes," *Pharmacy Practice Management Quarterly,* Vol. 17:3, Aspen Publishers, Inc., © 1997.

tions, symptoms, goals of therapy, and special considerations when choosing a therapeutic modality.

Risk Factors

The risk factors for NIDDM include physiological changes due to the aging process, a sedentary lifestyle, complications of other diseases, hereditary factors, female gender, parity, and obesity. (See "Risk Factors for NIDDM.") The physiological changes that occur during the aging process are numerous, some of which increase the development of NIDDM, while others affect the complications of the disease and the choice of treatment. Aging causes a decrease in insulin production by the pancreas and a decrease both in the number of insulin receptors and in the sensitivity of these receptors to the effect of insulin, which results in an inability to control the blood glucose level. Although these changes generally occur in all individuals, they are of greater significance in individuals with a family history of NIDDM. This decrease in glucose control is exacerbated by obesity, which may be a result of diets higher in carbohydrates and fat, and a more sedentary lifestyle, causing an even greater insulin requirement. Neurological changes of aging are associated with decreasing rate and amplitude of the nervous signals leading to compromised sensory input, decreased coordination, increased falls, and a slowing of mental function. These changes may become significantly worse in patients with NIDDM. Decreased thirst mechanism makes it more difficult to maintain adequate hydration when higher glucose levels produce an osmotic diuresis. Decreased visual acuity may compromise the patient's ability to monitor blood glucose levels and measure insulin doses, if use of insulin becomes necessary. The age-related slowing of renal glomerular filtration rate (GFR) and decreasing liver function may contraindicate the use of certain therapeutic modalities. The interaction of other diseases, such as dementia, depression, chronic renal failure, arthritis, and malnutrition, may make the evaluation and management of NIDDM much more difficult.

Complications of NIDDM

The long-term complications of NIDDM, although common to both types of diabetes, seem to occur more rapidly and more severely in the geriatric patient, possibly because the diagnosis is made at a later time in the course of the disease

---

Risk Factors For NIDDM

- physiological changes
- lifestyle changes
- complications of other diseases
- heredity
- female gender
- number of childbirths
- obesity

---

or the complications are superimposed on similar changes occurring due to the aging process. (See "Complications of NIDDM.") Chronic complications include vascular, neurological, metabolic, visual, and immunological. Acute complications that occur when blood glucose levels rise are slowing of mental function, blurring of vision, difficulty differentiating colors, polyuria, and polydypsia.

Vascular

Diabetes-induced vascular diseases are classified as either macrovascular (large vessel) or microvascular (small vessel) disease. These diseases are due to atherosclerotic changes that occur within the vessels and decreased blood flow to the affected areas. Macrovascular disease is accelerated by diabetes. NIDDM patients are more likely to have coronary artery disease with resultant angina and myocardial infarction; cerebrovascular disease producing decreased mental function and ischemic strokes; and peripheral vascular disease resulting in a decreased ability to combat local infections leading to possible gangrene with an accompanying amputation of toes, feet, or even legs. Macrovascular changes have also been implicated in sexual dysfunctions. In females, vaginal dryness is associated with painful intercourse and

---

Complications of NIDDM

- macrovascular disease
- microvascular disease
- neurological
- metabolic
- visual
- immunological

increased vaginal infections, and in males, erectile dysfunction, also caused by neurological complications, is the primary problem. Retinal abnormalities associated with steadily deteriorating visual acuity and renal disease producing decreased kidney function and protein loss are a result of the microvascular changes and neuropathies of NIDDM.

Neurological

Neurological complications of NIDDM include both central and peripheral effects. The central nervous system slowing causes cognitive impairment evidenced by a slowing of the thought process and memory retrieval. This effect may be exacerbated by the diabetic vascular changes and the aging process. Depression is also more common in diabetic older adults than the same age group without diabetes. Peripheral neuropathy produces significantly decreased sensory input leading to the patient's inability to feel pain. This decreased sensation allows foot cuts to go undetected and, in conjunction with peripheral vascular disease, may eventually lead to amputation of the extremity. Two thirds of amputations occur in patients over the age of 65, and two thirds of these are in individuals with diabetes. While pain sensation transmission is decreased in peripheral neuropathic neurons, the pain sensation of peripheral neuropathy is increased in patients with diabetes. One study showed that patients with diabetes complain of pain more frequently than nondiabetic controls exhibiting both an earlier stimulus detection and a decreased pain tolerance. The same study found similar results when blood glucose levels were increased in nondiabetic subjects.

Metabolic

Metabolic abnormalities include hyperlipidemia and atherosclerosis in NIDDM. These abnormalities lead to coronary artery disease and peripheral vascular disease.

Visual

Diabetic retinopathy, which can lead to decreased visual acuity and color blindness, increases with age from 10 percent at age 55 to about 30 percent at age 80. Cataracts and glaucoma also occur with greater frequency in patients with diabetes than in similarly aged nondiabetic patients. The color blindness produces a difficulty in differentiating shades of color. This may cause the misinterpretation of color-mediated tests in diabetes monitoring. Patients may also have blurring of vision intermittently when glucose levels are high because of increased glucose concentrations in the humors of the eye. Although the blurring can be corrected as the blood glucose levels are brought back to normal, it may have serious consequences when it occurs in patients who already have age-related visual changes.

Immunological

Immunological deficiency associated with NIDDM in older patients puts them at risk for the occurrence of a greater number of infections. These infections include pulmonary, genitourinary tract, cuts, and diabetic foot ulcers, which are more difficult to treat and take longer to heal.

Symptoms

The symptoms of diabetes in the older adult patient are similar to those in the young (i.e., polyuria, polydypsia, polyphagia, weakness, lethargy, and blurred vision). However, some differences do exist. Older patients frequently have nocturia as a result of benign prostatic hypertrophy (BPH), smaller bladder size, and other diseases due to the aging process or the more frequent use of diuretics. These other causes of nocturia must be distinguished from hyperglycemia. Polydypsia may not be obvious since decreased thirst sensitivity occurs with advancing age. Increased appetite may also not be noticeable since satiety occurs more readily in the geriatric patient. Weakness, lethargy, and blurred vision may appear as a result of aging, concurrent diseases, and/or medications consumed. It is, therefore, important to consider these differences when evaluating the geriatric patient.

Goals of Therapy

The primary goal for therapy of the geriatric patient with NIDDM is to maintain fasting blood glucose (FBG) levels below 140 mg/dL, all random blood glucose (RBG) levels below 200 mg/dL, and a hemoglobin A_{1c} (HbA$_{1c}$) below 8 percent. Achieving this goal will usually prevent the symptoms of hyperglycemia. Although the long-term advantage of treating asymptomatic hyperglycemia in the "old old" (older than 80 years of age) has not been documented, glycemic control does prevent acute symptoms. Tighter control may be necessary to prevent long-term complications (i.e., FBG less than 115 mg/dL and RBG less than 180 mg/dL, and HbA$_{1c}$ less than 7 percent). If the primary goal is accomplished, other goals, such as decreased incidence of symptoms, prevention of hyperosmolar coma, and prevention of ketoacidotic or lactic acidotic hyperglycemic coma will be achieved. The microvascular long-term complications may be prevented by glycemic control, but data do not support the prevention of macrovascular complications in Type II diabetes. (See "Goals of Therapy.") Above all, the goal should be

---

Goals of Therapy

- Control blood glucose levels.
- Decrease the incidence of symptoms.
- Prevent, reduce, or improve complications.
- Improve quality of life.

---

to improve the quality of life of the patient. The therapy or the monitoring procedure should not decrease the quality of life.

Special Considerations in Therapy

There are many age-related considerations that must be addressed when treating diabetes in the older adult patient, such as altered vision, dietary changes, musculoskeletal abnormalities, cognitive function impairment, decreased renal function, and other medications.

Altered Vision

Altered vision may make it more difficult, if not impossible, to perform self-monitoring procedures and drawing insulin into the syringe. It is imperative to watch older patients performing these functions to ensure their capability. This observing may be performed by any trained health professional and should not be limited to physicians or nurses. Pharmacists are ideally positioned to perform this role in hospitals, in home care, and especially in retail pharmacies when patients come to have their prescriptions filled. If patients are unable, family members can be trained or arrangements made for a visiting health professional to draw up the insulin and/or perform the monitoring tasks. Again, pharmacists could supply prefilled syringes and arrange the monitoring.

Dietary Changes

Decreased appetite may make it difficult for patients to maintain a diabetic diet and, if they are taking insulin or an oral hypoglycemic agent, may produce periods of hypoglycemia. A diary should be maintained for recording daily dietary intake, exercise involvement, blood glucose levels, and medication doses, if needed. The age-related decreased thirst sensitivity may result in dehydration, causing orthostatic hypotension and the possibility of sustaining an injury from a fall.

Musculoskeletal Abnormalities

Tremors and arthritis may also compromise patients' ability to take care of their therapy and monitoring. Poor dexter-

ity secondary to decreased joint mobility, muscle tremor, muscle weakness, and decreased coordination make it difficult to perform the mechanics of performing monitoring tests and, if necessary, drawing up insulin. As with the visual abnormalities, provision must be made to perform these functions for the patient.

Cognitive Function Problems

Impaired cognitive function and memory dysfunction may make it difficult for the patient to remember instructions and perform monitoring and therapeutic tasks. If the patient is unable to repeat instructions and perform monitoring and therapeutic activities, family members should be trained or arrangements made for a visiting health professional to draw up and administer the insulin and/or perform the monitoring tasks.

Decreased Renal Function

The decreased renal function associated with the aging process must be considered when choosing the therapeutic modality in the older adult diabetic patient. Since serum creatinine measurements in geriatric patients are usually within normal range despite a 30 to 50 percent decrease in GFR, a creatinine clearance should be measured or calculated to better determine kidney function prior to starting therapy.

Other Medications

Many older patients are taking other medications that may cause an increase in blood glucose levels or may interact with the diabetes therapy (e.g., diuretics, corticosteroids, beta blockers). These problems may be avoided by performing a thorough medication history prior to the initiation of any therapy. The same caution may be applied to the interaction between diabetes and other disease states since older individuals tend to have multiple maladies (e.g., decreased renal function, decreased neurological function, and Parkinson's disease).

Other Considerations

Other considerations include decreased physical activity, economics of therapy, medication interactions, and disease interactions. Decreased physical activity can lead to a lower requirement of glucose intake but an increased need for insulin. This combination is extremely difficult to control in a sedentary geriatric patient, who produces less insulin, and it may exacerbate the occurrence of NIDDM. Since many geriatric patients are living on low fixed incomes, the cost of the proposed therapy and monitoring should be carefully considered. Some choices of therapy and monitoring are less expensive than others. The least costly medication that will fit the patient's needs should be chosen, and monitoring tests should be done as infrequently as possible. For example, in a controlled patient, home glucose monitoring could be done once every other day or even less frequently, if deemed adequate. Performing the test at a different time each test day will eventually produce data to evaluate the patient's glycemic control over the whole day without the cost and trauma of multiple tests per day.

Therapy

Diabetes therapy in older adults requires a team approach in order to address all the issues involved. The input of physicians, nurses, pharmacists, dietitians, physical therapists, social workers, family, and friends must all be considered to maximize the patient's therapy for the attainment of the best possible outcome. The therapy also should have a multilayered approach. (See "Therapeutic Options.")

Nonpharmacological Therapy

The nonpharmacological aspects of therapy in the older adult diabetic patient with NIDDM are possibly more important to the achievement of the desired outcome than the medications. It is extremely important that a good base be established on which to apply the needed medication therapy. The components to the base are diet, exercise, lifestyle changes, and education.

Diet. Dietary therapy should be aimed at weight stabilization. If the patient is overweight, weight reduction will aid in the control of the hyperglycemia. NIDDM patients who are overweight and being treated with oral hypoglycemic agents have been able to discontinue the medications after weight reduction. Patients who are underweight due to decreased nutritional intake need to increase their body weight to a more ideal amount. Diets incorporating nutritional foods governed by the calorie intake to maintain the patient's ideal body weight, have been successful in producing weight stabilization and aiding in glucose control. The dietary program should also be low in fat since hyperlipidemia and atherosclerosis are more prevalent in patients with diabetes. Dietary therapy alone is not sufficient but must be used in conjunction with exercise and behavioral changes.

Exercise. A planned program of exercise developed specifically for each individual patient is the second leg of this therapeutic base. Exercise has multiple benefits for the patient. It improves the body's ability to move glucose into skeletal muscle cells with a decreased need for insulin, burns calories, improves tissue oxygenation, improves muscle strength, improves coordination, and ultimately improves the patient's quality of life. Although any amount of exercise is beneficial, it maybe difficult to achieve the necessary amount in the older patient due to underlying conditions (e.g., multiple disease states, arthritis, and osteoporosis).

Lifestyle. Lifestyle changes involve not only changing diet and starting an exercise program but also stopping smoking, drinking alcoholic beverages sparingly, adopting a less sedentary lifestyle, and avoiding stress-producing situations. It may be very difficult, however, to make some changes in the lifestyle of a 90-year-old patient. If smoking is this person's only "pleasure in life," it will be almost impossible, and maybe unnecessary, to stop that behavior. Each lifestyle change must be analyzed not only on its impact on disease therapy but also on how it will affect the patient's quality of life.

Education. If diet, exercise, and behavioral modification are the legs for the therapy base, education is necessary to stabilize them. Diabetes control is more likely to occur in patients who are well educated not only about their disease and the end results of the disease but also about all aspects of nonpharmacological and, if necessary, pharmacological therapy and monitoring procedures. (See "Therapeutic Options.") The patient must buy into the total package in order for the treatment to be successful. It is also very important to involve the patient's family in this process because they will be the patient's daily support and compliance advocates.

Pharmacological Therapy

Pharmacological therapy for NIDDM in the older adult patient should only be started in severe hyperglycemia or after nonpharmacological modalities have been unsuccessful in controlling the blood glucose levels. (See "Hypoglycemic Agents.")

Sulfonylureas. Sulfonylureas are usually the first choice of second generation medication therapy since they produce

---

Therapeutic Options

- diet
- exercise
- behavioral modification
- sulfonylureas
- metformin
- acarbose
- insulin

Hypoglycemic Agents

1. sulfonylureas
   - first generation
     - tolazamide (Tolinase)
     - tolbutamide (Orinase)
     - acetohexamide (Dymelor)
     - chlorpropamide (Diabinese)
   - second generation
     - glyburide (Micronase, Diabeta)
     - glipizide (Glucotrol, Glucotrol XL)
     - glimepiride (Amaryl)
2. Biguanide
   - metformin (Glucophage)
3. Alpha-glucosidase inhibitor
   - acarbose (Precose)
4. Insulin

a more predictable hypoglycemic response than the first generation. Chlorpropamide is the only sulfonylurea that should not be used in the geriatric patient because it has a very long half-life (t1/2) and multiple adverse reactions. The second generation sulfonylureas have equivalent hypoglycemic effects and differ primarily in their duration of hypoglycemic activity. In older adult patients glipizide usually needs to be administered twice a day, glyburide, is usually effective when given once daily due to a slightly longer half-life, while glimepiride should only be given once daily. The once-daily dosing of glyburide and glimepiride should produce a better compliance to therapy. Doses in older adult patients should always be started at the lowest dose and titrated upward based on the patient's response. The two primary concerns with sulfonylureas are weight gain and hypoglycemia, both of which can usually be kept to a minimum by good patient education and follow-up.

Biguanide. Metformin is usually prescribed as a second choice in older adult patients with NIDDM and may be added to or substituted for the sulfonylurea. The reason for this placement is the potential for lactic acidosis, which occurs in patients with decreased renal function (creatinine less than 60 ml/min.), a common finding in the geriatric patient. Metformin should be used with caution in patients with decreased GFR. Metformin also needs to be discontinued for any situation in which the patient has the potential of experiencing low blood pressure to the point of compromising renal function. It should not be administered to persons with cardiac failure, liver disease, and chronic acidosis. The possible advantages of metformin over sulfonylureas are no weight gain, more likely weight loss, and less potential for hypoglycemic episodes.

Alpha-glucosidase Inhibitor. Acarbose, due to its side effect profile, multiple daily dosing regimen, and lower efficacy, should not be used as initial therapy in the geriatric patient with diabetes but may be useful as an addition to a sulfonylurea, especially if the lack of control is due to postprandial hyperglycemia. Acarbose is not recommended for use in patients with cirrhosis or with renal impairment (serum creatinine greater than 2.0 mg/dL). Great caution must be used in the geriatric patient until creatinine clearance cautionary data are available, since normal serum creatinine levels may be obtained despite 50 to 60 percent renal function.

Insulin. Insulin should be used to treat older adult patients with NIDDM only after a trial of oral therapy has failed. Insulin may cause weight gain in NIDDM patients, which leads to the need for more insulin, causing more weight gain, resulting in steadily increasing doses of insulin in response to the patient's gain in weight. If used correctly, however, insulin is of benefit both in controlling hyperglycemia and preventing some end organ damage. Insulin self-administration by the geriatric diabetic patient may be compromised by decreased visual acuity, tremor, arthritis, and decreased cognitive function.

NIDDM treatment in the geriatric patient should be initiated with maximum nonpharmacological interventions followed by a sulfonylurea (glyburide or glipizide). If this regimen fails, the addition of metformin or acarbose, if they are not contraindicated, may improve glycemic control. Insulin therapy should be reserved until a program of nonpharmacological combined with oral hypoglycemic agents has been unsuccessful.

Monitoring

Disease and therapy monitoring in the older adult diabetic patient should be accomplished through a combination of laboratory and self-monitoring with a goal of achieving an FBG of less than 140 mg/dL, an RBG of less than 200 mg/dL, and a glycosylated hemoglobin of less than 8 percent. Self-monitoring by the geriatric with diabetes may be compromised by decreased visual acuity, tremor, arthritis, and decreased cognitive function.

MANAGING PERIODONTAL DISEASE*

Background

Definition. The term periodontal disease describes a group of localized infections that affect the tissue surrounding and supporting the teeth.

The two most common forms of periodontal disease are gingivitis and periodontitis. Gingivitis, an early and reversible condition, is an inflammation of the soft tissues surrounding the teeth. Persons with gingivitis have tender, edematous, red gums that may bleed upon gentle pressure, such as from toothbrushing.

Periodontitis is a progressive inflammatory condition that destroys periodontal ligament fibers and alveolar bone and can eventually cause tooth loss. Although gingivitis usually precedes periodontitis, not all gingivitis progresses to periodontitis.

For all persons, the keys to preventing periodontal disease are good oral hygiene and regular dental care. A third element crucial to persons with diabetes is good glycemic control; poorly controlled diabetes can invite or promote periodontal disease.

Occurrence. Disease is widely prevalent. Forty percent to 50% of US adults report gingival bleeding, and over 80% of adults have objective evidence of previous periodontal disease. The prevalence and severity of periodontal disease increase markedly with age. Eight percent of adults younger than age 65 and 34% of adults 65 and older have evidence of advanced periodontal destruction.

Among children and adolescents with poorly controlled insulin-dependent diabetes mellitus and among adults with poorly controlled non–insulin-dependent diabetes mellitus, the prevalence of periodontal disease is considerably greater than it is among their nondiabetic peers. The severity of periodontal disease is also usually greater among persons with diabetes.

Pathophysiology

- Disease is initiated by the toxic metabolic products of bacteria in dental plaque. Other associated factors include smoking, vitamin C deficiency, dental restorations, and prostheses.

- Disease appears to be aggravated by increased levels of blood glucose and by other conditions associated with poor glycemic control. Altered microbial flora, impaired immunity, vascular changes, and abnormal collagen metabolism may contribute to the development and severity of periodontal disease among persons with diabetes.

Prevention

Effective self-care is essential to periodontal health. To ensure that patients with diabetes are aware of the importance of maintaining good glycemic control as well as an effective regimen of oral hygiene, the health care provider should do the following:

- Inform patients of their increased risk of developing periodontal disease.
- Inform patients of the association between poor glycemic control and periodontal disease.
- Explain that severe periodontal disease and other oral infections may adversely affect glycemic control.
- Motivate patients to care for their teeth and gums.
- Explain how dental plaque contributes to periodontal disease.
- Inform patients that they can partly remove plaque by brushing and flossing their teeth at least twice a day.
- Explain that teeth lost to periodontal disease may be difficult to replace. Dentures often fit poorly over gums damaged by periodontitis; the resulting discomfort may limit a patient's dietary choices and may thus impede diabetes management.

To ensure that patients receive the regular professional dental care critical to preventing periodontal disease, the health care provider should do the following:

- Instruct patients to see a dentist at least every six months. Patients with periodontal disease will need to schedule more frequent appointments.
- Provide a list of recommended dentists or local dental clinics if the patient does not have a dentist.
- Urge patients to inform their dentist that they have diabetes. If possible, ask for the dentist's name and telephone number; you may need to alert this person to the special problems of treating a person with diabetes.

Efficient brushing and flossing remove the more superficial supragingival dental plaque. Subgingival plaque, as well as calculus (hard deposits of plaque, also called tartar), will require professional removal. For some patients, the dentist may prescribe antiplaque rinses, such as chlorhexidine.

---

*Source: *The Prevention and Treatment of Complications of Diabetes Mellitus: A Guide for Primary Care Practitioners,* Department of Health and Human Services, Public Health Service, Centers for Disease Control, National Center for Chronic Disease Prevention and Health Promotion, Division of Diabetes Translation, January 1, 1991.

To evaluate personal oral hygiene, the dentist or dental hygienist should ask patients to demonstrate how they remove plaque. Patients can then be shown, if necessary, how to more effectively care for their teeth.

Detection

To determine whether a patient is at increased risk for developing periodontal disease, the health care provider should ask about the patient's oral hygiene habits. Does the patient brush and floss twice daily? Does the patient use any other devices for cleaning teeth? When did the patient last see a dentist? Is the patient experiencing any of the following: bad taste in the mouth, bad breath, sore gums, swollen or red gums, bleeding gums, difficulty chewing, or oral pain?

The health care provider should inspect the patient's mouth for the following signs of dental disease:

- puffy, red gums
- a buildup of plaque
- obviously decayed teeth
- the characteristic bad breath of periodontitis

Patients showing these possible indicators of periodontal disease should be referred to a dentist.

Severe periodontal disease can be present without obvious inflammation. A complete dental examination, including periodontal probing of gum pockets, is necessary to determine the presence and severity of periodontal infection.

Treatment

The health care provider can treat periodontal disease by helping the patient achieve good glycemic control. Further measures fall to the dental health professional, who initially treats periodontal disease by removing plaque from infected areas of the patient's mouth. If infection or destruction has progressed too far, the dentist may prescribe antibiotic treatment, perform restorative procedures, perform surgery, or extract teeth.

The health care provider should work with the dentist in planning treatment and scheduling dental appointments. The health care provider should also be consulted before the patient is pretreated with an antibiotic or is hospitalized.

Patient Education Principles

- Help patients maintain good control of their blood glucose levels.

- Instruct patients to do the following to remove plaque:
  - brush their teeth with a soft toothbrush and a fluoridated toothpaste at least twice a day, especially before going to sleep
  - rinse their toothbrush thoroughly after each brushing, store it vertically (with the bristles at the top), and replace it at least every three months (toothbrushes can harbor bacteria)
  - use dental floss, bridge cleaners, water sprayers, or other cleaning aids recommended by their dentist
- Emphasize the importance of seeking regular preventive dental care at least every six months (or according to the dentist's recommended schedule).
- Encourage patients to ask their dentist for further instructions or advice on caring for their teeth.
- Instruct patients to see a dentist if they have bad breath, an unpleasant taste in the mouth, bleeding gums, sore gums or teeth, red or swollen gums, difficulty chewing, or loose teeth.
- Urge patients to inform their dentist that they have diabetes and to remind their dentist of this when they make appointments. Patients should also give their dentist their health care provider's name and telephone number.
- Stress the importance of scheduling dental appointments that do not interfere with the patient's insulin and meal schedule. The best time for an appointment may be a few hours after breakfast. Tell patients not to skip a meal or insulin before an appointment.

MANAGING EYE DISEASE*

Background

Diabetes mellitus is a major cause of blindness in the United States and is the leading cause of new blindness in working-aged Americans. Diabetic retinopathy alone accounts for at least 12% of new cases of blindness each year in the United States. People with diabetes are 25 times more at risk for blindness than the general population. The estimated annual incidence of new cases of proliferative diabetic retinopathy and diabetic macular edema are 65,000 and 75,000, respectively. Approximately 700,000 Americans have proliferative diabetic retinopathy—the most sight-threat-

*Source: *The Prevention and Treatment of Complications of Diabetes Mellitus: A Guide for Primary Care Practitioners,* Department of Health and Human Services, Public Health Service, Centers for Disease Control, National Center for Chronic Disease Prevention and Health Promotion, Division of Diabetes Translation, January 1, 1991.

ening form of retinopathy—and 500,000 have diabetic macular edema. Over a lifetime, 70% of people with insulin-dependent diabetes mellitus will develop proliferative diabetic retinopathy, and 40% will develop macular edema. Both complications, if untreated, frequently lead to serious visual loss and disability.

Diabetic retinopathy is often asymptomatic in its most treatable stages. Unfortunately, only about half of persons with diabetes receive adequate eye care. Early detection of diabetic retinopathy is critical.

The results of National Eye Institute–supported multicenter clinical trials of laser surgery and vitrectomy surgery have demonstrated that the risk of blindness from diabetes can be reduced.

- Timely laser surgery can reduce the risk of visual loss from high-risk proliferative diabetic retinopathy by approximately 60%.
- Timely laser surgery can reduce the risk of moderate visual loss from clinically significant diabetic macular edema by 50%.
- Vitrectomy can restore useful vision in some diabetic patients whose retinopathy is too advanced for laser surgery.

Diabetic retinopathy and macular edema. The process by which diabetes results in retinopathy and macular edema is not fully understood. It is known that diabetes causes the retinal capillaries to become functionally less competent. Five clinical pathological processes can be recognized in diabetic retinopathy:

- formation of microaneurysms (outpouchings of the capillary walls)
- increased vascular permeability of retinal capillaries
- closure of retinal capillaries and arterioles
- proliferation of new vessels and fibrous tissues
- contraction of fibrous tissue and hemorrhage and/or retinal detachment due to traction

Nonproliferative and proliferative diabetic retinopathy and macular edema have several clinical manifestations (see exhibit, "Clinical Manifestations of Eye Diseases"). Diabetic macular edema can be associated with any stage of diabetic retinopathy.

Cataracts. Cataracts are 1.6 times more common in people with diabetes than in those without diabetes. Furthermore, cataracts occur at a younger age and progress more rapidly in people with diabetes. Young people with IDDM occasionally develop snowflake or metabolic cataracts. These may lessen or resolve with improved glycemic control. Fortunately, cataract extraction with or without lens implantation is 90% to 95% successful in restoring useful vision, but the surgery is not without potential complications that are more frequent in patients with diabetes.

Open-angle glaucoma. Open-angle glaucoma is 1.4 times more common in the diabetic population. The prevalence of glaucoma increases with the patient's age and with the length of time the patient has had diabetes. Medical therapy for open-angle glaucoma is generally effective. Argon laser trabeculoplasty may normalize intraocular pressure in over 80% of patients in whom medical therapy has proven ineffective.

Neovascular glaucoma. Neovascular glaucoma is a more severe type of glaucoma that most commonly occurs among patients with severe proliferative diabetic retinopathy and retinal detachments. It occasionally follows vitrectomy or cataract surgery. Early recognition and emergency panretinal laser surgery may prevent full development of this devastating type of glaucoma. Diagnosis and evaluation require slit-lamp examination of the iris and gonioscopic evaluation of the filtration angle.

Prevention of Diabetic Retinopathy

Epidemiological studies have suggested that diabetic retinopathy and diabetic macular edema are associated with poorer glycemic control and higher blood pressure levels. Health care providers should work with their patients to achieve good blood glucose and blood pressure control. While the National Institutes of Health–sponsored Diabetes Control and Complications Trial is investigating whether very strict control of blood glucose levels is effective in preventing development of retinopathy and slowing its progression, it is prudent to maintain good control of blood glucose levels without causing significant hypoglycemia.

Because coexisting medical problems—including hypertension and renal disease—may affect the development and progression of diabetic retinopathy, blood pressure should be routinely measured. If hypertension exists even at borderline levels, it should be monitored and treated as needed. Aspirin treatment (650 mg per day) neither alters the progression of diabetic retinopathy nor increases the risk of vitreous hemorrhage. Therefore, diabetic retinopathy is not a contraindication for the medical use of aspirin.

Because diabetic retinopathy and diabetic macular edema cannot be prevented, routine early evaluation, timely laser surgery, and careful follow-up are critical.

CLINICAL MANIFESTATIONS OF EYE DISEASES

Nonproliferative Diabetic Retinopathy

- retinal microaneurysms
- occasional blot hemorrhages
- hard exudates
- one or two soft exudates

Preproliferative Diabetic Retinopathy

- presence of venous beading
- significant areas of large retinal blot hemorrhages
- multiple cotton wool spots (nerve fiber infarcts)
- multiple intraretinal microvascular abnormalities

Proliferative Diabetic Retinopathy

- new vessels on the disc (NVD)
- new vessels elsewhere on the retina (NVE)

- preretinal or vitreous hemorrhage
- fibrous tissue proliferation

High-Risk Proliferative Diabetic Retinopathy

- NVD with or without preretinal or vitreous hemorrhage
- NVE with preretinal or vitreous hemorrhage

Diabetic Macular Edema

- any thickening of retina <2 disc diameters from center of macula
- any hard exudate <2 disc diameters from center of macula with associated thickening of the retina
- any nonperfused retina inside the temporal vessel arcades
- any combination of the above

Source: *The Prevention and Treatment of Complications of Diabetes Mellitus: A Guide for Primary Care Practitioners*, Department of Health and Human Services, Public Health Service, Centers for Disease Control, National Center for Chronic Disease Prevention and Health Promotion, Division of Diabetes Translation, January 1, 1991.

Detection and Monitoring of Diabetic Retinopathy

Laser surgery, as defined by the National Eye Institute–sponsored Diabetic Retinopathy Study and Early Treatment Diabetic Retinopathy Study, can ameliorate the devastating effects of diabetic retinal disease, particularly when laser surgery is initiated at the most treatable stages. Emphasis, therefore, must be placed on early detection of diabetic retinopathy and timely referral to ophthalmologists experienced in the management of diabetic eye disease. Because mild, moderate, and even severe retinopathy may be present without any symptoms, the responsibility to screen or examine the patient with diabetes for retinopathy is significant.

The following examination schedule is designed to ensure the early detection and monitoring of diabetic eye disease:

- All patients with IDDM of more than five years' duration and all patients with non–insulin-dependent diabetes mellitus should have yearly eye examinations including a history of visual symptoms, measurement of visual acuity, measurement of intraocular pressure, and dilation of the pupils with thorough vitreous and retinal examination including stereoscopic examination of the macula.

- Retinopathy may progress more rapidly during puberty. Children in this developmental stage should have yearly eye examinations, regardless of how long they have had diabetes.
- Any woman who is planning pregnancy should be examined before pregnancy by a practitioner experienced in the diagnosis and classification of diabetic retinopathy. Any woman with known diabetes who becomes pregnant should be examined for retinopathy early in the first trimester. Retinopathy may progress very rapidly during pregnancy; close cooperation among the health care team is critical.

The practitioner may elect to perform the examination, but because proper stereoscopic examination requires dilation of the pupils and specialized techniques, such as binocular indirect ophthalmoscopy, referral to ophthalmologists or optometrists appropriately trained and skilled in the diagnosis and classification of diabetic eye disease is preferred.

After the initial eye examination, persons with diabetes should receive complete examinations once a year, unless more frequent examinations are indicated by the presence of abnormalities.

The patient should be under the care of a retinal specialist or ophthalmologist experienced in the treatment of diabetic retinopathy when any of the following conditions are identified (see exhibit, "Clinical Manifestations of Eye Diseases," for definitions):

- proliferative retinopathy
- macular edema
- preproliferative retinopathy (severe or very severe nonproliferative retinopathy)
- nonproliferative retinopathy in children during puberty or women during pregnancy

People with any degree of retinal disease—including those who have lost vision from retinopathy—should continue to receive regular eye care. Vitrectomy surgery may restore usable vision for some individuals who have lost sight from vitreous hemorrhage or fibrous tissue proliferation with traction detachment. Postsurgical treatment requires proper refraction, low vision evaluation, optical aids, and other techniques and devices to enable the person to use even severely limited vision. Referral to optometrists or ophthalmologists specializing in low vision may be appropriate. Support groups for the visually challenged and organizations providing vocational rehabilitation are available in most areas. All practitioners should be familiar with appropriate rehabilitative referral sources for their patients with visual impairment.

Treatment and Referral

Patients with high-risk proliferative diabetic retinopathy should receive immediate laser photocoagulation surgery. Some patients with diabetic macular edema are candidates for immediate macular laser surgery. If careful follow-up can be maintained, it is safe to defer treatment in those with severe nonproliferative diabetic retinopathy and non–high-risk proliferative retinopathy until it approaches or reaches the high-risk stage. Alternatively, in patients with bilateral non–high-risk proliferative retinopathy, one eye may be considered for laser surgery prior to the high-risk stage.

Certain patients with vitreous hemorrhage or recent traction retinal detachment may be candidates for vitrectomy. Laser surgery and vitrectomy surgery should be performed by a retinal specialist or other ophthalmologist experienced in laser surgery and the management of diabetic eye disease.

Patients with functionally decreased visual acuity should be referred for low vision evaluation and appropriate visual, vocational, and psychosocial rehabilitation.

Patient Education Principles

- Inform patients that sight-threatening eye disease is a common complication of diabetes and may be present even with good vision. Remind them to report all ocular symptoms, since essentially any symptoms may be diabetic in origin. Blurred vision while reading may indicate macular edema. The presence of floaters may indicate hemorrhage, and flashing lights may indicate retinal detachment. Inform patients that early detection and appropriate treatment of diabetic eye disease greatly reduce the risk of visual loss.
- Inform patients about the possible relationship between glycemic control and the subsequent development of ocular complications.
- Tell patients about the association between hypertension and diabetic retinopathy. Stress the importance of the diagnosis and continuing treatment of hypertension. Urge patients to work closely with their health care teams.
- Help patients understand the natural course and treatment of diabetic retinopathy and the importance of yearly eye examinations.
- Tell patients with diabetic retinopathy about the availability and benefits of early and timely laser photocoagulation therapy in reducing the risk of visual loss.
- Inform patients about their higher risks of cataract formation, open-angle glaucoma, and neovascular glaucoma.
- Tell all patients with any visual impairment (including blindness) about the availability of visual, vocational, and psychosocial rehabilitation programs.

MANAGING KIDNEY DISEASE*

Background

Description. Diabetic nephropathy represents a distinct clinical syndrome characterized by albuminuria, hypertension, and progressive renal insufficiency. Diabetic nephropathy can lead to end-stage renal disease (ESRD), a serious condition in which a patient's survival depends on either dialysis or kidney transplantation.

Occurrence. Among persons who have had insulin-dependent diabetes mellitus for 20 years, the incidence of ESRD approaches 40%. Among whites, the incidence of ESRD is lower among those with noninsulin-dependent diabetes mellitus than among those with IDDM. Because

*Source: *The Prevention and Treatment of Complications of Diabetes Mellitus: A Guide for Primary Care Practitioners*, Department of Health and Human Services, Public Health Service, Centers for Disease Control, National Center for Chronic Disease Prevention and Health Promotion, Division of Diabetes Translation, January 1, 1991.

NIDDM is much more common than IDDM, the number of whites with NIDDM who develop renal failure each year is about the same as for those with IDDM. In certain populations—including blacks, Hispanics, and Native Americans—persons with NIDDM have a higher incidence of ESRD.

About one third of new cases of ESRD in the United States are attributed to diabetes. These persons account for about one third of the $2.8 billion per year that is spent for the care of patients with ESRD.

Pathophysiology—IDDM

The natural history of renal involvement in persons with IDDM has been well characterized. When diabetes is first diagnosed, the histological appearance of the kidney is normal. Within three years, however, the typical changes of diabetic glomerulosclerosis appear: thickening of the glomerular basement membrane and mesangial expansion.

Renal blood flow and the glomerular filtration rate (GFR) are characteristically elevated, correlating with an increase in kidney size and weight. Mild albuminuria may be present if glycemia is not well regulated. Because of renal hyperfiltration, serum creatinine and urea nitrogen concentrations are usually slightly reduced.

After 10 to 15 years, the first laboratory evidence of renal damage may appear with the presence of persistent microalbuminuria (30 to 300 mg per 24 hours). In IDDM, the prevalence of hypertension increases markedly in patients with microalbuminuria, and hypertension clearly contributes to the progression of renal disease.

Clinical diabetic nephropathy is said to be present when a patient who has had diabetes for more than five years and has evidence of diabetic retinopathy develops clinically apparent albuminuria (>300 mg per 24 hours) and has no evidence of any other cause of kidney disease. When these criteria are fulfilled, a clinical diagnosis of diabetic nephropathy can generally be made without performing a renal biopsy.

About four years after the onset of clinical diabetic nephropathy, the serum creatinine level rises to 2 mg/dL or greater. Within an additional three years, about one half of patients will have developed ESRD.

Pathophysiology—NIDDM

The natural history of renal involvement in persons with NIDDM is not well established. Although microalbuminuria has been shown to be associated with the development of clinical diabetic nephropathy, the precise level of microalbuminuria that reliably predicts this condition has yet to be determined. Some individuals with low levels of albuminuria do not develop renal failure. In these persons, albuminuria may be due to the presence of other complicating renal diseases, such as obstructive uropathy, hypertension, or arteriolosclerosis, or may reflect an age-related increase in urinary albumin excretion.

Prevention

At present, strategies for preventing diabetic nephropathy must be viewed as limited in their effectiveness, since the exact pathogenic factors responsible for this condition are unknown.

In patients with albuminuria, blood pressure regulation is of critical importance in slowing the progression to renal failure. Other strategies that may slow the progression of renal disease include limiting the patient's protein intake, maintaining good glycemic control, promptly treating urinary tract infections, and avoiding potentially nephrotoxic drugs and radiographic dyes.

Detection

At the time of initial diagnosis, all diabetic patients should have a urinalysis performed. If bacteria or white blood cells are seen, a culture should be obtained.

Each year, obtain a sensitive quantitative measure of urinary albumin or protein excretion. In general, the protein excretion rate is about one third greater than that for albumin. Thus, a protein excretion rate of approximately 400 mg per 24 hours would correspond to an albumin excretion rate of 300 mg per 24 hours.

Measure renal function (serum creatinine and/or creatinine clearance) each year.

Before establishing a diagnosis of diabetic nephropathy, exclude other possible causes of renal disease, particularly obstructive uropathy and infection. If diabetic retinopathy is not present, suspect a nondiabetic cause of renal disease.

Hypertension is a common development with the onset of diabetic nephropathy or shortly thereafter. If the patient's initial blood pressure is higher than 140/90 mm Hg, at least three additional readings should be obtained over the next month.

Treatment

At present, no known interventions have been shown to reverse clinical diabetic nephropathy. However, practitioners can take several actions to monitor and perhaps slow the progress of this complication:

- Aggressively monitor and treat high blood pressure (>140/90 mm Hg) or significant increments in blood pressure (20/10 mm Hg or greater on careful follow-up) in patients with renal disease.
- Encourage all nonpregnant adults with diabetes, especially those with renal involvement, to limit their daily protein intake to 0.8 g/kg of body weight, as recommended by the American Diabetes Association.
- Strive to achieve good glycemic control, without undue side effects from hypoglycemia, in all diabetic patients, especially those with microalbuminuria.
- Recommend consultation with a diabetologist and/or a nephrologist if patients have microalbuminuria (30 to 300 mg per 24 hours), clinically overt albuminuria (>300 mg per 24 hours), nephrotic syndrome, elevated serum creatinine (>2 mg/dL), or diminished GFR (<50 mL per minute).
- Instruct patients with microalbuminuria or diabetic nephropathy to receive yearly eye examinations.
- Assess cardiovascular risk factors—particularly hypercholesterolemia and cigarette smoking—and provide appropriate treatment, especially for patients with NIDDM.
- Seek and treat other causes of renal disease, particularly obstructive uropathy and infection. Promptly treat any urinary tract infections. Repeat a urine culture after treatment to ensure resolution.

Patients who have developed ESRD will require kidney transplantation, hemodialysis, or peritoneal dialysis to prolong their lives. Because diabetic complications—especially retinopathy and neuropathy—progress more rapidly with the onset of renal failure, dialysis is usually instituted earlier (when the concentration of serum creatinine reaches about 6 mg/dL) for people with diabetes than for those without diabetes. Kidney transplantation is preferable to dialysis when a living relative of the patient is available as a donor; the patient's chances of survival are otherwise about equal among these three courses of treatment. The ultimate choice will require the input of the patient, the patient's family, the primary health care provider, and a nephrologist.

Patient Education Principles

- Inform patients about the potential renal complications of diabetes.
- Inform patients about the association between hypertension and accelerated renal disease. Discuss the need for regular blood pressure measurements and encourage patients to measure their own blood pressure at home. Stress the importance of treating hypertension.

- Explain the potential role that excessive protein in the diet may play in the pathogenesis and progression of diabetic nephropathy.
- Explain the possible relationship between poor glycemic control and the development of diabetic renal disease.
- Emphasize the importance of achieving and maintaining ideal body weight and of undertaking a regular physical exercise program as strategies for preventing hypertension and improving glycemic control.
- Review with patients the symptoms of urinary tract infection. Instruct patients to contact their health care providers if such symptoms occur.
- Review with patients which drugs are potentially nephrotoxic. Explain the danger of radiographic dye studies.
- Review the natural history of clinical diabetic nephropathy with patients who have this condition. Discuss the therapeutic options of dialysis versus transplantation for ESRD.

MANAGING CARDIOVASCULAR DISEASE*

Background

Occurrence. Cardiovascular disease is the leading cause of morbidity and mortality among persons with diabetes. In the United States in 1986, approximately 80,000 deaths from cardiovascular disease were associated with diabetes.

The annual risk for death from cardiovascular disease is two to three times greater for persons with diabetes than for persons without diabetes. For persons with diabetes, the risk for cerebrovascular disease and for coronary artery disease is two to three times greater, and the risk for peripheral vascular disease is five times greater. Among persons without diabetes, women have a lower rate of cardiovascular disease than men do; among persons with diabetes, women are not preferentially spared.

Risk factors. In persons with diabetes, smoking is a powerful risk factor for cardiovascular disease, and the prevalence of smoking appears to be higher in young people (less than 21 years old) with diabetes than in young people without diabetes.

---

*Source: *The Prevention and Treatment of Complications of Diabetes Mellitus: A Guide for Primary Care Practitioners*, Department of Health and Human Services, Public Health Service, Centers for Disease Control, National Center for Chronic Disease Prevention and Health Promotion, Division of Diabetes Translation, January 1, 1991.

Hypertension, also a strong risk factor for cardiovascular disease, occurs two to three times more often in persons with diabetes than in persons without diabetes. The risk for cardiovascular disease increases linearly with increases in blood pressure.

Abnormalities in the concentration of lipids and lipoproteins in plasma have been reported to occur in almost 30% of persons with diabetes. The risk for cardiovascular disease is directly proportional to the concentration of low-density lipoprotein (LDL) cholesterol and inversely proportional to the concentration of high-density lipoprotein (HDL) cholesterol. Although hypertriglyceridemia is common among persons with non–insulin-dependent diabetes mellitus, whether the triglyceride level independently predicts cardiovascular disease is uncertain.

The precise relationship between hyperglycemia and atherosclerosis is also unknown. Among persons with diabetes, several concomitant conditions may affect the etiology of atherosclerosis: obesity, inactivity, hyperinsulinemia, abnormalities in platelet function, and defects in blood coagulation and flow.

Among persons with diabetes, part of the increased likelihood of cardiovascular disease appears to be a consequence of the increased frequency of risk factors. Yet diabetes itself is an independent risk factor for cardiovascular disease.

Prevention

Although the benefit of controlling smoking, hypertension, and hypercholesterolemia has not been well studied in diabetic populations, there is no reason to believe that persons with diabetes will not benefit from controlling these risk factors. However, the precise benefit that can be achieved is not known.

Smoking. Smoking cessation may be the most important modification in behavior that can be made to reduce the risk for cardiovascular disease. Stress to patients the importance of not smoking. Encourage those who smoke to quit, and remind those who do not smoke not to start.

Blood pressure. Blood pressure should be closely monitored in patients with diabetes. When blood pressure is increased over 140/90 mm Hg, nonpharmacologic therapy should be instituted. Medication may need to be initiated early, depending on the blood pressure level. When selecting drugs for treating hypertension, consider their potential adverse effects on other risk factors for cardiovascular disease.

Plasma lipids. The incidence of atherosclerotic heart disease and the morbidity associated with this condition can be decreased in nondiabetic populations by reducing the plasma cholesterol level. When the total cholesterol is more than 200 mg/dL and the LDL cholesterol is more than 130 mg/dL, nonpharmacologic therapy should be instituted.

Plasma glucose. The relationship between plasma glucose and the development of cardiovascular disease is less clear. However, poor glycemic control is often associated with hyperlipidemia. Improved glycemic control has been shown to lower the concentration of cholesterol and triglycerides in plasma and to raise the concentration of HDL cholesterol in persons with diabetes who are either hyperlipidemic or normolipidemic.

Weight, exercise, and aspirin therapy. Additional recommendations for preventing cardiovascular disease in diabetic patients include weight loss (for obese persons) and an increased level of physical activity. For patients who have had cardiovascular events, aspirin therapy may help to prevent mortality or additional morbidity from cardiovascular disease.

Detection

The following guidelines may help in the detection of cardiovascular disease. At every office visit (at least four times a year):

- Measure the patient's blood pressure with a cuff appropriate for the patient's size.
- Ask patients whether they have had symptoms of the following conditions:

Condition	Symptoms
Cerebral vascular disease	Transient blindness, dysarthria, or unilateral weakness
Coronary artery disease, congestive heart failure	Chest pain or pressure, dyspnea, and orthopnea, paroxysmal nocturnal dyspnea, or edema (Painless myocardial infarction is common among diabetic patients, and they may have angina or myocardial infarction with atypical symptoms.)
Peripheral vascular disease	Intermittent claudication or foot ulcers that do not heal

At least once a year:

- Ask patients about their use of tobacco.
- Auscultate for bruits over all large arteries and palpate all peripheral pulses

Once a year:

- Measure triglycerides (TG), total cholesterol (TC), and HDL cholesterol levels in the fasting state, and calculate the level of LDL cholesterol. For TG under 400 mg/dL:

$$LDL = TC - HDL - (TG \backslash 5)$$

For children, consider measuring lipids every two years.
- Obtain a baseline electrocardiogram in all patients with diabetes and repeat the procedure yearly for those with clinically apparent cardiovascular disease.

Treatment

Smoking. Strongly advise patients who smoke to quit. Both the health hazards of smoking and the improved health that patients will enjoy when they stop smoking should be emphasized. Work with each patient to set a quit date, and follow up after that date. Nicotine gum may be used for physiological dependency. Behavioral treatment is recommended for psychological and social dependency. Health care providers should refer patients to smoking cessation programs in the community that are appropriate to patients' individual needs.

Hypertension. If the patient's blood pressure exceeds 140/90 mm Hg at two visits, begin nonpharmacologic therapy, including a low-sodium, alcohol-restricted diet designed for weight reduction. Regular exercise has also been shown to have a beneficial effect on blood pressure. Blood pressure should be maintained below 140/90 mm Hg. For individual patients, consider earlier pharmacologic intervention when indicated by clinical conditions (for example, diastolic blood pressure greater than 110 mm Hg) and the presence of other risk factors (such as albuminuria).

After three months of nonpharmacologic therapy, if the diastolic blood pressure remains above 90 mm Hg, begin pharmacologic treatment. Select drugs that do not worsen other risk factors for cardiovascular disease (including lipids) and that do not induce or worsen autonomic neuropathic complications of diabetes (including hypoglycemia unawareness, orthostatic hypotension, or impotence).

Hyperlipidemia. When the calculated LDL cholesterol level is greater than 130 mg/dL, consider the following guidelines for glycemic control, diet, and exercise.

Glycemic control. Glycemic control should be improved through diet, use of sulfonylureas, or insulin therapy. Weigh the benefits of improved glycemic control against the potential risk for hypoglycemia.

Dietary therapy. Dietary therapy should be instituted to reduce the weight of obese patients and to try to lower the LDL cholesterol level to below 130 mg/dL. Consider the following restrictions on diet:
- calorie restriction for weight reduction if obesity is present
- total fat less than 30% of total calories
- saturated fats less than 10% of total calories. Complex carbohydrates and fiber (especially soluble fiber) can be substituted for the usual intake of saturated fats. Preliminary studies suggest that some diabetic patients with hypertriglyceridemia may benefit by restricting carbohydrate intake to 40% to 45% of total calories. In those patients, monounsaturated fats may be used to maintain caloric balance.
- cholesterol less than 300 mg per day

Exercise. Weigh the potential benefits of exercise against the risks and recommend an exercise program, if appropriate. Regular aerobic exercise has been shown to be a useful adjunct to weight loss and to have a beneficial effect on lipids, especially levels of triglycerides and HDL cholesterol. Exercise may also cause a modest drop in the LDL cholesterol level. Before patients begin an exercise program, determine whether they have hypoglycemia unawareness, postural hypotension, proliferative retinopathy, painless myocardial ischemia, or insensitive feet. An exercise stress test is recommended for all diabetic patients over 40 years old who are considering an exercise program.

Reevaluation. After six months of therapy, if a patient's LDL cholesterol level is above 160 mg/dL, consider drug therapy. Drugs used to treat patients with hypercholesterolemia include bile acid sequestrants (cholestyramine or colestipol), HMG-CoA reductase inhibitors (lovastatin), fibric acid derivatives (gemfibrozil or clofibrate), nicotinic acid, and probucol. Drugs used to treat patients with hypertriglyceridema include fibric acid derivatives (gemfibrozil or clofibrate) and nicotinic acid.

Existing cardiovascular disease. Clinically apparent cardiovascular disease poses considerable diagnostic and therapeutic challenges to the practitioner. Consider consulting with specialists (such as cardiologists, neurologists, and vascular surgeons) early in the course of such disease. The guidelines below address some of the cardiovascular diseases common among persons with diabetes.

Cerebral vascular disease. Patients with signs and symptoms of cerebral vascular disease should be referred for specialized diagnostic tests, including noninvasive Doppler flow studies and, if necessary, carotid arteriography. Caution should be used with dye studies in patients with preexisting renal disease and/or dehydration. Patients with symptomatic cerebral vascular disease may be treated with aspirin and anticoagulants. If symptoms persist despite pharmacological treatment and if correctable vascular lesions are present, surgery may be considered.

Coronary artery disease. Heart disease due to coronary atherosclerosis is the most common cause of morbidity and mortality in patients with diabetes. Patients with signs or symptoms of coronary artery disease should receive a complete evaluation, including exercise testing and, if necessary, coronary arteriography. Contrast-dye studies should be used with caution because of the possible coexistence of diabetic nephropathy. Nitrates, calcium channel blockers, and beta-blockers may be prescribed for patients with angina. Consider coronary angioplasty or bypass surgery for patients with appropriate coronary lesions or intractable angina. Unless contraindicated, aspirin should be given for acute myocardial infarction. Because of their ability to prevent re-infarction in nondiabetic subjects, beta-blockers may be used in patients with diabetes after myocardial infarction—with attention to possible hypoglycemia and/or hyperlipidemia.

Peripheral vascular disease. Generally, no effective medical treatment is available for patients with peripheral vascular disease, although some patients may benefit from pentoxifylline. Patients who have incapacitating symptoms of peripheral vascular disease (such as rest pain) or who have foot lesions that are poorly healing require careful evaluation. To detect surgically correctable peripheral vascular disease, first use clinical examination of the pulses and then consider noninvasive means (Doppler flow study). Contrast-dye studies should be used with caution because of the possible coexistence of diabetic nephropathy. Refer patients for surgery, as appropriate.

Patient Education Principles

- Inform patients with diabetes that their risk of developing cardiovascular disease is higher than that of persons without diabetes.
- Inform patients of the absolute necessity of not smoking.
- Emphasize to patients the importance of following dietary principles appropriate for their conditions (such as hypertension or hyperlipidemia).
- Inform patients that hypertension and hyperlipidemia must be treated vigorously.
- Tell patients to immediately report symptoms of cardiovascular disease (for example, transient ischemic attack,

chest pain, and claudication) so that investigation and treatment can begin promptly.

MANAGING NEUROPATHY*

Background

Persons with diabetes who develop neuropathy may have no symptoms or may experience pain, sensory loss, weakness, and autonomic dysfunction. Neuropathy may result in significant morbidity and may contribute to other major complications, such as lower extremity amputation.

There are three major types of diabetic neuropathy:

- distal symmetrical polyneuropathy
- focal neuropathy
- autonomic neuropathy

Distal symmetrical polyneuropathy. This most common of the diabetic neuropathies is characterized by insidious onset, symmetrical distribution, and progressive course. Although its cause is unclear, distal symmetrical polyneuropathy is believed to result from abnormal neural metabolism, generalized neural ischemia, or both. The onset and course of illness cannot be predicted for an individual patient, but increasing age, male sex, increasing height, longer duration of diabetes, poorer glucose control, hypertension, alcohol consumption, and smoking may be independent risk factors.

Estimates of the prevalence of distal symmetrical polyneuropathy differ greatly, but approximately 12% of patients have this condition when diabetes is diagnosed, and nearly 60% have it after 25 years.

Three overlapping clinical syndromes have been described:

1. Acute painful neuropathy, an uncommon but extremely unpleasant complication of diabetes, often occurs without evidence of other significant neurologic impairment. It may occur early or late in the course of diabetes and may be associated with the institution of insulin treatment or with abrupt or considerable weight loss. Patients develop dysesthesia and paresthesia in the lower extremities. The severe, burning pain is often associated with cutaneous hyperesthesia and is worse at

*Source: *The Prevention and Treatment of Complications of Diabetes Mellitus: A Guide for Primary Care Practitioners,* Department of Health and Human Services, Public Health Service, Centers for Disease Control, National Center for Chronic Disease Prevention and Health Promotion, Division of Diabetes Translation, January 1, 1991.

night. Objective evidence of neuropathy may be minimal. Symptoms generally resolve slowly, within months of achieving good glycemic control. Relapses are rare.

2. Small fiber neuropathy may occur after only a few years of diabetes. Patients have varying degrees of pain and sensory loss; they usually feel a burning pain and may develop dysesthesia. Prominent features of small fiber neuropathy are distal loss of temperature sensation and of pinprick or pressure sensation. Vibratory sensation, position sense, muscle strength, and ankle reflexes are generally unimpaired. Neuropathic ulcers occasionally occur at sites of trauma.

3. Large fiber neuropathy generally occurs in the setting of small fiber neuropathy. Patients have impaired distal vibration sensation and impaired distal position sense. Ankle reflexes are reduced or lost. In most severe instances, patients develop sensory ataxia and have a positive Romberg's test. Large fiber neuropathy is most strongly associated with the development of neuropathic foot ulcers and neuropathic arthropathy affecting the interphalangeal, metatarsophalangeal, and ankle joints.

Focal neuropathy. Focal neuropathy is an uncommon condition believed to occur after the acute occlusion of a blood vessel produces ischemia in a nerve or group of nerves. The characteristics of focal diabetic neuropathy are sudden onset, an asymmetrical nature, and a self-limited course. Near total recovery generally occurs within two weeks to 18 months. Examples of focal diabetic neuropathies are cranial neuropathies, truncal neuropathies, mononeuropathies, radiculopathies, and plexopathies. Both sensory and motor components may be present.

Autonomic neuropathy. This troubling complication of diabetes encompasses multiple disturbances affecting the following systems: sudomotor (possible symptoms include heat exhaustion), pupillary (poor night vision), adrenomedullary (hypoglycemia unawareness), cardiovascular (orthostatic hypotension and painless myocardial ischemia), gastrointestinal (gastroparesis, constipation, diarrhea, and fecal incontinence), and urogenital (bladder dysfunction and sexual dysfunction).

The box below indicates complications that can occur with autonomic neuropathy.

Detection

Interview. The practitioner should conduct an interview at each visit—at least four times a year—to determine whether the patient is experiencing the following:

Condition	Description
Orthostatic hypotension	Suspect this condition when a patient reports having postural faintness, weakness, visual impairment, or syncope. In patients whose intravascular volume is not depleted, autonomic neuropathy may be diagnosed if the systolic blood pressure falls more than 30 mm Hg or if the diastolic blood pressure falls more than 10 mm Hg when the patient changes from a lying to a standing position.
Gastroparesis	May be associated with symptoms of anorexia, early satiety, bloating, abdominal pain, nausea, and vomiting. Signs may include weight loss and erratic glycemic control.
Constipation	A common manifestation that may be difficult to treat.
Diabetic diarrhea	May last from a few hours to several weeks. May be severe and watery, is generally worse at night, and is often preceded by abdominal cramps. During remissions, the patient may report constipation.
Fecal incontinence	Associated with a reduced threshold of conscious rectal sensation, low basal internal sphincter pressure, and reduced voluntary control of the external anal sphincter.
Diabetic bladder dysfunction	Associated with defective perception of bladder filling and decreased reflex bladder emptying. Patients may strain to initiate a stream, may be unable to completely void, may dribble when urinating, and may have recurrent urinary tract infections.
Sexual dysfunction	Men may experience impotence. Women may experience decreased vaginal lubrication and dyspareunia.

- peripheral pain, paresthesia, or numbness
- weakness
- hypoglycemia awareness
- orthostatic light-headedness
- gastrointestinal symptoms, such as bloating, nausea, vomiting, constipation, diarrhea, and loss of bowel control
- urogenital symptoms, such as loss of bladder control and sexual dysfunction

Physical examination. The practitioner should inspect the feet at each visit —at least four times a year. At least once a year, the practitioner should perform a physical examination to assess neurologic function. The practitioner should measure blood pressure and pulse rate—both when the patient is lying down and standing—and should assess the patient's muscle strength, deep tendon reflexes, and sense of touch. Four modalities of touch should be assessed.

Distal temperature sensation. Touch a cool piece of metal (such as a tuning fork) to the patient's foot; ask the patient to describe the object's temperature. Another method is to alternately touch the patient's foot with a test tube containing cool water and another containing warm water; ask the patient to distinguish between these objects.

Distal pinprick or pressure sensation. Have the patient close his or her eyes. Hold a pin lightly between your thumb and forefinger and touch it to the patient's foot. Ask the patient to say when a sensation is felt and whether the sensation is sharp or dull. Clarify a doubtful response by alternately touching the patient with the point and the head of the pin. As an alternative, pressure sensation can be assessed with a monofilament.

Distal vibratory sensation. Tap a 128-Hz tuning fork and place the end of the handle on a bony surface of the patient, such as the distal first metatarsal head or the malleoli of the ankles. Ask the patient to say when the vibration ceases.

Position sense. Have the patient close his or her eyes. Grasp between your thumb and index finger the lateral and medial sides of the patient's toe. Ask the patient to describe the toe's position as you alternately flex and extend it.

Differential Diagnosis

The practitioner should exclude other potential causes of neuropathy before attributing a patient's neuropathy to diabetes.

Distal Symmetrical Polyneuropathy

The differential diagnosis of distal symmetrical polyneuropathy includes the following:

- medications
- exposure to toxins, including ethanol, organic solvents, and heavy metals
- uremia
- hypothyroidism
- pernicious anemia
- intoxication from vitamin B_6
- syphilis
- gammopathy or myeloma
- malignancy
- collagen vascular disease
- porphyria
- hereditary neuropathy

Focal Neuropathy

The differential diagnosis of focal neuropathy includes the following:

- cranial neuropathy
  - increased intracranial pressure
  - aneurysm
  - tumor
- truncal neuropathy
  - cardiopulmonary disease
  - degenerative joint disease
  - disc disease
  - tumor
  - Paget's disease
- mononeuropathy
  - trauma
  - hemorrhage
  - tumor
  - multiplex

Autonomic Neuropathy

The differential diagnosis of autonomic neuropathy includes the following for the manifestations indicated:

- hypoglycemia unawareness
  - medications
  - lack of knowledge about hypoglycemia
- orthostatic hypotension
  - medications
  - hypovolemia
  - panhypopituitarism
  - pheochromocytoma
  - Shy-Drager syndrome
- gastroparesis
  - medications
  - ketoacidosis
  - gastric or intestinal obstruction

- constipation
  - medications
  - dehydration
  - intestinal obstruction
- diarrhea
  - medications
  - dietary sorbitol or lactose
  - enteric pathogens
  - bacterial overgrowth
  - primary intestinal diseases
  - pancreatic exocrine insufficiency
- impotence
  - medications
  - hormonal abnormalities
  - vascular disease
  - psychogenic disease

Treatment

Distal symmetrical polyneuropathy. Often the pain resolves. For patients with painful neuropathy, the practitioner should institute rigorous glucose control. If pain continues, consider using pharmacologic agents such as amitriptyline, imipramine, nortriptyline plus fluphenazine, carbamazepine, mexiletine, or capsaicin.

Inform patients with distal sensory or motor abnormalities about foot care. Tell patients who have lost sensation in their feet to wear special protective footwear and to avoid activities (such as jogging) that can traumatize the feet (see the section, Managing Foot Problems).

If painful neuropathy persists or worsens, consider referring the patient to a diabetologist.

Focal neuropathy. After other causes are excluded (see preceding discussion of differential diagnosis), management is palliative. Spontaneous resolution generally occurs within a period of months but may persist over years.

Autonomic neuropathy. Various treatments are available for autonomic neuropathy. If signs or symptoms of autonomic neuropathy are present, consider referring the patient to a diabetologist.

Hypoglycemia unawareness. If necessary, alter patients' targeted goals for glycemic control. Encourage patients to monitor their blood glucose regularly. Instruct patients to carry with them a source of simple sugar and to wear a necklace or bracelet that identifies them as having diabetes. Patients should also have glucagon available; their families and friends need to know how and when to use it.

Orthostatic hypotension. Patients may benefit from improved glycemic control (to reduce glycosuria), from volume and salt repletion, and from mechanical support with waist-high elastic stockings. Vasoconstrictors may be indicated.

Gastroparesis. Patients may benefit from correction of metabolic abnormalities (including hyperglycemia, ketosis, and hypokalemia), from dietary modification (eating small, liquid, low-fiber, low-fat meals), and from a prokinetic agent such as metoclopramide.

Constipation. Patients may benefit from correction of glycosuria, adequate hydration, a high-fiber diet, and psyllium.

Diarrhea. Patients may benefit from a bowel program that includes ingesting dietary fiber and making regular efforts to move the bowels. Another possible treatment is a short-term trial of an antidiarrheal agent (such as loperamide or diphenoxylate hydrochloride and atropine sulfate) or a broad-spectrum antibiotic with anaerobic coverage (such as tetracyline or metronidazole hydrochloride). Metoclopramide may occasionally be beneficial.

Fecal incontinence. Patients may be candidates for biofeedback training.

Diabetic bladder dysfunction. Patients may benefit from treatment to improve bladder emptying and to reduce the risk of urinary tract infection.

Impotence. Patients may benefit from noninvasive devices to assist erection, from a semirigid or inflatable penile prosthesis, or from papaverine injections.

Patient Education Principles

- Inform patients about the relationship between poor glycemic control and the subsequent development of diabetic neuropathy.
- Stress that because sensory or motor neuropathy may be asymptomatic, routine evaluation is necessary even for patients who have no symptoms of neuropathy.
- Explain that diabetic neuropathy can contribute to the development of other complications, including loss of limb.
- Inform patients who have lost sensation in their feet about the importance of caring for their feet, wearing proper shoes, and getting appropriate exercise.
- Discuss the signs and symptoms of autonomic neuropathy.
- Explain the benefits of treatment to patients with autonomic neuropathy.

MANAGING FOOT PROBLEMS*

Background

Persons with diabetes are at significant risk for lower extremity amputations; such procedures are 15 times more common among persons with diabetes than among those without diabetes. Yet if patients whose feet are particularly at risk are aggressively sought out and treated, up to 50% of amputations can be prevented.

Pathophysiology

Peripheral neuropathy, peripheral vascular disease, and infection all may contribute to amputation in patients with diabetes. Peripheral neuropathy may contribute to loss of sensation in the feet and to the development of foot deformities. In insensitive feet, deformities can cause pressure points that are vulnerable to ulceration. Inadequate blood supply and infection can then lead to osteomyelitis and gangrene.

Many persons with diabetes who undergo a lower extremity amputation have an amputation of the contralateral leg within a few years. This occurs not only because of peripheral neuropathy and peripheral vascular disease but also because the remaining foot bears increased pressure and frequently develops ulceration and infection.

The in-hospital mortality rate for diabetic patients who receive an amputation is higher than the rate for nondiabetic patients. In general, morbidity and mortality are high among diabetic patients who have amputations. All diabetic patients who undergo amputation require close supervision for other medical problems, particularly coronary artery disease.

Occurrence. Persons with diabetes account for approximately 50,000 (or 50%) of all nontraumatic amputations performed in the United States each year. The risk is greater for patients over 40 years old who have had diabetes for more than 10 years.

Cost. Although there is some variation, the average hospital stay for an amputation is approximately 25 days, and the average in-hospital cost is $25,000.

Prevention

Saving the diabetic foot and preventing amputation requires the following:

*Source: *The Prevention and Treatment of Complications of Diabetes Mellitus: A Guide for Primary Care Practitioners*, Department of Health and Human Services, Public Health Service, Centers for Disease Control, National Center for Chronic Disease Prevention and Health Promotion, Division of Diabetes Translation, January 1, 1991.

- identification of feet at risk
- prevention of foot ulcers
- treatment of foot ulcers
- prevention of recurrence of foot ulcers

Achieving these goals requires patient and family education in the care of the foot, frequent foot inspection, and teamwork among medical disciplines.

Identification of feet at risk. The diabetic patient with distal symmetrical polyneuropathy and peripheral vascular disease has feet at risk for problems. At each visit, the health care provider should inquire for symptoms of peripheral neuropathy, including pain, burning, tingling, and numbness. Patients with insensitive feet may not be aware of ulcerations or lesions. Therefore, the shoes and stockings must be removed at every visit—at least four times a year—and the feet inspected for dryness, calluses, corns, and ulcers. The health care provider should also inspect between the toes and inspect for deformities. At least once a year, the health care provider should assess the patient's ability to sense temperature, pinprick or pressure, touch, and vibration and should test muscle strength and deep tendon reflexes (see the section, Managing Neuropathy).

At every visit, the health care provider should also ask the patient about symptoms of intermittent claudication. In persons with diabetes and neuropathy, severe ischemia may exist without symptoms. At least once a year, the health care provider should palpate the following pulses: dorsalis pedis, posterior tibial, popliteal, and femoral.

Prevention of foot ulcers. Diabetic patients with feet at risk must learn foot hygiene and how to protect their feet. Changes in activity may be needed. Patients with foot deformities almost always require specially molded, extra-depth shoes. Deformed feet will not fit into ordinary shoes, although the patient, because of loss of sensation, may think they fit. The wearing of ordinary shoes on deformed feet may result in abrasions, ulcerations, and infection, which can lead to gangrene and amputation. If the patient's circulation is good, prophylactic correction of foot deformities should be considered.

Peripheral polyneuropathy may have a number of etiologies, such as drugs, alcohol, chemical toxins, and uremia. These must always be considered in the differential diagnosis of neuropathy in the patient with diabetes.

Factors that contribute to peripheral vascular disease should be avoided or treated. Smoking, the most significant risk factor for peripheral vascular disease, is associated with atherosclerosis, and even one cigarette can cause vasoconstriction that lasts for an hour or longer. Other risk factors for peripheral vascular disease should be treated, including hypertension, hypercholesterolemia, and perhaps hyperglycemia.

Rest pain and night pain are major indications for vascular surgery. Other indications are ulcers that will not heal, infections resistant to treatment, and incipient gangrene. In recent years, there has been an increase in the success of vascular surgical procedures. There are, however, risks to persons with diabetes who undergo vascular surgery, including the risk of angiography. Conservative measures should thus always be considered before vascular surgery. Pentoxifylline may improve the circulation in patients with peripheral vascular disease; aspirin and dipyridamole have not been conclusively shown to be effective. Oral vasodilators are ineffective in improving blood flow, and sympathectomy is not helpful in these patients.

Treatment of foot ulcers. Carefully evaluate and vigorously debride foot ulcers to establish the depth of the ulcer. Use X-ray studies to help exclude the possibility of embedded foreign objects or osteomyelitis. If osteomyelitis is suspected, use follow-up radiographs and appropriate scans to help establish the diagnosis. Where there is significant infection, use parenteral antibiotics. Since anaerobes frequently occur in the foot ulcers of diabetic patients, take both aerobic and anaerobic bacterial cultures to help select antibiotics.

Ulcers that occur in areas other than the usual plantar area, that cannot be explained by previous trauma or ill-fitting shoes, or that do not respond to aggressive treatment should be biopsied.

Ensure that patients do not put weight on the affected foot. Patients who do not feel pain will likely continue to walk; the resulting pressure on the foot will prevent healing. Total bed rest or the use of crutches may be required. Total-contact casts have been shown to help patients with foot ulcers ambulate while ulcers heal; the casts redistribute pressure so that the area of the ulcer bears much less weight than it would otherwise.

Good glycemic control also may help the patient's foot to heal. Topical use of hyperbaric oxygen, however, is not effective.

If foot ulcers do not respond to therapy, vascular surgery must be considered.

Prevention of recurrence of foot ulcers. Without special postulcer care, recurrence of the ulcer is almost certain. Such care may entail a change in job, a change in walking habits, and, most important, special shoes. Extra-depth shoes with molded plastic insoles help redistribute weight and may prevent recurrent ulcers. In one study, ulcers recurred in only about 20% of patients who wore these special shoes, whereas ulcers recurred in 80% of patients who resumed wearing ordinary shoes.

If ulcers recur despite protective shoes, the most likely cause is a bony deformity. If the patient's circulation is good,

orthopedic procedures to repair such deformities may help prevent recurrence of the ulcer.

Detection and Monitoring

All patients with diabetes should be given a complete foot examination at each visit (or at least four times a year).

The health care provider should ensure that these patients are instructed in proper foot care. A member of the health care team should instruct patients to do the following:

- wash their feet daily
- inspect their feet daily
- use foot creams or lubricating oil
- cut their toenails correctly
- never cut calluses or corns
- avoid self-medication and extremes of temperature
- never walk barefooted
- wear appropriate shoes
- inspect the inside of the shoes daily
- seek medical care for all skin lesions

If these patient instructions cannot be give during regular office visits, the health care provider should arrange to collaborate with another qualified specialist.

Treatment

Calluses. Assess the shoes of patients who have calluses. Teach patients to manage calluses with an emery board, callus file, or pumice stone—but strongly caution patients against trying to perform "home surgery" on calluses.

Deformities. If the foot is deformed, the patient will likely need consultation and should benefit from having specially molded shoes. Surgical correction should be considered for bunions, claw toes, or hammer toes—if the patient's circulation is good.

Neuropathic ulcers. When a neuropathic ulcer is present, consultation may be necessary, and the patient may need to be hospitalized where resources for proper treatment are available. Whenever a patient is hospitalized for any reason or is put at bed rest, heel protection should be used; the heels must be checked daily for evidence of pressure injury.

Additional considerations. Caring for the feet of persons with diabetes is complex. The expertise of professionals from many disciplines is often required. Health care providers may not be able to manage all aspects of foot care by themselves and may need to consult with other professionals:

- A diabetes nurse educator can teach about foot care.
- A pedorthist can provide special shoes for the patient with foot deformities.
- A podiatrist can help with the design and selection of special shoes and shoe inlays and can teach the patient how to manage calluses, corns, toenails, and minor foot deformities.
- A neurologist can help with the differential diagnosis of complicated peripheral neuropathies.
- A vascular surgeon can help improve peripheral blood flow in cases of peripheral vascular disease.
- An expert in infectious diseases can advise on the treatment of infected foot ulcers (with or without osteomyelitis).
- An orthopedist may be needed to treat major foot deformities or perform amputation.
- A social worker and a rehabilitation expert can help with the various socioeconomic problems, including loss of job, that may result from foot problems and particularly from amputation.

Patient Education Principles

- Instruct patients on the importance of regular foot care.
- Inform patients about the relationship between neuropathy, peripheral vascular disease, and foot ulcers.
- Urge patients to avoid risk factors associated with worsening of neuropathy.
- Urge patients not to smoke—particularly if they have peripheral vascular disease.
- Inform patients about special shoes for preventing or treating foot problems.
- Refer patients to a certified pedorthist if they have foot deformities or otherwise need special shoes.
- Inform patients about the availability of podiatric services; encourage patients to use these services.

MANAGING HYPERTENSION IN PATIENTS WITH DIABETES*

Approximately three million Americans have both hypertension and diabetes. For patients with noninsulin dependent diabetes mellitus (NIDDM), the incidence of essential hypertension increases with age and exists in about one out of every two patients. In patients with both insulin-dependent diabetes mellitus (IDDM) and NIDDM, diabetic nephropathy is also an important factor for the development of hypertension. Uncontrolled hypertension and diabetes are risk factors for cardiovascular mortality and morbidity, renal dysfunction, and retinopathy. In patients with diabetes, the presence of hypertension may lead to premature and more severe cardiovascular events as well as perpetuate renal and retinal dysfunction. The relationship between diabetes and hypertension is not fully understood, but it is clear that these diseases are interrelated. Hyperinsulinemia (insulin resistance) may affect the sympathetic and renin-angiotensin systems sodium excretion by the kidneys and interfere with peripheral vasodilation. These effects may contribute, in part, to elevations in blood pressure. Furthermore, hyperinsulinemia may contribute to or is associated with dysplipidemia and obesity. Although the exact interrelation between hypertension and diabetes is unknown, patients with both conditions are at increased risk for associated morbidity and mortality than with either hypertension or diabetes alone. For these reasons, patients with hypertension and diabetes should be treated early and aggressively.

Consensus Statements

A number of expert panels and government agencies have offered consensus statements with respect to the detection, management, and treatment of hypertension and diabetes. To this end, the goal of these efforts, in general, is to increase awareness of the impact of hypertension and diabetes as well as guide health care providers to provide optimal care for patients with diabetes and hypertension.

The goal blood pressure to be attained in hypertensive diabetic patients is less than 130/85 mm Hg. To achieve this goal, nondrug therapies and lifestyle modifications should be employed for three months. If an inadequate response or considerable progress has not been achieved, drug therapy should be initiated. Drugs from various classes that include angiotensin converting enzyme (ACE) inhibitors, alpha blockers, calcium channel antagonists, and low-dose diuretics may be initially considered while continuing nondrug and lifestyle modification efforts. Due to the compelling and growing evidence for the renal protective effects of ACE inhibitors, they are now considered the drugs of choice in insulin-dependent and noninsulin-dependent diabetic patients who have albuminuria or proteinuria. If initial monotherapy with any of the above agents does not provide an adequate response, the dose may be increased, another agent may be tried, or a second agent may be added to the therapy. Failing this, a second or third antihypertensive agent may be added to attain the desired blood pressure. If not prescribed for initial therapy, low-dose diuretic therapy should be included in subsequent therapy. Beta blockers, although effective in controlling blood pressure, are reserved for those hypertensive diabetic patients who have a clear indication other than hypertension for beta-blocker therapy. This treat-

*Source: Bradley G. Phillips, PharmD, "Treatment of Hypertension in Patients with Diabetes," *Managing the Patient with Type II Diabetes*, Aspen Publishers, Inc., © 1997.

ment algorithm outlines general treatment strategies that should be considered along with other patient and drug-related issues and considerations before a specific treatment plan is formulated for each diabetic patient.

Therapy Considerations

Selection of the optimal antihypertensive agent in each patient with diabetes should be based on the agent's impact on morbidity and mortality, glucose, electrolytes, insulin resistance, and lipids, as well as the cost of therapy and associated drug-induced adverse effects. Thiazide diuretics and beta blockers have been shown to reduce cardiovascular morbidity and mortality in patients with hypertension. For these reasons, they are considered the initial drugs of choice in the treatment of hypertension by the Joint National Committee on the Detection, Evaluation, and Treatment of High Blood Pressure (JNC). However, no study to date has evaluated the impact of these agents, or others, on cardiovascular morbidity and mortality in the diabetic population. It is assumed that diuretics and beta blockers will indeed confer the same beneficial effect on morbidity and mortality in hypertensive diabetic patients as they do in nondiabetic patients. There are several studies to give support to or possibly refute this presumption. The Systolic Hypertension in the Elderly Program (SHEP) evaluated the efficacy of low-dose diuretic, with atenolol and reserpine if needed, with placebo in 4,736 patients with an average baseline systolic blood pressure of 160 mm Hg or greater and a diastolic blood pressure of less than 90 mm Hg. The study found that with an average of four and a half years of active treatment, there was a 36 and 27 percent decrease in fatal and nonfatal strokes and myocardial infarctions, respectively, compared to those patients receiving placebo. A subsequent analysis to compare study outcomes in patients with NIDDM to patients without diabetes enrolled in SHEP revealed that both groups had a 34 percent reduction in cardiovascular disease rate at five years. Further, the absolute risk reduction for treatment compared to placebo in patients with NIDDM was twice as great compared to patients without diabetes. Conversely, studies found an increase in cardiovascular mortality in 759 hypertensive diabetic patients receiving diuretic therapy. This finding is supported by another study, which reported a similar outcome for hypertensive diabetics receiving diuretic therapy.

These conflicting results have fostered, in part, divergent opinions on the role of diuretic and beta-blocker therapies in patients with diabetes. Regardless, many consensus statements support low-dose diuretics for the treatment of hypertension in the diabetic population. Other antihypertensive therapies (e.g., ACE inhibitors, calcium channel antagonists, and alpha blockers) are currently being evaluated in ongoing trials that are designed to evaluate the impact of treatment on morbidity and mortality in hypertensive patients.

The clinical implications of insulin resistance are a possible effect on blood pressure, lipids, and obesity. Antihypertensive agents have varying effects on insulin sensitivity. In general, ACE inhibitors, alpha blockers, and calcium channel antagonists improve insulin sensitivity and lipidemia, or are lipid neutral. Conversely, beta blockers and diuretics may worsen insulin sensitivity and the lipid profile (see Table 1). Electrolyte imbalances may be provoked by ACE inhibitors and diuretics. Although it is unclear if these possible drug-induced changes produce clinically relevant changes in the long-term, it would seem prudent to consider these effects in each diabetic patient at the time the decision is made to initiate a specific agent to treat high blood pressure. For example, in a patient with documented hyperinsulinemia or insulin resistance, it may be prudent to select an agent that does not worsen insulin sensitivity.

Pharmacologic selection to treat blood pressure in patients with diabetes should also take into consideration the patient's concomitant disease states, medical history, and ability to pay for medications. In doing so, an antihypertensive that has a proven beneficial impact on other disease states, independent of its effect on blood pressure, may be prescribed. For example, an ACE inhibitor may be considered over other antihypertensive therapies in a patient who has diabetes and also has congestive heart failure or left ventricular hypertrophy. Similarly, an alpha blocker may be favored if the patient suffers from benign prostatic hypertrophy. Therefore, the efficacy of the agent to control blood pressure and its effect on body chemistry should be considered in concert with its documented benefit in other disease states (see Table 2). Ultimately, drug therapy will be doomed to failure, regardless of its efficacy and beneficial effects on other disease states, if the patient cannot afford to pay for the medication.

Perhaps the most important consideration is to treat hypertension, diabetes, and dyslipidemia aggressively, as each is associated with significant morbidity and mortality. Therefore, in striving to attain optimal blood pressure control, the same effort should be directed to maintain glycemic control. Intensive insulin therapy in IDDM has been reported to delay the onset and slow the progression of diabetic neuropathy, retinopathy, and nephropathy. It is unknown, however, if intensive insulin therapy in NIDDM would produce similar outcomes. As insulin resistance may play more of a role in the progression and severity of diabetic complications in patients with NIDDM, insulin therapy may be withheld until oral agents have been initiated and optimized. To this end, patients with NIDDM may be prescribed oral sulfonylureas and, now, newer agents like metformin and acarbose in an attempt to control glycemia without aggravating insulin resistance.

Table 1. The impact of various classes of antihypertensive agents on body chemistry

	ACE inhibitors	Alpha blockers	Beta blockers	Calcium channel antagonists	Diuretics
Insulin sensitivity	↑	↑	↓	− ↑	− ↓
Electrolytes	− ↑	−	−	−	↓ ↑
Lipidemia	−	↓	− ↑	−	↑
Glycemia	− ↓	−	↑	−	↑

Notes: ↑ = increase, ↓ = decrease, − = neutral.

Specific treatment measures and unique issues common to each specific class of antihypertensive drugs are delineated below with specific reference to the hypertensive diabetic population.

Nondrug Therapy

Nondrug treatment measures should always be employed prior to initiating drug therapy in diabetic patients with mild to moderate hypertension or in concert with drug therapy in diabetic patients with more severe hypertension. Nondrug therapy, in general, should focus on the modification of lifestyle to include regular aerobic activity, an attempt to attain and maintain ideal body weight, cessation of smoking, and moderation of alcohol intake. Dietary changes and physical activity can lead to improvements in glycemic, lipemic, and blood pressure control. For example, restricting sodium intake to less than 2.3 and or attaining up to a 10 lb. weight loss has been shown to lower blood pressure and improve glycemic control. Daily alcohol intake should be limited to no more than 1 oz. of ethanol (equivalent to 24 oz of beer, 8 oz. of wine, or 2 oz. of hard liquor). Patients should be encouraged to and assisted in smoking cessation. Lifestyle modifications may be tried for three months in order to control and maintain blood pressure before drug therapy is initiated.

Antihypertensive Therapy

ACE Inhibitors

ACE inhibitors decrease the progression of diabetic nephropathy independent of their blood–pressure-lowering properties. In patients with IDDM and renal disease, ACE inhibitor therapy has been shown to reduce the combined endpoint of death, dialysis, or renal transplant by 50 percent. These beneficial effects on the progression of diabetic nephropathy are also apparent in patients with NIDDM. In two recent, randomized, double-blind, placebo-controlled studies, ACE inhibitor therapy was associated with a decline in the loss of glomerular infiltration rate (GFR), albuminuria, and maintenance of serum creatinine levels. The retardation of declining GFR was observed for patients with mild (no more than 300 mg/24 hours) and overt (more than 300 mg/24 hours) proteinuria present at the start of the study. These findings are in accordance with a metaanalysis that reported that ACE inhibitors decrease proteinuria independent of the type of diabetes, stage of renal disease, or duration of therapy. Other

Table 2. Treatment considerations with various disease states or conditions

Coexisting condition	ACE inhibitor	Alpha blocker	Beta blocker	Calcium channel antagonist	Diuretic
DM	++	++	−	+	+/−
Aged	+/−	+	+/−	++	++
CHF	+++	+/−	−	−	++
CAD	+	+	++	+/−	+/−
LVH	+	+/−	+	+	+/−

Notes: DM = diabetes mellitus; CHF = congestive heart failure; CAD = coronary artery disease; LVH = left ventricular hypertrophy; + = treatment benefit; − = treatment detriment; +/− = treatment neutral.

reasons that may predicate ACE inhibitor therapy in diabetic patients include the improvement in insulin sensitivity and the neutral effect on lipids. For these reasons, ACE inhibitors are the preferred antihypertensive agents in diabetic patients with microalbuminuria or overt diabetic nephropathy.

The potential beneficial effects for ACE inhibitor therapy do, however, need to be considered along with several important associated adverse effects. Perhaps most important is that ACE inhibitors may worsen renal insufficiency. This is particularly important in those patients who have preexisting renal dysfunction and in those who are more dependent on the reninangiotensin system to maintain adequate renal perfusion. For example, patients with severe congestive heart failure or renal artery disease should be monitored more frequently for an increase in serum creatinine. Likewise, ACE inhibitors may cause a dramatic and abrupt decline in renal function in patients with bilateral renal artery stenosis, a condition that is more common in patients with diabetes. Caution should also be exercised when initiating therapy in patients with diabetes who are on diuretic therapy to avoid a more pronounced decline in blood pressure when these agents are prescribed together. As part of patient follow-up, serum electrolytes should be monitored to avoid hyperkalemia, which is associated with ACE inhibitor therapy.

Alpha-1 Blockers

Alpha-1 blockers are attractive antihypertensive medications for diabetic patients as they may produce a beneficial effect on lipids, improve insulin sensitivity, and possess a favorable adverse effect profile. In addition, the longer-acting alpha-1 blockers can be administered once daily, which may lead to a better compliance rate. The main drawback associated with this class of agents is that they may provoke orthostatic hypotension. To limit this unwanted side effect, the lowest dose should be initially prescribed and the dose titrated slowly after sitting and standing blood pressures have been measured and evaluated. In addition, the first dose may be given just prior to bedtime. Unlike the central acting alpha agonists, peripheral alpha antagonists are less likely to be associated with a more pronounced or severe orthostatic hypotension in diabetics with known or suspected autonomic dysfunction.

Beta Blockers

Beta blockers should be considered for the treatment of hypertension in patients with diabetes under select conditions where there is a clear benefit (i.e., myocardial infarction or angina). The reasons for limiting beta-blocker therapy to those patients who would obtain a demonstrable benefit from therapy are secondary to drug-related effects on metabolism and on the cardiovascular and nervous systems. Beta blockers without intrinsic sympathomimetic activity (ISA; e.g., atenolol and metoprolol) may aggravate lipids and decrease insulin sensitivity. In addition, by blunting the sympathetic response to a hypoglycemic event, beta blockers can prolong recovery and mask symptoms the patient may rely on to signal an event. Further, beta blockers can increase claudication in patients with diabetes with peripheral vascular disease. However, these potential drug adverse effects may be outweighed in patients with diabetes following myocardial infarction, as acute and long-term beta-blocker therapy (without ISA) can improve morbidity and mortality. Although beta blockers with ISA may have fewer of the above-mentioned adverse effects, they offer no clear advantage over other agents. There is also some evidence that when beta-blocker and diuretic therapies are combined in older adult obese patients, the risk of developing NIDDM is increased compared to controls. For these reasons, beta-blocker therapy is usually reserved for those patients with diabetes for whom the benefits of therapy outweigh the risks and in select hypertensive diabetic patients for whom other antihypertensives are contraindicated, ineffective, or not tolerated.

Calcium Channel Antagonists

Calcium channel antagonists (CCAs), alone or in combination with other antihypertensive agents, are viable treatment options to control blood pressure in the diabetic population. In general, these agents are lipid neutral and do not interfere with diabetic control, CCAs, as a class, tend to be more effective with age, which make them an attractive therapy in older patients with NIDDM. In addition, studies have shown that CCAs, with the exception of nifedipine, may improve diabetic nephropathy by decreasing proteinuria and microalbuminuria. However, not all studies are in agreement with this finding, and it is unknown if this beneficial effect is maintained with continued long-term therapy. It has also been proposed that an additive effect may be produced by combining a CCA with an ACE inhibitor in patients with diabetic nephropathy. Clearly, more well-controlled studies are needed to clarify the impact of specific CCAs on diabetic renal disease and to determine if combination therapy with an ACE inhibitor produces a synergistic effect.

Orthostatic hypotension, constipation, and peripheral edema are the main side effects associated with CCAs. Initiating therapy at the lowest possible dose and titrating slowly may be the best means of curtailing these unwanted side effects. Also, extra caution should be exercised to avoid orthostatic hypotension in diabetes with known or suspected neuropathy. As highlighted recently in the literature, short-acting agents (e.g., nifedipine) should be avoided in general for the chronic treatment of hypertension secondary to a possible increase in the risk of myocardial infarction.

Diuretics

Thiazide diuretics have been shown to provoke adverse effects on lipid metabolism, blood glucose, and blood chemistry (e.g., potassium, magnesium, and urea). However, when prescribed in low dose (25 mg or less a day of hydrochlorothiazide), these unwanted side effects may not be as pronounced and may be of little clinical importance. Of note, loop diuretics have not been shown to have these effects and are preferred over thiazides when a patient's renal function worsens (serum creatinine greater than 2.5 mg/dL). As patients with diabetes can be described as having an expanded plasma volume, diuretic therapy may be a necessary and effective therapy to control blood pressure in this population. Further, combination therapy with an ACE inhibitor can produce a synergistic effect in lowering blood pressure and therefore can be considered for patients with diabetes who require more than one antihypertensive agent to control blood pressure.

Example of an Office Guide

The office guide is a brief synopsis of the recommendations contained in the body of the text and is designed so that it may be photocopied and placed in the patient's medical record.

Patient's Name:_____

Address:_____

Phone: home (   ) _____

             work (   ) _____

Date of birth: _____/_____/_____
                    mo   day   year

Year of diagnosis: _____

Type of diabetes: IDDM _____   NIDDM _____   Other _____

Diet: calories _____
        meals and snacks (circle)
            breakfast   snack   lunch   snack   dinner   snack   snack

Exercise: type _____   frequency _____/week
             duration _____ minutes   time of day _____

Monitoring: blood glucose _____   urine glucose _____   urine ketones _____
              frequency _____/day

Oral hypoglycemia agent:_____

Insulin:_____

Other medications:_____

Source: *The Prevention and Treatment of Complications of Diabetes Mellitus: A Guide for Primary Care Practitioners*, Department of Health and Human Services, Public Health Service, Centers for Disease Control, National Center for Chronic Disease Prevention and Health Promotion, Division of Diabetes Translation, January 1, 1991.

HPHC Adult Diabetes Guideline:
For Screening and Prevention of Complications

Mohammed Ally, MD; Karen Bell, MD; Barbara Burchard, NP; Helene Clayton, RN, BSN, CDE; Peter Connolly, MD; Vera Fajtova, MD; Rick Flannery; Jeffrey Garber, MD; Nancy Sokol, MD.
For additional information, contact Karen Bell, MD at 617-731-7392.

**Harvard Pilgrim
Health Care**

Name _____   Date of Birth _____

Date _____   Date Diagnosed _____

Medical Record # _____

INITIAL ASSESSMENT—DIABETES MELLITUS ✔ box if positive

Symptoms of: ☐ polyuria ☐ polydipsia ☐ polyphagia ☐ weight loss ☐ nocturia

☐ fatigue ☐ pruritis ☐ ketoacidosis ☐ visual change ☐ hypoglycemia

Notes: _____

_____

_____

Complications: ☐ neuropathy ☐ retinopathy ☐ cardiovascular disease _____

☐ nephropathy ☐ peripheral vascular disease _____

Diet Awareness (describe) _____

Exercise (describe) _____

Self-Monitors: ☐ Blood: frequency _____ ☐ Urine: frequency _____

(✔ if done)   targets _____   results _____

results _____

Medications (all) _____

Smoking   ☐ No ☐ Yes How much? _____   ☐ Encouraged to quit

Substance Abuse/Alcohol/Other _____

Contraception _____   ☐ N/A

Foot Care (done by) _____   Last checked by clinician _____

Dental Care—Dentist _____   Last Seen _____

Eye Care—Ophthalmologist _____   Last Seen _____
       (Optometrist, if dilated exam done)

Family History (Diabetes mellitus) _____

PSYCHOSOCIAL explore

Stressful events ☐ Changes in job ____ ☐ Family life ____ ☐ Other ____

Social and family support _____

_____

_____

Adaptation to Diabetes _____

_____

_____

(Please turn over)

HPHC clinical guidelines are designed to assist clinicians by providing an analytical framework for the evaluation and treatment of the more common problems of HPHC patients. They are not intended to either replace a clinician's judgement or to establish a protocol for all patients with a particular condition. It is understood that some patients will not fit the clinical conditions contemplated by a guideline and that a guideline will rarely establish the only appropriate approach to a problem.

continues

HPHC Adult Diabetes Guideline continued

PHYSICAL EXAM ✔ box if within normal limits; note if not

Height _____   Weight _____   Blood Pressure (with orthostatic measurements when indicated) _____

HEENT:
- ☐ Fundi _____
- ☐ Teeth _____
- ☐ Thyroid _____
- ☐ Pupils _____
- ☐ Gums _____
- ☐ Other _____
- ☐ EOMs _____

Cardiovascular:
- ☐ Heart _____
- ☐ Peripheral pulses _____
- ☐ Carotids _____

Neurological exam:
- ☐ Touch _____
- ☐ Temperature sensation _____
- ☐ Proprioception _____
- ☐ Reflexes _____
- ☐ Vibratory sensation _____

Skin/Foot:
- ☐ Foot color _____
- ☐ Injection sites _____
- ☐ Toenails _____

Notes: _____
_____
_____
_____
_____

MANAGEMENT PLAN AND PATIENT INSTRUCTIONS

At first visit:

Provide Diabetes Manual ☐   Medication recommendation _____

Nutrition recommendation (including calories) _____

Recommended follow-up appointments (Primary Care/Eye/Other) _____
_____

LAB ✔ box if ordered/record results (optional)

☐ Fasting serum glucose (random if not possible) _____   ☐ Glycohemoglobin

☐ Fasting cholesterol (random if not possible) _____   ☐ HDL _____   ☐ LDL _____   ☐ Fasting triglycerides _____

☐ Urinalysis _____

☐ Microalbumin (if indicated) _____

☐ Creatinine (if urinalysis or albumin abnormal or comorbidity) _____

☐ TSH (Type I patients only) _____

☐ EKG (if patient 40+ years or diagnosed DM for at least 10 years) _____

NOTES

_____
_____
_____
_____
_____
_____
_____
_____
_____
_____
_____
_____
_____

Signature _____

continues

HPHC Adult Diabetes Guideline continued

DIABETES PATIENT INFORMATION

The management plan should be individualized, emphasizing patient self-management. Ideally, the plan should be formulated in collaboration with the patient, incorporating long- and short-term goals.

I BASIC ANATOMY AND PHYSIOLOGY OF DIABETES MELLITUS

   1. Understands basic pathophysiology   ____/____ Date/initials

   2. Understands the importance of glycemic control   ____/____ Date/initials

II MEDICATIONS

   1. Oral hypoglycemic agents

      a. type/dose _____

      b. frequency _____

      c. action _____

      d. side effects _____

   2. Insulin

      a. type/dose _____

      b. duration of action _____

      c. injection technique, including mixing, storage, site selection _____

      d. dosage adjustment algorithms _____

   3. Other medications that may affect blood glucose levels _____

III NUTRITION

   1. States caloric level for ideal body weight   ____/____ Date/initials

   2. Understands carbohydrates, proteins, fats   ____/____ Date/initials

   3. Knows own specific meal plan and how to select foods in appropriate portion sizes, including dining out and special occasions.   ____/____ Date/initials

   4. Knows diet for associated conditions(i.e., cardiac, renal, pregnancy)   ____/____ Date/initials

IV MONITORING CONTROL

   1. Self Blood Glucose Monitoring (SBGM)

      a. frequency   ____/____ Date/initials

      b. adequate record keeping   ____/____ Date/initials

   2. Tests urine ketones with hyperglycemia and sick days   ____/____ Date/initials

   3. Understands specific goals of treatment   ____/____ Date/initials

V HYPOGLYCEMIA

   1. Understands causes and symptoms of hypoglycemia   ____/____ Date/initials

   2. Knows strategies for managing hypoglycemia   ____/____ Date/initials

   3. Carries I.D. card or bracelet   ____/____ Date/initials

   4. Significant other knows use of Glucagon, if appropriate   ____/____ Date/initials

continues

HPHC Adult Diabetes Guideline continued

VI   HYPERGLYCEMIA/SICK DAYS

    1. Understands causes and symptoms of hyperglycemia and/or DKA   ____/____ Date/initials

    2. Follows "Sick Day Guidelines" on day of illness

       a. q 4 hr. monitoring   ____/____ Date/initials

       b. check urine ketones if glucose is 240 or higher   ____/____ Date/initials

       c. push fluids   ____/____ Date/initials

       d. supplemental insulin   ____/____ Date/initials

       e. notify health care professional   ____/____ Date/initials

VII EXERCISE

    1. Understands and incorporates effective aerobic exercise habits.   ____/____ Date/initials

VIII FOOT CARE

    1. Understands potential for foot problems   ____/____ Date/initials

    2. Checks feet daily   ____/____ Date/initials

    3. Knows proper foot care, including first aid   ____/____ Date/initials

    4. Sees podiatrist if necessary   ____/____ Date/initials

IX   COMPLICATIONS

    1. Understands and practices health care measures to prevent or manage the following:

       a. Neuropathy   ____/____ Date/initials

       b. Nephropathy   ____/____ Date/initials

       c. Retinopathy   ____/____ Date/initials

       d. Sexual Dysfunction   ____/____ Date/initials

       e. Cardiovascular Disease   ____/____ Date/initials

X   CONTRACEPTION

    1. Women of childbearing age understand the necessity of optimal blood glucose control
before conception and during pregnancy   ____/____ Date/initials

    2. Knows options for and is offered acceptable and effective methods of contraception ____/____ Date/initials

XI   PSYCHOSOCIAL ISSUES

    1. Understands effects of stress on diabetes management   ____/____ Date/initials

    2. Employs appropriate methods for dealing with the emotional stress of a chronic disease ____/____ Date/initials

    3. Is aware of available HPHC programs and community resources
(ADA, Medic, Alert, Support Groups)   ____/____ Date/initials

XII FAMILY EDUCATION

    1. Family and/or "significant other" is aware of diabetes management and
participates in patient care as necessary   ____/____ Date/initials

continues

HPHC Adult Diabetes Guideline continued

Name _____   Date of Birth _____

Date _____   Date Diagnosed _____

Medical Record # _____

ADULT DIABETES INTERVAL FOLLOW-UP TYPE I—q3 MONTHS TYPE II—q6 MONTHS	Blue shaded areas should be done annually unless otherwise indicated				
INTERIM HISTORY YEAR →					
(✔ if positive and describe evaluation in notes) MONTH →					
Symptoms of hypo-/hyperglycemia					
Symptoms of complications					
Diabetic therapy (define) (✔ if changed)					
Self-monitoring					
Patient adjusts own insulin (if applicable)					
Cardiovascular: symptoms of CAD, PVD					
Problems with adherence					
Other illnesses					
Psychosocial issues					
Concerns about exercise, tobacco, diet, conception planning					

Notes: _____

_____

_____

PHYSICAL EXAM					
Complete Physical Exam (✔ if done, record elsewhere)					
Pulses (auscultate carotid and femoral) (✔ if normal)					
Blood Pressure (actual)					
Weight (actual)					
Neurological Exam					
Sensation (vibration, proprioception, light touch, temperature, DTR's [including ankle]) (✔ if normal)					
Dental Exam					
Gums/Gingival Exam (✔ if normal)					
Ophthalmologic Exam—by ophthalmologist/optometrist to include:					
test of visual acuity: (intraocular pressure; dilation with stereoscopic exam of macula) (✔ if done)					
Fundoscopic Exam (✔ if normal)					
Foot Exam					
Skin (interdigital cracking) (✔ if normal)					
Nails (✔ if normal)					
Deformities (✔ if normal)					

Notes: _____

_____

_____

continues

HPHC Adult Diabetes Guideline continued

ADULT DIABETES INTERVAL FOLLOW-UP TYPE I—q3 MONTHS TYPE II—q6 MONTHS	Blue shaded areas should be done annually unless otherwise indicated				
LABORATORY (write in values)					
Glucose Control					
Fasting Serum Glucose (random if not possible)					
Glycohemoglobin (more frequent if status of control is unknown)					
Cardiovascular (annual unless abnormal)					
Fasting Cholesterol					
HDL					
LDL					
Triglycerides					
Renal					
Urinalysis					
Microalbuminuria determination (when indicated)					
Serum creatinine if (+) albumin, hypertension, or other risks of renal disease					

Notes: _____
_____
_____
_____
_____
_____
_____
_____

VACCINATION					
Influenza	yearly (date)				
Pneumococcal	once (unless high risk) (date)				
TD	q 10 years (date of last injection)				
OTHER (if indicated)					
Pap Smear					
Mammogram					
Digital Rectal Exam					
FOBT					

Notes: _____
_____
_____
_____
_____
_____
_____

NUTRITIONAL MANAGEMENT OF DIABETES*

The *1994 Nutrition Recommendations and Principles for People with Diabetes Mellitus*, published by the American Diabetes Association, lists five specific goals of medical nutrition therapy:

1. Maintenance of optimal blood-glucose levels by balancing food intake with insulin, oral glucose-lowering medications, and activity levels (normal fasting plasma glucose: <115 mg/dL; normal postprandial glucose: <140 mg/dL; normal glycosylated hemoglobin: HbA1c <6%)
2. Achievement of optimal lipid levels (to reduce the risk of macrovascular disease)
3. Provision of appropriate calories for maintaining or achieving reasonable body weight for adults, normal growth and development rates in children and adolescents, increased needs in pregnancy and lactation, and increased needs in recovery from illness
4. Prevention, delay, or treatment of nutrition-related complications such as hypoglycemia (acute) and long-term complications such as renal disease, autonomic neuropathy, hypertension, and cardiovascular disease
5. Improvement of overall health through optimal nutrition. The principles of healthy eating can be taught from the Food Guide Pyramid and Dietary Guidelines for Americans

Principles of Nutrition Therapy

The basic principles of nutrition therapy and Type I diabetes (IDDM) are to integrate insulin therapy into the patient's usual eating and exercise patterns. Meal plans should be developed based on one's usual food intake, taking into consideration food preferences and ethnic, religious, and cultural factors. Individuals need to monitor blood glucose and to adjust insulin for the amount of food usually eaten. Daily consistency of eating and exercise habits is important, as is consistent timing of insulin injections. Patients on intensive insulin therapy have more flexibility with schedules and timing and amounts of food eaten at meals.

Nutrition therapy and Type II diabetes (NIDDM) stress the importance of achieving optimal glucose, lipid, and blood pressure (BP) goals. About 80% of people with NIDDM are obese and would benefit from moderate weight loss of 10 to 20 pounds. Weight loss is often difficult and requires behavior modification strategies to change behaviors and the encouragement of exercise as determined safe for the patient. A reduction and modification of fat in the diet and a realistic decrease in calories to help with long-term success are important considerations. Diet should always be considered the most important way of normalizing blood glucose, even if oral agents are being used.

The *1994 Nutrition Recommendations* also concludes that there is no such thing as an "American Dietetic Association (ADA) diet." Each person needs to have an individual diet tailored for his or her specific needs, based on metabolic, nutrition, and lifestyle requirements. Specific nutrient recommendations are suggested:

- **Protein.** About 10% to 20% of total calories should come from protein. There is controversial evidence supporting higher or lower intakes. With the onset of nephropathy, protein should be restricted to the recommended dietary allowance (RDA) (0.8 g/kg/ideal body weight [IBW]/day). Giving protein less than this amount may be detrimental.
- **Fat.** For people with normal weight and lipid levels, the American Hospital Association (AHA) guidelines of less than or equal to 30% of total calories from fat and less than 10% of energy from saturated fat can be followed. Dietary cholesterol intake should be less than 300 mg/day. For persons with elevated low-density lipoprotein cholesterol, the National Cholesterol Education Program (NCEP) Step II diet of less than 7% saturated fat, less than 200 mg/day of cholesterol, and less than 30% fat calories is recommended.
- **Carbohydrates.** The percentage of calories from carbohydrates will vary, and should be individualized based on eating habits, glucose, and lipid goals.
- **Fiber.** The amount of fiber needed for persons with diabetes is the same as for the general public: 25 to 30 g/day. While soluble fibers (eg, beans, oat bran) may improve lipid levels, fiber intake has an insignificant effect on blood glucose levels. Dietary fiber has also shown to have a beneficial effect in treating or preventing some gastrointestinal (GI) disorders, including colon cancer.
- **Sucrose.** Scientific evidence does not justify restriction of sucrose in the diet. Sucrose produces a glycemic response similar to bread, rice, and potatoes. New guidelines state that sucrose and sucrose-containing foods can be substituted for other carbohydrates in meals and should be consumed as part of a healthy meal. It should also be remembered that many foods high in sucrose are also high in fat and empty calories and should not be used instead of other foods needed for a healthy meal plan.

*Source: Karen Sachs, "Nutritional Management of Diabetes in Home Care," *Home Health Care Management & Practice*, Vol. 8:6, Aspen Publishers, Inc., © 1996.

- **Nutritive sweeteners.** Examples of nutritive sweeteners are fructose, honey, corn syrup, molasses, fruit juice or fruit juice concentrate, dextrose, maltose, and hydrogenated starch hydrolysate. These sweeteners frequently contain the same calories per gram as sucrose. Other sweeteners are mannitol and sorbitol. If these sugar alcohols are taken in large amounts, they may cause diarrhea.
- **Nonnutritive sweeteners.** Saccharin, aspartame, and acesulfame K have been approved for use in the United States by the FDA and are safe for people with diabetes to use as sugar substitutes.
- **Sodium.** Intake recommendations for sodium for people with diabetes are the same as for the general public. The recommendations are for 2,400 mg sodium/day, and less than 2,400 mg/day if hypertension exists.
- **Alcohol.** For insulin users, a limit of 2 drinks/day, taken with food, is suggested. Food intake should not be reduced to compensate for alcohol ingestion. For those with NIDDM, 1 oz of alcohol equals two fat exchanges. Weight and triglyceride levels should be monitored in those with frequent alcohol consumption.

Medical Nutrition Therapy Process

Due to the complexity of medical nutrition therapy, the *1994 Nutrition Recommendations* stresses the team approach to help each patient obtain good metabolic control. The home health care diabetes management team should include a registered dietitian, a registered nurse, a physician, the patient with diabetes, a home health care aide if needed, and other staff as appropriate.

The recommendations also suggest a four-step model for medical nutrition therapy for diabetes:

1. **Assessment.** This step involves obtaining the results of clinical data such as blood sugar records, results of HbA1c tests, total cholesterol levels, high-density lipoprotein cholesterol, and triglycerides. Height and weight are taken (or caretakers are asked to supply this information if a patient is bedbound and unable to be assessed). A dietary history or 24-hour recall is done, and then a nutrient intake analysis is computed. An assessment also includes analysis of medical, lifestyle, and psychosocial data, and cultural, religious, and ethnic food preferences. Information obtained from the assessment will be used to decide what nutrition intervention is needed, what nutrition problems and misinformation exist, and what the patient's health beliefs and ideas of self-management are.
2. **Goal setting.** The second step of providing medical nutrition therapy involves helping the patient to set reasonable goals for nutrition management of diabetes. Goals should be realistic and specific and should be determined by the patient.
3. **Nutrition intervention.** This intervention is based on the goals determined by the patient and information obtained from the assessment. The purpose of the intervention is to provide the patient with self-management tools to control diabetes, improve metabolic outcomes, and increase knowledge and skills necessary to change or maintain eating habits. A meal plan is developed that is individualized for the patient's nutritional needs, nutrition risk factors, food preferences, lifestyle, and budget. Intervention involves two stages: basic and in-depth.
4. **Evaluation.** This is the final step of the medical nutrition therapy process. Without evaluation, it is impossible to determine if any teaching has occurred and if the results of the intervention have improved outcomes and have met the patient's needs. The patient may need help in problem solving to achieve established goals, or new goals may need to be developed to reflect the patient's new level of self-management. Further nutrition intervention may be necessary if the patient's goals and metabolic status have changed.

Integrating Nutrition in Home Health Care

What are some of the barriers and benefits of providing medical nutrition therapy in home health care? Is it possible to really teach patients what they need to know and to be able to follow the four-step medical nutrition therapy process in the home? The answer is "it depends." It depends on the dietitian's or other health care provider's ability to be flexible, resourceful, creative, and quick thinking. It depends on having a good knowledge of barriers to nutrition education that may be faced in the home and on having creative solutions that allow one to circumvent these barriers to provide the therapy needed, instead of being blocked by them.

When you knock on a new patient's door, you never know who or what will be inside. Meeting new patients, new caretakers, new living situations can be seen as a wonderful challenge that makes being a home health care professional exciting and worthwhile. When you enter a patient's home it is important to remember that you are a guest. Respect, courtesy, and kindness go a long way in establishing a rapport with the patient that will facilitate the teaching you are there to provide. Being able to tune out distractions, to rise above dysfunctional family systems, and to work with resources available will help you to most effectively help the patient to choose the goals most important to him or her and to reach his or her best possible level of self-management. Home health care providers of medical nutrition therapy need to teach the patient what he or she needs to know to be able to manage once they no longer come into the home. Patients who can follow their meal plan (by themselves or with a caretaker's help), who are aware of the importance of nutrition within the context of their diabetes care plan, who understand the importance of self–blood glucose monitoring, and who have improved outcomes as documented by lower HbA1c levels have been able to learn and internalize the education provided to them.

Some of the barriers to providing medical nutrition therapy in the home include the following:

- The patient/caretaker cannot read.
- The patient/caretaker can read but cannot *see* to read.
- The patient/caretaker will not tell you he or she cannot see the print or has never learned to read. (Never make assumptions in home health care!)
- The patient is on medication affecting mental status.
- The patient lives alone and is either bedbound or unable to ambulate and has no one to help prepare meals.
- The patient is blind.
- The patient has a low functional ability and needs assistance with meal preparation and shopping.
- There is no stove or refrigerator in the home.
- The shared cooking facilities are "down the hall" and the patient is unable to walk to them.
- There is no food in the kitchen.
- The patient cannot chew food because his or her dentures either do not fit or do not exist.
- The patient cannot swallow.
- The patient is anorexic and will not eat.
- The patient has altered mental status and forgets to eat or forgets when he or she has already eaten.
- The patient has no money for food.
- The patient's "caretaker" discussed at hospital discharge lives 20 miles away and works during the day.
- There is no glucometer in the home.
- The patient forgets to take insulin.
- The patient is in denial about the disease process and will not listen to you.
- Family members understand that the patient has diabetes and needs to follow a meal plan, but they don't care because they are just too busy with their own lives.

- The family is abusive and withholds food from the patient and mistreats him or her.
- The patient's physician does not want you to increase calories for wound healing because the "blood sugar may go up," and the physician does not understand the importance of nutrition intervention.
- The patient has IDDM and is on the wrong kind or wrong amount of insulin.
- The physician finds nothing wrong with a fasting blood sugar of 300 because it is "normal" for the patient.
- The patient knows he or she has diabetes, does not care that he or she has diabetes, and would rather die early than follow a meal plan.

There are also benefits to providing medical nutrition therapy in the home. The main benefit is the possibility of providing lasting change for the patient within his or her family system that will lead to improved outcomes, reduction of risk factors, and an improved quality of life. When providing education in the home, the health care provider knows exactly what he or she has to work with. And if the provider does not have enough resources to help the patient achieve his or her goals, referrals can be made to other disciplines for additional resources or patient care. Social workers can help patients obtain food stamps, meals-on-wheels, and help in the home or can provide intervention to other agencies to help alleviate abusive home situations. Speech therapists can help evaluate a patient's swallowing to see if a tube feeding may be needed or if swallowing exercises and alterations in food texture will help a patient consume more food. Occupational therapists can help the patient to self-feed or can show the caretakers how to help the patient. Home health care aides can help prepare food for the patient and can help teach the family the basics of shopping, cooking, and serving food once their services are completed. Physicians can be consulted if changes in medication are needed, and the more dietitians consult with physicians as to the progress of the patient's nutritional status, the more physicians will realize the value of medical nutrition therapy in the patient's treatment plan. Feedback to the patient's nurse will facilitate the changes needed in the nursing plan and will help the nurse to be able to check the patient's progress and compliance with the nutrition care plan to let the dietitian know when goals have been met and when new interventions may be necessary.

3. Clinical Pathway and Care Planning Forms

Teaching Plan for Noninsulin-Dependent Diabetes Mellitus— Type II

Teaching is complete when patient and/or caregiver can do the following:

DEFINITION AND OVERVIEW

☐ Describe the difference between Type I and Type II diabetes.

☐ Verbalize the difference between NIDDM and the nondiabetic state.

☐ State the normal range for blood glucose.

☐ List possible causes of NIDDM.

☐ List the signs and symptoms of uncontrolled diabetes (hyperglycemia).

☐ State that optimal care of NIDDM involves efforts to achieve near-normal blood glucose levels.

☐ State that blood glucose control is achieved through a regimen of diet, exercise, and medication if necessary.

☐ If patient is obese, state that diet and weight loss are the main components of treatment of NIDDM.

ORAL DIABETES MEDICATION

☐ State that oral diabetes medication helps the pancreas release insulin to lower blood glucose.

☐ State when oral diabetes medication is to be taken.

☐ State that oral diabetes medication is not effective in the absence of a meal plan.

☐ List potential problems associated with the use of oral diabetes medication.

DIABETES MONITORING

Blood Glucose Monitoring

☐ State that blood glucose monitoring is the most accurate home method of assessing blood glucose control.

☐ Demonstrate accuracy in using reagent strips and/or blood glucose meter.

☐ Describe/demonstrate correct maintenance of blood glucose meter.

☐ Verbalize when blood glucose tests are to be done.

☐ State that monitoring results should be recorded and brought to follow-up appointments.

Urine Testing

☐ State that blood glucose monitoring is the most accurate home method of assessing blood glucose control.

☐ List indications for testing urine for ketones.

Laboratory Tests

☐ Discuss the relationship of the glycosylated hemoglobin test to diabetes control.

☐ Discuss the relationship of blood lipids to diabetes control/complications.

PSYCHOLOGICAL ASPECTS OF HAVING NIDDM

☐ Recognize impact of NIDDM on daily living.

☐ Recognize the need to accept responsibility for diabetes.

continues

Teaching Plan for NIDDM—Type II continued

☐ List resources/sources of support available to individuals with diabetes.

INSULIN

☐ Verbalize that insulin is a hormone that lowers blood sugar by transferring glucose into body cells.

☐ State that insulin injections are necessary when the pancreas is unable to produce sufficient insulin.

☐ Verbalize species, type, action of individual insulin prescription.

☐ State that insulin doses can be tailored to meet individual's needs.

☐ State the times the individual's insulin prescription should be taken.

☐ Verbalize the rationale for consistency in timing of meals and in amount of food eaten.

☐ Verbalize that insulin or food intake may need to be adjusted for exercise.

☐ Demonstrate accurate method of drawing up and administering insulin.

☐ Demonstrate accurate method of drawing up a mixed insulin dose.

☐ List appropriate injection sites and appropriate site rotation.

☐ Measure/inject insulin correctly with an assistive device/injection aid.

☐ Describe the care/storage of insulin.

☐ Accurately describe adjustment of the insulin dose.

EXERCISE

☐ State that a regular program of daily exercise will lower blood glucose and sustain fitness.

☐ State that exercise should be initiated slowly and increased gradually.

☐ List guidelines for preventing hypoglycemia.

☐ Discuss exercise precautions if complications are present.

ACUTE COMPLICATIONS

Hyperglycemia

☐ Verbalize causes of hyperglycemia.

☐ State that the physician should be notified if hyperglycemia persists and/or acetone is present.

Hypoglycemia

☐ State that hypoglycemia occurs when blood glucose falls below 70 mg/dL.

☐ List causes of hypoglycemia.

☐ List symptoms of hypoglycemia.

☐ Describe the treatment of hypoglycemia.

☐ Describe how hypoglycemia can be prevented.

☐ Wears medical ID or verbalizes intent to wear ID.

CHRONIC COMPLICATIONS

☐ Describe daily care of skin, teeth, and gums.

☐ List the chronic complications associated with diabetes.

☐ List risk factors for atherosclerotic vascular disease.

☐ State that good diabetes control may prevent disease of the eye, kidney, and nerves.

☐ Discuss the importance of an annual ophthalmologic examination.

☐ Discuss the importance of prompt recognition and treatment of bladder infections.

continues

Teaching Plan for NIDDM—Type II continued

FOOT CARE

- [ ] List factors that contribute to the development of foot problems in diabetes.
- [ ] Describe/demonstrate daily foot care.

RESEARCH

- [ ] List areas of active research in diabetes related to treatment, cure, and prevention.

NUTRITION

- [ ] State principles of diabetic diet.
- [ ] Name appropriate sweeteners.
- [ ] Name various forms of hidden sugars in food.
- [ ] Discuss different ways of reducing dietary fats.
- [ ] Evaluate nutrition information on a food label.
- [ ] Discuss appropriate food selections when dining out.

Source: Joanne Scharnak and Janis Corcoran Bartel, "Loyola Group Develops Standardized Teaching Plans," *Inside Ambulatory Care*, Special Insert, Vol. 2:12, Aspen Publishers, Inc., © 1996.

Diabetes Teaching Sheet

Follow-Up Dates			Material Covered	Method	Verbalization/Return of Knowledge	Emotional Status	Learner: Patient/Family		Comments	Evaluation of Learning	Initials
			Explanation of diabetes mellitus								
			Symptoms and signs of hypo- and hyperglyce-mia								
			Importance of skin/foot care								
			Importance of activity and exercise								
			Stress management								
			Medications								
			Type, dosage, time, insulin								
			Mixing different types								
			Self-administration								
			Site selection and rotation								
			Proper technique								
			Proper disposal of equipment								
			Oral hypoglycemia agents								
			Proper dosage and time								
			Blood glucose meter instruction								
			Location for purchase of meter								
			Diabetes outpatient classes								
			Diabetes support group								
			Nutrition education								

Date	Circle videos shown to patient and/or family	Comments
_____	Diabetes Basics	
_____	In Balance, In Control	
_____	Understanding Your Diabetes	
_____	Food Facts of Diabetes	
_____	Diabetes Medication as Directed	
_____	When Control Gets out of Balance	
_____	Exercise	
_____	Know Your Diabetes	
_____	Other Videos	

continues

Diabetes Teaching Sheet continued

Teaching Methods	Emotional Status	Evaluation of Learning	Teacher Signature/Title	Initials
A = Audiovisual	1. Accepting	1. Communication/understands		
D = Demonstration	2. Alert and responsive	2. Unable to understand/communicate		
E = Evaluation	3. Calm	3. Return demonstration with much assistance		
H = Handout	4. Confused	4. Return demonstration with minimal assistance		
C = Class	5. Uninterested	5. Return demonstration without assistance		
	6. Anxious	6. Introduction of concept/no response required		
		7. Refused teaching		
Learner: Patient, Family, Significant Other				

Courtesy of Midwest Regional Medical Center, Midwest City, Oklahoma.

Diabetes Flow Sheet

Name   I.D. No.   DOB:

Date													
Basic Guidelines of Diabetes Care													
Review Self Blood Glucose Results (every visit)													
Blood Pressure (every visit) Target													
Weight (every visit) Target													
Foot Exam (every visit)													
HbA$_{1c}$ (every 3 months) Lab Range Target													
Microalbuminuria (every year if urine protein negative)													
Dilated Eye Exam (yearly)													
Cholesterol (every year)/Triglycerides (every year) Target													
HDL (every year)/LDL (every year) Target													
Influenza (every yr)/Pneumonia Vaccination (at least once; see CDC recommendations)													
DM Health Record Review													
Self-Management Training													
Smoking Cessation													
Self Blood Glucose Monitoring													
Nutrition/Weight Management													
Physical Activity													
Sick Day Management													
Hypo/Hyperglycemia													
Foot Care													
General Care													
Periodic H&P													
Mammogram/CXR													
Stool for Occult Blood or FlexaSig.													
PPD/Tetanus													
EKG													
Medication Adherence													

Source: Copyright © 1995 Diabetes Coalition of California, Sacramento, California.

Diabetes, Type I, Pediatric—Provider Pathway, Office Setting

	First Visit after Initial Episode	Second Visit Second Week	Third Visit Third to Fourth Week	Fourth Visit Fifth to Seventh Week	Monthly Visit for 3 Months or PRN
Date					
Assessment	Head to toe physical exam with special emphasis on following systems: • Cardiovascular • Respiratory • Gastrointestinal • Neurological • Ophthalmic • Nephrological	Reassess systems: • Cardiovascular • Respiratory • Gastrointestinal • Neurological Review blood glucose diary Assess growth and development	Review blood glucose diary	Reassess the following systems: • Cardiovascular • Respiratory • Gastrointestinal • Neurological Review blood glucose diary	Assess the following systems: • Cardiovascular • Respiratory • Gastrointestinal • Neurological Review blood glucose diary Assess growth and development
Diagnostics and Treatments	CBC SMA UA RBG Cholesterol and triglycerides Weight and height Urine dip for ketones	RBG Urine dip for ketones Weight	RBG Urine dip for ketones Weight	RBG Urine dip for ketones Weight	RBG Urine dip for ketones Weight and height Hba1c
Teaching and Counseling	Proper insulin injection Storage and preparation of insulin Blood glucose monitoring S&S hyperglycemia S&S hypoglycemia ADA diabetic diet Blood glucose diary	Construct treatment plan Discuss rotation of insulin injections Review S&S of hypo/hyperglycemia Plan exercise program Discuss preparation and administration of glucagon	Modify and review treatment plan Reinforce knowledge base on insulin use, diet, and exercise	Modify and review treatment plan Reinforce knowledge base on insulin use, diet, and exercise	Modify and review treatment plan Reinforce knowledge base on insulin use, diet, and exercise

continues

Note: RBG, random blood glucose.

Diabetes, Type I, Pediatric continued

	First Visit after Initial Episode	Second Visit Second Week	Third Visit Third to Fourth Week	Fourth Visit Fifth to Seventh Week	Monthly Visit for 3 Months or PRN
Date					
Medications	Regular and NPH insulin Dosage: 0.5–0.9 U/kg/day	Adjust insulin based on RBG, weight, and blood glucose diary	Adjust insulin based on RBG, weight, and blood glucose diary	Adjust insulin based on RBG, weight, and blood glucose diary	Adjust insulin based on RBG, weight, and blood glucose diary
Consults	Dietitian				Annual ophthalmic exam Semiannual dental exam
Physiological Outcomes	Normal physiologic exam No ketonuria	Minimal polyuria, polydypsia, and polyphagia Blood glucose <200 mg/dL	No polyuria, polydypsia, polyphagia Maintaining or appropriate ↑ in weight Blood glucose <180 mg/dL	No symptoms Maintaining or appropriate ↑ in weight Blood glucose <150 mg/dL	No ED visits Appropriate weight Appropriate growth and development Blood glucose <120 mg/dL
Educational Outcomes	Demonstrates insulin injection Properly tests for blood glucose Knows S&S of hypo/hyperglycemia Has base knowledge of ADA diet	Family gaining confidence in checking blood glucose and administering insulin Knows when to seek medical attention based on S&S of hypo/hyperglycemia Knows when to administer glucagon	Patient and family modify treatment plan with provider/team Patient and family express confidence in managing mild/moderate hypo/hyperglycemic events at home	Patient and family more involved in self-care Patient and family fully manage mild/moderate hypo/hyperglycemic events at home	Patient and family understand diabetes mellitus, self-care treatments Patient and family know when to come to health care center or ED
Psychosocial Outcomes	Patient and family are no longer in denial and have begun acceptance of the diagnosis Patient knowledge base for control and treatment has begun	Patient and family accept diagnosis and show increased involvement in treatment Patient and family have increased knowledge and skills for control and treatment	Patient and family initiate self-care via treatment plan	Level of self-care by patient and family has increased	Self-care with health center backup

continues

Diabetes, Type I, Pediatric continued

	First Visit after Initial Episode	Second Visit Second Week	Third Visit Third to Fourth Week	Fourth Visit Fifth to Seventh Week	Monthly Visit for 3 Months or PRN
Date					
Medication Outcomes	Knows difference between regular and NPH insulin Knows handling and storage of insulin Knows how to prepare and inject with syringe	Patient and family have increased confidence in storing, preparing, and injecting insulin	Decreased insulin need due to better control with diet and exercise	Less fluctuation in insulin needs due to better control with diet and exercise	Insulin needs appropriate for height and weight No lipodystrophy
Comments					
Initials/Date					

Source: Rufus S. Howe, *Clinical Pathways for Ambulatory Care Case Management*, Aspen Publishers, Inc., © 1996.

Diabetes, Type I, Pediatric—Provider Pathway, Posthospitalization Setting

	First Visit after Initial Hospitalization	Second Visit 1 Month after Hospitalization	Third Visit Second Month and Every 2–3 Months	Annually
Date				
Assessment	Complete history and physical Measurement of height and weight recorded on growth chart Funduscopic exam Vital signs Assessment of home glucose monitoring, diary, and meds	BP General physical exam with special attention to signs of lipodystrophy, neuropathy, retinopathy, thyroid size, and foot care Assess Tanner's scale development Measurement of height and weight recorded on growth chart Psychological/social adaptation to diabetes Review of home monitoring, meds, diary Review food diary and exchanges	BP General physical exam with special attention to signs of lipodystrophy, neuropathy, retinopathy, thyroid size, and foot care Assess Tanner's scale development Measurement of height and weight recorded on growth chart Psychological/social adaptation to diabetes Review of home monitoring, meds, diary	Complete physical exam Complete eye and visual exam by an ophthalmologist Foot exam Assess adaptation and compliance to diabetic regimen Examination of injection sites
Diagnostic Tests	Chemistry profile 24-hour urine for creatinine clearance, protein, and glucose excretion Thyroid function tests Antithyroid antibodies Microalbuminuria Hba1c	BS Urine ketones/glucose	BS Urine ketones/glucose Hba1c	BUN Thyroid tests Antithyroid antibodies Chemistry profile 24-hour urine HDL/LDL Hba1c

Note: CDE, certified diabetic educator.

continues

Diabetes, Type I, Pediatric continued

continues

	First Visit after Initial Hospitalization	Second Visit 1 Month after Hospitalization	Third Visit Second Month and Every 2–3 Months	Annually
Date				
Teaching	Review all previous inpatient education including: • Educating patient and family regarding the pathophysiology and potential complications of diabetes • Management techniques including causes and symptoms of hypo/hyperglycemia and management • Fingersticks for glucose monitoring, urine glucose and ketone checks, and recording in diary • When to seek medical intervention • Dietary instructions • Instructions of family members on glucagon use • Injection procedure and site rotation • Insulin action, peaks, and side effects • Effects of illness, exercise, and stress on glucose levels • Honeymoon phase	Reinforce all previous teaching Educate family/patient about self-management Educate family/patient to various fast food exchanges Provide literature on diabetes for patient/family Test patient/family on questions of diabetes and management	Continue to reinforce needed areas of diabetic teaching focusing on patient's needs Encourage question list for each visit Continue education on family/patient self-management	Review diet yearly to eliminate problems associated with caloric need alteration during growth and development
Medications	Rx for: • Syringes • Regular and NPH insulin according to protocol • Glucagon • Sliding scale approach to insulin—have patient call with blood sugars and adjust PRN	Review diary and sliding scale Make adjustments as needed in insulin regimen Patient will call with abnormal glucose values for insulin dosage adjustments	Review diary and sliding scale Make adjustments as needed in insulin regimen	Review diary and sliding scale Make adjustments as needed in insulin regimen Consider insulin pump or using pork insulin in brittle diabetics

Diabetes, Type I, Pediatric continued

	First Visit after Initial Hospitalization	Second Visit 1 Month after Hospitalization	Third Visit Second Month and Every 2–3 Months	Annually
Date				
Consults/Referrals	Nutritional consult with registered dietitian Management team approach should include endocrinologist, psychologist, nutritionist nurse-practitioner, and CDE School personnel and/or school nurse should be informed by parents of child diabetic	Diabetic support group for parent/child Family/individual counseling if psychological problem and poor adaptation Follow up with registered dietitian	Follow up with registered dietitian as needed	Ophthalmologist Follow up with registered dietitian for caloric increases Physiological outcomes
Physical exam WNL	Recurrent hospital admissions and diabetic ketoacidosis are avoided Hyper/hypoglycemic attacks are less frequent or avoided Blood glucose levels are fluctuating	Near normal glucose levels are maintained with fluctuations Physical exam WNL Normal growth and development are evidenced by appropriate rise in growth chart Patient will attain normal sexual maturation Physical exam WNL	Near normal glucose levels are maintained 100–150 mg/dL Hyper/hypoglycemic attacks are avoided Hba1c is decreasing Normal growth and development are evidenced by appropriate rise in growth chart Patient will be euglycemic	Physical exam is WNL Hba1c is less than 8 Complications of diabetes are averted (ie, neuropathy/retinopathy) Normal growth, development, and sexual maturation are achieved Laboratory tests are WNL Injection sites are free of lipodystrophy

continues

Diabetes, Type I, Pediatric continued

	First Visit after Initial Hospitalization	Second Visit 1 Month after Hospitalization	Third Visit Second Month and Every 2–3 Months	Annually
Date				
Educational Outcomes	Patient will be able to verbalize understanding of pathophysiology of diabetes and potential complications Family/patient will be able to demonstrate insulin injection technique, fingerstick technique, and use of glucometer and urine testing for glucose and ketones Utilization of home monitoring will be evidenced by blood sugar diary Patient/family will recognize early symptoms of hypoglycemia (ie, hunger, tiredness) so immediate intervention can avert profound hypoglycemia Family will know SE and peaks of insulin Family seeks frequent advice from medical personnel Family/patient adheres to diet recommended by nutritionist Family will verbalize understanding of glucagon usage	Patient and family become more comfortable with diabetic management Family asks appropriate questions and identifies areas of knowledge deficits Family knows when to seek medical care Family shows increasing knowledge of diabetes by answering questions (ie, test)	Patient and family are capable of accepting all aspects of diabetic care needed to develop excellent control Medical care is sought when needed Advances in diabetic care are shared with patient/family	Patient and family can verbalize understanding of disease and self-care treatments including insulin peaks and signs and symptoms of hyper/hypoglycemia Diabetic education has enhanced long-term compliance and control
Psychosocial Outcomes	Family/patient takes a positive approach to diabetes Open discussions with family and good rapport will ease the trauma of lifestyle adaptations for the patient Continue patient knowledge of disease and treatment	Early recognition of psychological denial or deterioration is made and appropriate referrals are instituted Patient and family will institute proper lifestyle adaptation Increase of patient/family understanding and knowledge of disease/meds	Patient and family begin self-care with medical backup and phone calls between visits Family seeks psychological support when needed	Self-sufficiency is attained that will allay feelings of dependency in child Health care visits are maintained every 3 months Long-term compliance is achieved

continues

Diabetes, Type I, Pediatric continued

	First Visit after Initial Hospitalization	Second Visit 1 Month after Hospitalization	Third Visit Second Month and Every 2–3 Months	Annually
Date				
Medication Outcomes	Review insulin dosages: Maintain or modify Frequent contact with patient provides for insulin adjustment Honeymoon phase—insulin dosage may need to be lowered to prevent hypoglycemia Instability of blood glucose levels is a regular feature of children and adolescents; as a result frequent changes in insulin dosages are needed	Sliding scale is reviewed Insulin dosages: Maintained or modified Decreasing contact with provider via phone for insulin adjustments	Patient/family will begin to adjust sliding scale to blood glucose levels, exercise, and meals Lesser need for frequent contact with provider via phone concerning insulin adjustments	Self-adjustment in insulin dosage is ultimate goal Contact with provider during illness or emergency Insulin pump is used for control of brittle diabetes Insulin dosages begin to stabilize
Comments	Extensive inpatient education regarding the management of the disease is required prior to outpatient teaching Child should wear identification band for diabetes Children over 9 years old should be encouraged to take over as many self-management tasks as possible including blood and urine testing and injections Child should carry sugar product or oral preparation at all times	Inform child/parent about camps for diabetic children	Patient may need more frequent visits if poor control or knowledge deficit is evident	
Initials/Date				

Source: Rufus S. Howe, *Clinical Pathways for Ambulatory Care Case Management*, Aspen Publishers, Inc., © 1996.

Diabetes, Type I, Adult—Provider Pathway, Clinic Setting

	First Visit after Initial Episode	Second Visit Second Week	Third Visit Third Week	Fourth Visit Fourth Week
Date				
Assessment	H&P FBS Knowledge of diabetic management	PE Lab values Review diary of blood values and diet/insulin compliance	FBS	FBS
Diagnostics and Treatments	FBS, Hba1c, SMA 12, CBC, UA, BUN, creatinine, cholesterol, ECG	FBS via glucometer	FBS via glucometer	FBS via glucometer
Teaching/Counseling	Importance of home glucose monitoring, exercise regimen, diet, and insulin compliance Use of One-Touch Diet restrictions Proper technique in insulin administration Blood level parameters Insulin site rotation S&S of hypo/hyperglycemia Universal precautions	Complications of diabetes (heart, stroke, kidney) Return demonstration of insulin technique Review teaching to evaluate understanding from previous visit Instruct regarding diet/exercise/insulin relationship	PVD complications Importance of routine foot care Initiate One-Touch calibration Review understanding of diet/exercise/insulin relationship	Visual and neurological complications of diabetes Importance of routine eye exam Importance of continued follow-up and diabetes mellitus management
Medications	Humulin N insulin 20 U SQ AM	Continue insulin dose according to blood sugar	Insulin adjusted based on blood levels	Adjust insulin accordingly
Consults/Referrals			Podiatrist	Ophthalmologist
Physiological Outcomes	Blood sugar in acceptable range Lab values WNL	Blood sugar in acceptable range	Blood sugar WNL	Blood sugar WNL

Note: PVD, peripheral vascular disease.

continues

Diabetes, Type I, Adult continued

	First Week after Initial Episode	Second Visit Second Week	Third Visit Third Week	Fourth Visit Fourth Week
Date				
Educational Outcomes	Able to perform return demonstration of One-Touch Able to administer insulin with supervision Able to verbalize method of disposal of supplies Able to demonstrate accurate site rotation Able to repeat S&S of hypo/ hyperglycemia, normal blood values	Able to verbalize relationship between diet/exercise/insulin Knowledgeable of ADA diet exchange Knowledgeable of complications of diabetes	Can independently demonstrate insulin administration and One-Touch monitor use Can verbalize understanding of importance of foot care, routine eye exam Knowledgeable of PVD complications Can demonstrate One-Touch calibration	Able to verbalize visual and neurological complications of diabetes
Psychosocial Outcomes	Begin knowledge of disease process and management	Continue knowledge of disease process and management	Patient has significant knowledge of disease process and management	Discuss continued feedback with health care provider
Medication Outcomes	Review insulin dose, response	Can continue on insulin without complication	Control of hyperglycemia with insulin	Maintain on present insulin dose
Comments				
Initials/Date				

Source: Rufus S. Howe, *Clinical Pathways for Ambulatory Care Case Management*, Aspen Publishers, Inc., © 1996.

Diabetes, Type II—Nonambulatory Provider Pathway

	Follow-Up Week 1	Follow-Up Weeks 2–3	Follow-Up Weeks 5–6	Follow-Up 3 Months
Date				
Assessment	VS, weight, skin, diet history, family support, and resources	VS, weight, skin, review of 2-week diary of events	Same as visit for weeks 2–3	Same as visit for weeks 2–3
Diagnosis and Treatments	Home glucose monitoring, urine dip	Same	Same	Hba1c, blood sugar, urine dip
Teaching and Counseling	Importance of accepting diagnosis Importance of diet, exercise, medication, and glucose monitoring Knowledge of the warning signs of hypoglycemia Treatment of hypoglycemia with simple sugars	Continue diet teaching, meal selection Review topics presented at first visit	Foot and skin care, exercise, and review of topics presented at first visit	Encourage avoidance of smoking and alcohol Encourage regular eye examinations
Medications	Oral hypoglycemics—side effects and drug interactions OTC meds that contain sugar	Same	Same	Same
Consults and Referrals				Ophthalmologist, podiatrist, or endocrinologist PRN
Physiological Outcomes	Blood glucose is WNL	Same Minimal S&S of hypoglycemia	Same Weight closer to normal range	Hba1c is WNL
Educational Outcomes	Correct definition of diagnosis and list of S&S of hypoglycemia	Knows dosage and side effects of meds	Patient can manage diet regimen, begin exercise program, and manage mild hypoglycemia	Patient and significant other express understanding of disease

continues

Diabetes, Type II continued

	Follow-Up Week 1	Follow-Up Weeks 2–3	Follow-Up Weeks 5–6	Follow-Up 3 Months
Date				
Psychosocial Outcomes	Begin understanding of diet modifications, weight, and activity changes	Review of same	Increase knowledge of lifestyle modifications through support groups, literature, and seminars	Patient and family can understand meal selection and preparation and can resume normal activities with minor necessary modifications
Medication Outcomes	Accept and understand dosage and side effects of oral hypoglycemics, if prescribed	Same Knowledge of proper storage of pills	Same	Plan for renewal of meds before prescription is completed
Comments	Remind patient to plan for snacks and emergencies and to increase dietary intake before exercise	Have patient check insurance coverage to obtain home blood glucose monitoring kit and meds as easily as possible	Knowledge of foot care, prevention of calluses, and infection	
Initials/Date				

Source: Rufus S. Howe, *Clinical Pathways for Ambulatory Care Case Management*, Aspen Publishers, Inc., © 1996.

Diabetes, Type II—Provider Pathway, Ambulatory Setting

	Initial Visit	1 Month	3 Months	6 Months	9 Months	Annual
Date						
Assessment	Complete history and physical Height and weight, BP, pulse, RR Ophthalmoscopic exam Foot exam	Examine skin, heart, and lungs Palpate pulses Foot exam H/O S&S hyper/ hypoglycemia Weight, BP, pulse, RR	Examine skin, heart, and lungs Palpate pulses Foot exam H/O S&S hyper/ hypoglycemia Weight, BP, pulse, RR	Examine skin, heart, and lungs Palpate pulses Foot exam H/O S&S hyper/ hypoglycemia Weight, BP, pulse, RR	Examine skin, heart, and lungs Palpate pulses Foot exam H/O S&S hyper/ hypoglycemia Weight, BP, pulse, RR	Complete history and physical Height, weight, BP, RR, pulse Ophthalmoscopic exam Foot exam
Diagnostics and Treatments	Hba1c Random plasma glucose Lipid profile, UA, CBC Microalbuminuria SMA 20 Thyroid function tests ECG	Random plasma glucose	Hba1c Random plasma glucose	Random plasma glucose	Random plasma glucose	Hba1c Random plasma glucose Lipid profile, UA, CBC Microalbuminuria SMA 20 Thyroid function tests
Teaching and Counseling	Importance of dietary management and exercise S&S hyper/hypogly- cemia Foot care Basic pathophysi- ology of diabetes and long-term complications Home glucose monitoring Educational, nutritional, exercise counseling	Develop treatment plan Teach home glucose monitoring Manage low blood sugar Establish degree of glycemic control	Review and modify treatment plan Review home glucose monitoring diary	Review and modify treatment plan	Review and modify treatment plan	Review and modify treatment plan

continues

Diabetes, Type II continued

	Initial Visit	1 Month	3 Months	6 Months	9 Months	Annual
Date						
Medications			Initiate oral hypoglycemic medications if not adequately controlled by diet	Modify medication according to blood glucose and home monitoring diary	Modify medication according to blood glucose and home monitoring diary	Modify medication according to blood glucose and home monitoring diary
Consults/Referrals	Ophthalmologist Dietitian	MD if blood glucose ≥400 Consider smoking cessation Consider support group MD for complications	MD for diabetes complications	MD for diabetes complications	MD for diabetes complications	MD for diabetes complications
Physiological Outcomes	Minimal/no symptoms of hyperglycemia Elevated blood glucose Physical exam MNL	No symptoms	No symptoms Glycemic control	No symptoms Glycemic control	No symptoms Glycemic control	No symptoms Glycemic control
Educational Outcomes	Knows S&S of hyper/ hypoglycemia Knows proper foot care Knows diabetes exchange lists	Demonstrates correct use of glucose meter Establishes degree of glycemic control	Confident managing hypoglycemia Manages diabetes Confident in menu plan Knows when to seek medical attention Understands that exercise helps control blood sugar Expresses understanding of disease, S&S hyper/hypoglycemia when comes to clinic	Confident in managing hypoglycemia Can take home self-care interventions and manage low blood sugar and menu planning	Can manage dietary restrictions when eating at a restaurant Can modify treatment plan	Understands disease and its management Confident with skills to manage disease

continues

Diabetes, Type II continued

	Initial Visit	1 Month	3 Months	6 Months	9 Months	Annual
Date						
Psychosocial Outcomes	Beginning knowledge base of disease, control, and treatment	Increase patient knowledge and understanding of disease, control, treatment. Make necessary lifestyle changes. Acceptance of living with chronic disease	Patient involved in self-care, management of diabetes, and in treatment plan. Positive lifestyle change maintained	Increased self-care with provider backup	Increased self-care with provider backup	Self-care with provider backup
Medication Outcomes			May initiate oral hypoglycemic agents	Review meds. Maintain or modify meds as necessary	Review meds. Maintain or modify meds as necessary	Review meds. Maintain or modify meds as necessary
Comments				Consider insulin therapy if unable to control blood sugar on oral agents	This approach would necessitate insulin administration teaching	Maintenance visits of 3–6 months
Initials/Date						

Source: Rufus S. Howe, *Clinical Pathways for Ambulatory Care Case Management*, Aspen Publishers, Inc., © 1996.

Diabetes, Type II—Provider Pathway

	Initial Visit	Second Visit 3 Days	Third Visit 1 Week from Second	Fourth Visit 2 Weeks from Third	Monthly Visits
Date					
Assessment	Measure height and weight Examine skin and feet Perform ophthalmoscopic exam, cardiac assessment, neuro exam, and psychosocial assessment Palpate thyroid, auscultate lungs, evaluate pulses			Auscultate heart and lungs Evaluate pulses Examine feet	Same as initial visit
Diagnostics	Measure BP FBS, CBC, SMA 12, TFT, Hba1c, fasting lipids, UA	Measure weight and BP Fasting fingerstick ECG	Measure weight and BP Fingerstick	Measure weight and BP Fingerstick	Measure weight and BP Fingerstick Hba1c q 3 months CBC, SMA 12, fasting lipids, TFT, UA, and ECG q year
Teaching	Discuss: S&S of hyper- and hypoglycemia and long-term complications of diabetes mellitus Discuss role of familial history and obesity Discuss diet and exercise therapy with possible addition of oral hypoglycemic	Discuss results of lab tests and normal BG range Discuss possible SE of oral hypoglycemics	Reinforce information patient obtained from nutritionist Administer Medic-Alert card	Discuss progress with diet; foot care regimen; home BG monitoring	Discuss "sick day routine" Review patient BG log q visit

continues

Note: ADA, American Diabetes Association; BG, blood glucose; DTRs, deep tendon reflexes.

Diabetes, Type II continued

	Initial Visit	Second Visit 3 Days	Third Visit 1 Week from Second	Fourth Visit 2 Weeks from Third	Monthly Visits
Date					
Medications/Treatment	Pending results of tests	Diet and exercise therapy as first line with addition of oral meds if indicated Will start at glyburide 2.5 mg PO qd	Adjust accordingly	Adjust accordingly	Adjust accordingly
Consults		Refer to nutritionist	Refer to ophthalmologist and podiatrist	Refer to dental clinic Refer to ADA to contact for support group information	
Physiological Outcomes	Patient slightly obese, C/O polyuria, polydypsia, polyphagia, fatigue Ophthalmoscopic exam WNL, thyroid WNL, lungs clear, normal S_1 and S_2, pulses palpable in all extremities, feet WNL, BP WNL, DTRs WNL Fingerstick = 200, 2 hour postprandial	Patient C/O polyuria, polydypsia, polyphagia, and fatigue FBS = 162 mg/dL Labs from last visit: FBS = 179 mg/dL UA = 100 mg/dL glucose All other labs WNL	Patient C/O occasional polyuria/polydypsia FBS = 132 mg/dL BP WNL Weight remains the same	Patient denies polyuria, polydypsia, or fatigue FBS = 109 mg/dL BP WNL Weight loss of 2 lb	Patient denies polyuria, polydypsia, or fatigue FBS = 129 mg/dL BP WNL Patient continues to lose weight
Educational Outcomes	Patient verbalizes understanding of S&S of hypo- and hypergly-cemia, and long-term complications of the disease Patient verbalizes importance of diet and weight loss	Patient verbalizes understanding of normal BG range	Patient verbalizes importance of following diet and losing weight Patient states that he/she has begun a slow walking program	Patient expresses desire to self-manage disease and is gaining increasing knowledge of self-care	Patient expresses ever-increasing knowledge of self-care Patient home monitoring BG fasting and 2 hours postprandial after largest meal of day

continues

Diabetes, Type II continued

	Initial Visit	Second Visit 3 Days	Third Visit 1 Week from Second	Fourth Visit 2 Weeks from Third	Monthly Visits
Date					
Psychosocial Outcomes		Patient begins to understand what it means to be diabetic		Patient begins to incorporate self-care regimen into daily life	Patient manages disease at home with backup primary care provider
Medication Outcomes	Diet and exercise therapy with addition of oral hypoglycemics if indicated	Same	Same	Same	Same
Comments					
Initials/Date					

Source: Rufus S. Howe, *Clinical Pathways for Ambulatory Care Case Management*, Aspen Publishers, Inc., © 1996.

Diabetes Home Health Clinical Pathway

Clinical Path—Dx _Insulin-Dependent Diabetes Mellitus (IDDM)_ Pt. Name _____

Goals: To attain normoglycemic levels (within one week)

To become independent with glucose monitoring device (within one week)

To become independent with insulin administration (within one week)

To be knowledgeable regarding disease process (within two weeks)

To be knowledgeable about, and therefore compliant with, medications (within two weeks)

To be knowledgeable about, and therefore compliant with, diabetic diet (within one week)

KEY

✓ = Done I = Instructed/Reinstructed

Ø = None

N/A = Not Applicable

V = Variance A = Achieved

Signature _____ Initials _____

_____

_____

Date																
Initials																
EVERY VISIT																
1. Assess for signs of hypoglycemia																
2. Assess for signs of hyperglycemia																
3. Assess blood glucose level (if applicable)																
4. Assess nutritional intake																
5. Administer insulin (in absence of capable caregiver)																
6. Assess effectiveness of medications																
7. Assess untoward effects of medication																

continues

Diabetes Home Health Clinical Pathway continued

INSTRUCTION	Date																								
1. Patient rights and responsibilities																									
2. Patient financial liability for home care																									
3. Patient/home safety																									
4. Expectations of home care																									
Use of clinical pathway																									
Role of patient																									
Role of significant other																									
Role of home care staff																									
Payer criteria/discharge plan																									
5. Plan for care (discuss/collaborate)																									
6. Written visit schedule																									
7. Medication regimen																									
8. Pertinent telephone numbers																									
Physician																									
Agency																									
Department of Health hotline																									
Pharmacy																									
Durable medical equipment																									
9. When to notify the physician																									
10. Insulin administration																									
11. Diet																									
12. Use of glucose monitor																									
13. Disease process																									
Signs of hypoglycemia																									
Treatment of hypoglycemia																									
Definition of IDDM																									
Steps to control																									
Relationship of activity to insulin needs																									
Signs of hyperglycemia																									
Treatment of hyperglycemia																									
Complications attributed to poor compliance																									

continues

Diabetes Home Health Clinical Pathway continued

INSTRUCTION	Date																													
Importance of foot care																														
Importance of eye care																														
Sick day management																														
Use of identification bracelet																														
14. Medications																														
15. Discharge instructions																														

Source: Barbara Stover Gingerich and Deborah Anne Ondeck, *Clinical Pathways for the Multidisciplinary Home Care Team*, Aspen Publishers, Inc., © 1996.

Skilled Nursing Facility Interdisciplinary Plan of Care: Diabetes Mellitus

PROBLEM	GOALS	INTERVENTIONS	DISCIPLINES

Diabetes Mellitus or Potential for Complications, that is Hypoglycemia or Hyperglycemia and/or Nutrition Impaired and/or Skin Integrity Impaired (especially feet/legs) and/or Vision Impaired (diabetic retinopathy)
 	
R/T
 	
___ Diabetes mellitus
___ _____
    _____
	___ Will remain free of diabetes mellitus s/s AEB
	A. Hyperglycemia
	  ___ Appetite loss
	  ___ Nausea
	  ___ Skin hot/dry/flushed
	  ___ Urination, frequent
	  ___ Vomiting
	  ___ Weight loss
	B. Hypoglycemia
	  ___ Confused
	  ___ Diaphoresis
	  ___ Dizziness
	  ___ Headache
	  ___ Hunger
	  ___ Irritability
	  ___ Paleness
	  ___ Pulse increased
	  ___ Respirations shallow
	  ___ Restlessness
	  ___ Stupor
	  ___ Vision blurred
	  ___ Weakness
	
	by/through: _____
	
	And/or
	___ _____
	    _____
	    _____
	    _____
	
	by/through: _____
		___ Assess/record/report to MD prn s/s of
		  ___ Hyperglycemia
		    ___ Appetite loss
		    ___ Nausea
		    ___ Skin hot/dry/flushed
		    ___ Urination, frequent
		    ___ Vomiting
		    ___ Weight loss
		  ___ Hypoglycemia
		    ___ Confused
		    ___ Diaphoresis
		    ___ Dizziness
		    ___ Headache
		    ___ Hunger
		    ___ Irritability
		    ___ Paleness
		    ___ Pulse increased
		    ___ Respirations shallow
		    ___ Restlessness
		    ___ Stupor
		    ___ Vision blurred
		    ___ Weakness
		
		___ Lab/diagnostic work: Monitor/report results to MD
		  ___ See lab work on MD orders or
		  ___ Check applicable labs or
		  ___ FBS
		    _____
		  ___ See lab section of chart or
		Date/frequency/results: ____
		    _____
		Report any recommendations for diet changes to nursing/MD prn
			N
			
			N D

Resident's name: _____ Date: _____

continues

SNF Interdisciplinary Plan of Care continued

PROBLEM	GOALS	INTERVENTIONS	DISCIPLINES
		___ Provide/serve/monitor intake of diet: _____ _____	D N NA
		___ No concentrated sweets ___ No added sugar	
		___ If resident becomes hypo-glycemic ___ Administer: _____ ___ Call MD _____	N
		___ Accu check blood sugar ___ Frequency _____ ___ Hyperglycemia/hy-poglycemia s/s prn	N
		___ Provide foot care; observe circulation and integrity and communicate to nursing/MD prn	N NA
		___ Meet with resident/family to discuss any concerns R/T the diabetes mellitus	S
		___ Arrange ophthalmology examination Communicate with nursing to ensure resident is ready for the appointment	S
		___ Provide a program of ac-tivities that accommodates resident's problem: _____ ___ Encourage exercise program ___ Offer food that complies with diet at food-related activities Invite/escort to: _____ _____	A

continues

SNF Interdisciplinary Plan of Care continued

PROBLEM	GOALS	INTERVENTIONS	DISCIPLINES
		___ Meds: Administer/monitor effectiveness/side effects ___ See physician order sheet, or ___ List: _____	N
		___ Resident education ___ Disease process ___ Foods to avoid ___ Foot care ___ Infection avoidance and s/s ___ Smoking cessation ___ Stress management ___ _____	N D S
		___ _____ _____ _____ _____	__ __

Source: Janie L. Krechting and Victoria E. Koper, *Interdisciplinary Care Plans for Long-Term Care*, Aspen Publishers, Inc., © 1996.

PART II

Self-Management of Diabetes: Patient Education

About Diabetes

Almost every one of us knows someone who has diabetes. An estimated 16 million people in the United States have diabetes mellitus—a serious, lifelong condition. About half of these people do not know they have diabetes and are not under care for the disorder. Each year, about 650,000 people are diagnosed with diabetes.

Although diabetes occurs most often in older adults, it is one of the most common chronic disorders in children in the United States. About 127,000 children and teenagers age 19 and younger have diabetes.

WHAT IS DIABETES?

Diabetes is a disorder of metabolism—the way our bodies use digested food for growth and energy. Most of the food we eat is broken down by the digestive juices into a simple sugar called glucose. Glucose is the main source of fuel for the body.

After digestion, the glucose passes into our bloodstream where it is available for body cells to use for growth and energy. For the glucose to get into the cells, insulin must be present. Insulin is a hormone produced by the pancreas, a large gland behind the stomach.

When we eat, the pancreas is supposed to automatically produce the right amount of insulin to move the glucose from our blood into our cells. In people with diabetes, however, the pancreas either produces little or no insulin, or the body cells do not respond to the insulin that is produced. As a result, glucose builds up in the blood, overflows into the urine, and passes out of the body. Thus, the body loses its main source of fuel even though the blood contains large amounts of glucose.

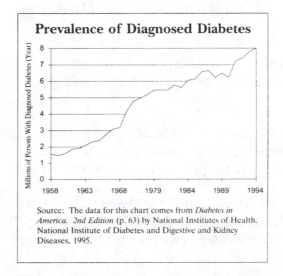

Prevalence of Diagnosed Diabetes

Source: The data for this chart comes from *Diabetes in America. 2nd Edition* (p. 63) by National Institutes of Health, National Institute of Diabetes and Digestive and Kidney Diseases, 1995.

continues

continued

WHAT ARE THE DIFFERENT TYPES OF DIABETES?

The three main types of diabetes are:

- Insulin-dependent diabetes mellitus (IDDM) or Type I diabetes
- Noninsulin-dependent diabetes mellitus (NIDDM) or Type II diabetes
- Gestational diabetes

INSULIN-DEPENDENT DIABETES

Insulin-dependent diabetes is considered an autoimmune disease. An autoimmune disease results when the body's system for fighting infection (the immune system) turns against a part of the body. In diabetes, the immune system attacks the insulin-producing beta cells in the pancreas and destroys them. The pancreas the produces little or no insulin.

Someone with IDDM needs daily injections of insulin to live. At present, scientists do not know exactly what causes the body's immune system to attack the beta cells, but they believe that both genetic factors and viruses are involved. IDDM accounts for about 5 to 10 percent of diagnosed diabetes in the United States.

IDDM develops most often in children and young adults, but the disorder can appear at any age. Symptoms of IDDM usually develop over a short period, although beta cell destruction can begin months, even years, earlier.

Symptoms include increased thirst and urination, constant hunger, weight loss, blurred vision, and extreme tiredness. If not diagnosed and treated with insulin, a person can lapse into a life-threatening coma.

Noninsulin-Dependent Diabetes

The most common form of diabetes is noninsulin-dependent diabetes. About 90 to 95 percent of people with diabetes have NIDDM. This form of diabetes usually develops in adults over the age of 40 and is most common among adults over age 55. About 80 percent of people with NIDDM are overweight.

In NIDDM, the pancreas usually produces insulin, but for some reason, the body cannot use the insulin effectively. The end result is the same as for IDDM—an unhealthy buildup of glucose in the blood and an inability of the body to make efficient use of its main source of fuel.

The symptoms of NIDDM develop gradually and are not as noticeable as in IDDM. Symptoms include feeling tired or ill, frequent urination (especially at night), unusual thirst, weight loss, blurred vision, frequent infections, and slow healing of sores.

continues

continued

Gestational Diabetes

Gestational diabetes develops or is discovered during pregnancy. This type usually disappears when the pregnancy is over, but women who have had gestational diabetes have a greater risk of developing NIDDM later in their lives.

WHAT IS THE SCOPE AND IMPACT OF DIABETES?

Diabetes is widely recognized as one of the leading causes of death and disability in the United States. According to death certificate data, diabetes contributed to the deaths of more than 169,000 persons in 1992.

Diabetes is associated with long-term complications that affect almost every major part of the body. It contributes to blindness, heart disease, strokes, kidney failure, amputations, and nerve damage. Uncontrolled diabetes can complicate pregnancy, and birth defects are more common in babies born to women with diabetes.

Diabetes cost the United States $92 billion in 1992. Indirect costs, including disability payments, time lost from work, and premature death, totaled $47 billion; medical costs for diabetes care, including hospitalizations, medical care, and treatment supplies, totaled $45 billion.

WHO GETS DIABETES?

Diabetes is not contagious. People cannot "catch" it from each other. However, certain factors can increase one's risk of developing diabetes. People who have family members with diabetes (especially NIDDM), who are overweight, or who are African American, Hispanic, or Native American are all at greater risk of developing diabetes.

IDDM occurs equally among males and females, but is more common in whites than in nonwhites. Data from the World Health Organization's Multinational Project for Childhood Diabetes indicate that IDDM is rare in most Asian, African, and Native American populations. On the other hand, some northern European countries, including Finland and Sweden, have high rates of IDDM. The reasons for these differences are not known.

NIDDM is more common in older people, especially older women who are overweight, and occurs more often among African Americans, Hispanics, and Native Americans. Compared with non-Hispanic whites, diabetes rates are about 60 percent higher in African Americans and 110 to 120 percent higher in Mexican Americans and Puerto Ricans. Native Americans have the highest rates of diabetes in the world. Among Pima Indians living in the United States, for example, half of all adults have NIDDM. The prevalence of diabetes is likely to increase because older people, Hispanics, and other minority groups make up the fastest growing segments of the U.S. population.

continues

continued

HOW IS DIABETES MANAGED?

Before the discovery of insulin in 1921, all people with IDDM died within a few years after the appearance of the disease. Although insulin is not considered a cure for diabetes, its discovery was the first major breakthrough in diabetes treatment.

Today, daily injections of insulin are the basic therapy for IDDM. Insulin injections must be balanced with meals and daily activities, and glucose levels must be closely monitored through frequent blood sugar testing.

Diet, exercise, and blood testing for glucose are also the basis for management of NIDDM. In addition, some people with NIDDM take oral drugs or insulin to lower their blood glucose levels.

People with diabetes must take responsibility for their day-to-day care. Much of the daily care involves trying to keep blood sugar levels from going too low or too high. When blood sugar levels drop too low—a condition known as hypoglycemia—a person can become nervous, shaky, and confused. Judgment can be impaired. Eventually, the person could pass out. The treatment for low blood sugar is to eat or drink something with sugar in it.

On the other hand, a person can become very ill if blood sugar levels rise too high, a condition known as hyperglycemia. Hypoglycemia and hyperglycemia, which can occur in people with IDDM or NIDDM, are both potentially life-threatening emergencies.

People with diabetes should be treated by a doctor who monitors their diabetes control and checks for complications. Doctors who specialize in diabetes are called endocrinologists or diabetologists. In addition, people with diabetes often see ophthalmologists for eye examinations, podiatrists for routine foot care, dietitians for help in planning meals, and diabetes educators for instruction in day-to-day care.

The goal of diabetes management is to keep blood glucose levels as close to the normal (nondiabetic) range as safely possible. A recent government study, sponsored by the National Institute of Diabetes and Digestive and Kidney Diseases (NIDDK), proved that keeping blood sugar levels as close to normal as safely possible reduces the risk of developing major complications of diabetes.

The 10-year study, called the Diabetes Control and Complications Trial (DCCT), was completed in 1993 and included 1,441 people with IDDM. The study compared the effect of two treatment approaches—intensive management and standard management—on the development and progression of eye, kidney, and nerve complications of diabetes. Researchers found that study participants who maintained lower levels of blood glucose through intensive management had significantly lower rates of these complications.

continues

continued

Researchers believe that DCCT findings have important implications for the treatment of NIDDM, as well as IDDM.

WHAT IS THE STATUS OF DIABETES RESEARCH?

NIDDK supports basic and clinical research in its own laboratories and in research centers and hospitals throughout the United States. It also gathers and analyzes statistics about diabetes. Other institutes at the National Institutes of Health also carry out research on diabetes-related eye diseases, heart and vascular complications, pregnancy, and dental problems.

Other government agencies that sponsor diabetes programs are the Centers for Disease Control and Prevention, the Indian Health Service, the Health Resources and Services Administration, the Bureau of Veterans Affairs, and the Department of Defense.

Many organizations outside of the government support diabetes research and education activities. These organizations include the American Diabetes Association, the Juvenile Diabetes Foundation International, and the American Association of Diabetes Educators.

In recent years, advances in diabetes research have led to better ways to manage diabetes and treat its complications. Major advances include:

- New forms of purified insulin, such as human insulin produced through genetic engineering
- Better ways for doctors to monitor blood glucose levels and for people with diabetes to test their own blood glucose levels at home
- Development of external and implantable insulin pumps that deliver appropriate amounts of insulin, replacing daily injections
- Laser treatment for diabetic eye disease, reducing the risk of blindness
- Successful transplantation of kidneys in people whose own kidneys fail because of diabetes
- Better ways of managing diabetic pregnancies, improving chances of successful outcomes
- New drugs to treat NIDDM and better ways to manage this form of diabetes through weight control
- Evidence that intensive management of blood glucose reduces and may prevent development of microvascular complications of diabetes
- Demonstration that antihypertensive drugs called ACE-inhibitors prevent or delay kidney failure in people with diabetes

WHAT WILL THE FUTURE BRING?

In the future, it may be possible to administer insulin through nasal sprays or in the form of a pill or patch. Devices that can "read" blood glucose levels without having to prick a finger to get a blood sample are also being developed.

continues

continued

Researchers continue to search for the cause or causes of diabetes and ways to prevent and cure the disorder. Scientists are looking for genes that may be involved in NIDDM and IDDM. Some genetic markers for IDDM have been identified, and it is now possible to screen relatives of people with IDDM to see if they are at risk for diabetes.

The new Diabetes Prevention Trial—Type I, sponsored by NIDDK, identifies relatives at risk for developing IDDM and treats them with low doses of insulin or with oral insulin-like agents in the hope of preventing IDDM. Similar research is carried out at other medical centers throughout the world.

Transplantation of the pancreas or insulin-producing beta cells offers the best hope of cure for people with IDDM. Some pancreas transplants have been successful. However, people who have transplants must take powerful drugs to prevent rejection of the transplanted organ. These drugs are costly and may eventually cause serious health problems.

Scientists are working to develop less harmful drugs and better methods of transplanting pancreatic tissue to prevent rejection by the body. Using techniques of bioengineering, researchers are also trying to create artificial islet cells that secrete insulin in response to increased sugar levels in the blood.

For NIDDM, the focus is on ways to prevent diabetes. Preventive approaches include identifying people at high risk for the disorder and encouraging them to lose weight, exercise more, and follow a healthy diet. The Diabetes Prevention Program, another new NIDDK project, will focus on preventing the disorder in high-risk populations.

WHERE IS MORE INFORMATION AVAILABLE?

For more information about IDDM, NIDDM, and gestational diabetes, as well as diabetes research, statistics, and education, contact:

National Diabetes Information Clearinghouse
1 Information Way
Bethesda, MD 20892-3560
(301) 654-3327

The following organizations also distribute materials and support programs for people with diabetes and their families and friends:

American Association of Diabetes Educators
444 North Michigan Avenue, Suite 1240
Chicago, IL 60611
(800) 832-6874
(312) 644-2233

continues

continued

American Diabetes Association
ADA National Service Center
1660 Duke Street
Alexandria, VA 22314
(800) 232-3472
(703) 549-1500

Juvenile Diabetes Foundation International
120 Wall Street
19th Floor
New York, NY 10005
(800) 223-1138
(212) 785-9500

Points To Remember

What Is Diabetes?
- A disorder of metabolism—the way the body digests food for energy and growth

What Are the Different Types of Diabetes?
- Insulin-dependent diabetes (IDDM)
- Noninsulin-dependent diabetes (NIDDM)
- Gestational diabetes

What Is the Scope and Impact of Diabetes?
- Affects 16 million people
- A leading cause of death and disability
- Costs $92 billion per year

Who Gets Diabetes?
- People of any age
- More common in older people, African Americans, Hispanics, and Native Americans

---

Source: "Diabetes Overview," National Institute of Diabetes and Digestive and Kidney Diseases," National Institutes of Health.

What Is Diabetes?

The two types of diabetes, insulin-dependent and noninsulin-dependent, are different disorders. While the causes, short-term effects, and treatments for the two types differ, both can cause the same long-term health problems. Both types also affect the body's ability to use digested food for energy. Diabetes doesn't interfere with digestion, but it does prevent the body from using an important product of digestion, glucose (commonly known as sugar), for energy.

GLUCOSE

After a meal the digestive system breaks some food down into glucose. The blood carries the glucose or sugar throughout the body, causing blood glucose levels to rise. In response to this rise, the hormone insulin is released into the bloodstream to signal the body tissues to burn the glucose for fuel, causing blood glucose levels to return to normal. A gland called the pancreas, found just behind the stomach, makes insulin. Glucose the body doesn't use right away goes to the liver, muscle or fat for storage. In someone with diabetes, this process doesn't work correctly.

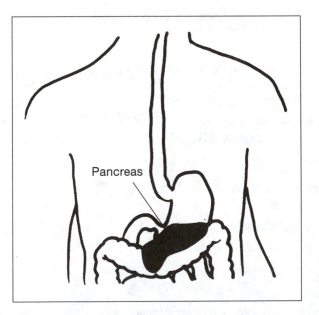

Pancreas

Insulin-Dependent Diabetes

In people with insulin-dependent diabetes, the pancreas doesn't make insulin. This condition usually begins in childhood and is also known as Type I (formerly called juvenile-onset) diabetes. People with this kind of diabetes must have daily insulin injections to survive.

continues

continued

Insulin Resistance

In people with noninsulin-dependent diabetes the pancreas usually produces some insulin. But the body's tissues don't burn the glucose properly. Insulin resistance is an important factor in noninsulin-dependent diabetes.

REMEMBER

- Diabetes interferes with the body's use of food for energy.
- While noninsulin-dependent diabetes and insulin-dependent diabetes are different disorders, they can cause the same complications.

NOTES:

Source: "Noninsulin-Dependent Diabetes," National Institutes of Health, NIH Publication No. 95–241, September 1992.

Diabetes Mellitus

WHAT IS DIABETES? HOW DOES THE BODY WORK?

To understand diabetes, it is important to know how the body works. Much of the food eaten is changed by the body into sugar. The sugar is carried to the cells of the body by the blood.

The sugar is used by the body for

- Short-term use: instant energy
- Later use: stored in the liver and muscles
- Long-term use: changed into fat and stored

INSULIN

In order for the cells to use the sugar, insulin is needed. Insulin is key a key that opens the cells, letting the sugar get from the bloodstream into the cells.

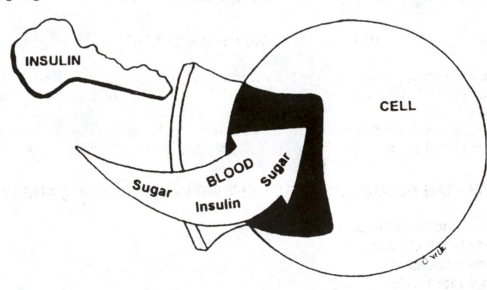

Once this happens, the body is then able to work, play, think, talk, run, and do the many things it wants to do.

Insulin is a hormone or chemical. Insulin is made by a part of the body called the pancreas. The pancreas is found behind the stomach.

continues

continued

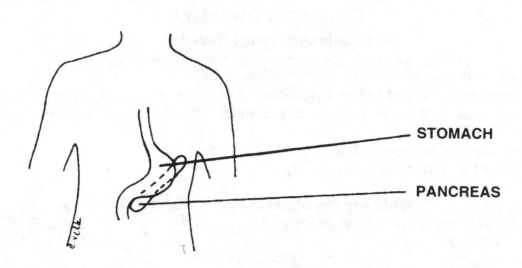

Diabetes happens when the sugar cannot get into the cells; either there is not enough insulin or the insulin is not being used properly. When the sugar is unable to get into the cells to be used as energy, too much sugar builds up in the bloodstream.

WHY TAKE CARE OF DIABETES?

Many problems may result if diabetes is not cared for. To prevent or delay these problems, KEEP THE BLOOD SUGAR WITHIN THE NORMAL RANGE.

All people have sugar in their bloodstream. In diabetes, this blood sugar can become high. The normal range for blood sugar is 70 to 130 mg/dL (milligrams per deciliter).

HOW CAN BLOOD SUGAR BE KEPT WITHIN A NORMAL RANGE?

- Eat the right amount of food at the right time.
- Eat the right types of food.
- Follow an exercise plan.
- Test blood sugar levels.
- Take insulin and/or diabetes pills (oral hypoglycemic agents) as ordered by doctor.

WHAT IS TYPE I DIABETES (INSULIN-DEPENDENT DIABETES MELLITUS)?

Type I diabetes is present when the sugar cannot get into the cells because the pancreas makes little or no insulin.

continues

continued

People with Type I Diabetes

- Are usually young at the time of diagnosis (under 35)
- Have normal body weight before diagnosis
- May or may not have a family history of diabetes
- Will need insulin for life
- Are more likely to develop diabetic coma (ketoacidosis)
- Have signs of diabetes come on quickly

What Are the Signs of Type I Diabetes?

- Frequent urination
- Extreme hunger
- Extreme thirst
- Extreme and sudden weight loss
- Weakness and tiredness
- Nausea and vomiting
- High blood sugar (glucose)
- High amount of sugar in urine
- Ketones in urine
- Dry skin

WHAT IS TYPE II DIABETES (NONINSULIN-DEPENDENT DIABETES MELLITUS)?

Type II diabetes is present when the sugar cannot get into the cells because

- The pancreas does not make enough insulin.
- The cells are not able to use the insulin in the right way.

People with Type II Diabetes

They are usually

- Over the age of 35
- Overweight
- Able to control the diabetes with diet and exercise
- Have a family history of diabetes
- Signs come on slowly

continues

continued

What Are the Signs of Type II Diabetes?

- Increased
  1. Thirst
  2. Urination
  3. Tiredness
  4. Appetite
  5. Weight loss
- More likely to develop infection
- Cuts and sores that take a long time to heal
- Blurred vision

When Type II diabetes cannot be controlled by diet and exercise, diabetes pills may be needed. There may also be a time when insulin will be needed to keep the blood sugar under good control.

NOTES:

Source: St. Joseph Rehabilitation Hospital and Outpatient Center, *Patient Education and Discharge Planning Manual for Rehabilitation,* Aspen Publishers, Inc., © 1995.

Symptoms of Diabetes

The symptoms of diabetes may begin gradually and can be hard to identify at first. They may include

- fatigue
- a sick feeling
- frequent urination, especially at night
- excessive thirst

When there is extra glucose in blood, one way the body gets rid of it is through frequent urination. This loss of fluids causes extreme thirst. Other symptoms may include

- sudden weight loss
- blurred vision
- slow healing of skin, gum, and urinary tract infections. Women may notice genital itching.

A doctor also may suspect a patient has diabetes if the person has health problems related to diabetes. For instance, heart disease, changes in vision, numbness in the feet and legs or sores that are slow to heal, may prompt a doctor to check for diabetes. These symptoms do not mean a person has diabetes, but anyone who has these problems should see a doctor.

REMEMBER

- The symptoms of diabetes can develop gradually and may be hard to identify at first.
- Symptoms may include feeling tired or ill, excessive thirst, frequent urination, sudden weight loss, blurred vision, slow healing of infections, and genital itching.

NOTES:

Source: "Noninsulin-Dependent Diabetes," National Institutes of Health, NIH Publication No. 95–241, September 1992.

What Causes Noninsulin-Dependent Diabetes?

There is no simple answer to what causes noninsulin-dependent diabetes. While eating sugar, for example, doesn't cause diabetes, eating large amounts of sugar and other rich, fatty foods can cause weight gain. Most people who develop diabetes are overweight. Scientists do not fully understand why being overweight increases someone's chances of developing diabetes. But they believe being overweight is a major factor leading to noninsulin-dependent diabetes.

A major cause of diabetes is insulin resistance. Scientists are still searching for the causes of insulin resistance, but they have identified two possibilities. The first could be a defect in insulin receptors on cells. Like an appliance that needs to be plugged into an electrical outlet, insulin has to bind to a receptor to function. Several things can go wrong with receptors. There may not be enough receptors for insulin to bind to, or a defect in the receptors may prevent insulin from binding.

A second possible cause involves the process that occurs after insulin plugs into the receptor. Insulin may bind to the receptor, but the cells don't read the signal to metabolize the glucose. Scientists are studying cells to see why this might happen.

REMEMBER

- In people with noninsulin-dependent diabetes, insulin does't lower blood sugar, a condition called insulin resistance.
- Obesity is a risk factor for diabetes.

NOTES:

Source: "Noninsulin-Dependent Diabetes," National Institutes of Health, NIH Publication No. 95–241, September 1992.

Who Develops Noninsulin-Dependent Diabetes?

Age, sex, weight, physical activity, diet, lifestyle, and family health history all affect someone's chances of developing diabetes. The chances that someone will develop diabetes increase if the person's parents or siblings have the disease.

Experts now know that diabetes is more common in African Americans, Hispanics, Native Americans, and Native Hawaiians than in whites. They believe this is the result of both heredity and environmental factors, such as diet and lifestyle. The highest rate of diabetes in the world is in an Arizona community of Native Americans called the Pimas.

While the chances of developing diabetes increase with age, gender isn't a risk factor, although African American women are more likely to develop diabetes than African American men.

While people can't change family history, age, or race, it is possible to control weight and physical fitness. A doctor can decide if someone is at risk for developing diabetes and offer advice on reducing that risk.

POINTS TO REMEMBER

The following factors increase someone's chances of developing diabetes

- obesity
- family history of diabetes
- advancing age

NOTES:

Source: "Noninsulin-Dependent Diabetes," National Institutes of Health, NIH Publication No. 95–241, September 1992.

Diagnosing Diabetes

URINE TEST

A doctor can diagnose diabetes by checking for symptoms such as excessive thirst and frequent urination and by testing for glucose in blood or urine. When blood glucose rises above a certain point, the kidneys pass the extra glucose in the urine. However, a urine test alone is not sufficient to diagnose diabetes.

SIMPLE BLOOD TEST

A second method for testing glucose is a blood test, usually done in the morning before breakfast (fasting glucose test) or after a meal (postprandial glucose test).

ORAL GLUCOSE TOLERANCE TEST

The oral glucose tolerance test is a second type of blood test used to check for diabetes. Sometimes it can detect diabetes when a simple blood test does not. In this test, blood glucose is measured before and after a person has consumed a thick, sweet drink of glucose and other sugars. Normally, the glucose in a person's blood rises quickly after the drink and then falls gradually again as insulin signals the body to metabolize the glucose. In someone with diabetes, blood glucose rises and remains high after consumption of the liquid.

DECIDING WHETHER YOU HAVE DIABETES

A doctor can decide, based on these tests and a physical exam, whether you have diabetes. If a blood test is borderline abnormal, the doctor may want to monitor your blood glucose regularly. If you are overweight, you will be advised to lose weight. The doctor also may monitor your heart, since diabetes increases the risk of heart disease.

POINTS TO REMEMBER

A doctor will diagnose diabetes by looking for four kinds of evidence:

- risk factors like excess weight and a family history of diabetes
- symptoms such as thirst and frequent urination
- complications like heart trouble
- signs of excess glucose or sugar in blood and urine tests

Source: "Noninsulin-Dependent Diabetes," National Institutes of Health, NIH Publication No. 95–241, September 1992.

Treating Diabetes

CONTROLLING BLOOD GLUCOSE

The goals of diabetes treatment are to keep blood glucose within normal range and to prevent long-term complications.

Short-Term Effects of Diabetes

Why control blood glucose? Diabetes can cause short-term effects: some are unpleasant and some are dangerous. These include thirst, frequent urination, weakness, lack of ability to concentrate, loss of coordination, and blurred vision. Loss of consciousness is possible with very high or low blood sugar levels, but is more of a danger in insulin-dependent than in noninsulin-dependent diabetes.

Long-Term Effects of Diabetes

Long-term complications of diabetes may result from many years of high blood glucose. If people with diabetes keep their blood glucose levels under control, they reduce the risk of complications.

DIET AND EXERCISE

In 1986, a National Institutes of Health panel of experts recommended that the best treatment for noninsulin-dependent diabetes is a diet that helps the person maintain normal weight. In people who are overweight, losing weight is the one treatment that is clearly effective in controlling diabetes. In some people, exercise can help keep weight and diabetes under control.

MEDICINES

When diet and exercise alone can't control diabetes, two other kinds of treatment are available: oral diabetes medications and insulin. The treatment a doctor suggests depends on the person's age, lifestyle, and the severity of the diabetes.

POINTS TO REMEMBER

- Diabetes treatment can reduce symptoms, like thirst and weakness, and the chances of long-term problems, like heart and eye disease.
- If treatment with diet and exercise isn't effective, a doctor may prescribe oral medications or insulin.
- There is no known cure for diabetes; daily treatment must continue throughout a person's lifetime.

Source: "Noninsulin-Dependent Diabetes," National Institutes of Health, NIH Publication No. 95–241, September 1992.

Diabetes Diet

The proper diet is critical to diabetes treatment. It can help you:

- achieve and maintain desirable weight. Many people with diabetes can control their blood glucose by losing weight and keeping it off.
- maintain normal blood glucose levels.
- prevent heart and blood vessel diseases, conditions that tend to occur in people with diabetes.

A doctor will usually prescribe diet as part of diabetes treatment. A dietitian or nutritionist can recommend a diet that is healthy, but also interesting and easy to follow. You don't have to be limited to a preprinted, standard diet. You can get assistance in the following ways:

- A doctor can recommend a local nutritionist or dietitian.
- The local American Diabetes Association, American Heart Association, and American Dietetic Association can provide names of qualified dietitians or nutritionists and information about diet planning.
- Local diabetes centers at large medical clinics, hospitals, or medical universities usually have dietitians and nutritionists on staff.

DIABETIC DIET PLANNING

Guidelines for diabetes diet planning include the following:

- Many experts, including the American Diabetes Association, recommend that 50 to 60 percent of daily calories come from carbohydrates, 12 to 20 percent from protein, and no more than 30 percent from fat.
- Spacing meals throughout the day, instead of eating heavy meals once or twice a day, can help a person avoid extremely high or low blood glucose levels.
- With few exceptions, the best way to lose weight is gradually: one or two pounds a week. Strict diets must never be undertaken without the supervision of a doctor.
- People with diabetes have twice the risk of developing heart disease as those without diabetes, and high blood cholesterol levels raise the risk of heart disease. Losing weight and reducing intake of saturated fats and cholesterol, in favor of unsaturated and monounsaturated fats, can help lower blood cholesterol.

Meats and dairy products are major sources of saturated fats, which should be avoided; most vegetable oils are high in unsaturated fats, which are fine in limited amounts; and olive oil is a good source of monounsaturated fat, the healthiest type of fat. Liver and other organ meats and egg yolks are particularly high in cholesterol. A doctor or nutritionist can advise you on this aspect of diet.

continues

continued

OTHER DIET TIPS

- Studies show that foods with fiber, such as fruits, vegetables, peas, beans, and whole-grain breads and cereals may help lower blood glucose. However, it seems that a person must eat much more fiber than the average American now consumes to get this benefit. A doctor or nutritionist can advise you about adding fiber to a diet.
- Exchange lists are useful in planning a diabetes diet. They place foods with similar nutrients and calories into groups. With the help of a nutritionist, you plan the number of servings from each exchange list that you should eat throughout the day. Diets that use exchange lists offer more choices than preprinted diets. More information on exchange lists is available from nutritionists and from the American Diabetes Association.

FOOD AND BLOOD GLUCOSE LEVELS

Continuing research may lead to new approaches to diabetes diets. Because one goal of a diabetes diet is to maintain normal blood glucose levels, it would be helpful to have reliable information on the effects of foods on blood glucose. For example, foods that are rich in carbohydrates, like breads, cereals, fruits, and vegetables break down into glucose during digestion, causing blood glucose to rise. However, scientists don't know how each of these carbohydrates affect blood glucose levels.

Research is also under way to learn whether foods with sugar raise blood glucose higher than foods with starch. Experts do know that cooked foods raise blood glucose higher than raw, unpeeled foods. You can ask a doctor or nutritionist about using this kind of information in diet planning.

NOTES:

Source: "Noninsulin-Dependent Diabetes," National Institutes of Health, NIH Publication No. 95–241, September 1992.

Why Is Diet Important?

Diet helps to keep the balance between sugar and insulin in the body. The goal of any treatment of diabetes is to keep the blood sugar at normal level (70 to 130 mg/dL). A good diet may help keep this balance. No matter how the diabetes is being treated, diet is important.

WHAT TO EAT

Some foods change to sugar quickly, while others take a longer time. The best choices are foods that raise the blood sugar more slowly.

Foods That Raise Blood Sugar Slowly

1. FOODS HIGH IN FIBER	Fresh fruit, vegetables, cereals, whole-grain breads, beans, rice, oats, and lentils
2. STARCHES & GRAINS	Breads, cereals, pastas, potatoes, and rice
3. FRUITS & VEGETABLES	Fresh or frozen are best, but canned foods are OK. If using canned foods, eat • Fruit packed in water or in its own juices. • Vegetables low in salt.
4. FOODS LOW IN SUGAR	Do not eat or drink regular soda, candy, desserts, or pastries.
5. FOODS LOW IN FAT	Eat and drink low-fat dairy products and low-fat meats.

IMPORTANT FACTS ABOUT THE DIET

- Let the food and insulin work together. To do this
   1. Eat at the same time every day.
   2. Eat three balanced meals every day.
   3. Eat about the same amount of food every day.
- Limit alcohol intake.
- Limit salt intake if told by doctor.

continues

continued

Foods To Avoid

Problem Foods	Foods To Substitute
Alcohol—all types of sweet wines, liquors, cordials, beer, malt liquor	Dry white wine (in limited amounts)
Butters—apple, cherry, peach	
Breakfast bars	
Cakes	
Candy	Candy sweetened with sugar substitute
Carbonated beverages with sugar	Sugar-free sodas
Carnation Instant Breakfast	
Cereal (sugar coated)	Plain cereals (i.e., Rice Krispies, Cheerios)
Chewing gum with sugar	Sugar-free chewing gum
Chocolate powdered drink mix	Chocolate drinks with artificial sweeteners
Cookies	
Corn syrup/starch	
Danishes	
Donuts	
Fruit—candied fruit, canned fruit (light or heavy syrup), dried fruit	Fresh fruit or fruit packed in own juice
Fructose	
Granola bars	
Hershey chocolate (all choc. syrups)	Sugar-free chocolate syrup
Honey	
Hot chocolate	Hot chocolate with artificial sweeteners
Ice Cream—ice cream soda, ice cream sundaes, ice milk	Plain (i.e., vanilla or frozen yogurt with artificial sweeteners)
Jams	Jams with artificial sweeteners
Jelly	Jellies with artificial sweeteners
Jell-O (gelatin desserts)	Sugar-free gelatin desserts

continues

continued

Problem Foods	Foods To Substitute
KoolAid	Sugar-free KoolAid
Life Savers	Sugar-free Life Savers and hard candies
Marshmallows	
Milk (sweetened condensed)	Unsweetened condensed milk
Malted milk	
Molasses	
Pastries	
Pie	
Preserves	
Pudding	Sugar-free pudding
Sherbet	
Sugars—brown, cinnamon with sugar, confectioners (powdered), cubes, decorative, white	Saccharine, Sweet /n/ Low, Sucaryl, Sweet 10, Aspartame, Equal, NutraSweet
Syrups—blueberry, boisenberry, maple, sucrose	Syrup artificially sweetened

Source: St. Joseph Rehabilitation Hospital and Outpatient Center, *Patient Education and Discharge Planning Manual for Rehabilitation,* Aspen Publishers, Inc., © 1995.

Alcoholic Beverages and Diabetes

Most people with diabetes can drink alcohol safely if they drink in moderation (one or two drinks occasionally). In higher quantities alcohol can cause health problems:

- Alcohol has calories without the vitamins, minerals, and other nutrients that are essential for maintaining good health. A doctor can discuss whether it's safe for a person with diabetes to drink. People who are trying to lose weight need to account for the calories in alcohol in diet planning. A dietitian also can provide information about the sugar and alcohol content of various alcoholic drinks.
- Alcohol on an empty stomach can cause low blood glucose or hypoglycemia. Hypoglycemia is a particular risk in people who use oral medications or insulin for diabetes. It can cause shaking, dizziness, and collapse. People who don't know someone has diabetes may mistake these symptoms for drunkenness and neglect to seek medical help.
- Oral diabetes medications—tolbutamide and chlorpropamide—can cause dizziness, flushing, and nausea when combined with alcohol. A doctor can advise patients on the safety of drinking when taking these and other diabetes medications.
- Frequent, heavy drinking can cause liver damage over time. Because the liver stores and releases glucose, blood glucose levels may be more difficult to control in a person with liver damage from alcohol.
- Frequent heavy drinking also can raise the levels of fats in blood, increasing the risk of heart disease.

NOTES:

Source: "Noninsulin-Dependent Diabetes," National Institutes of Health, NIH Publication No. 95–241, September 1992.

Exercise and Diabetes

BENEFITS OF EXERCISE

Exercise has many benefits, and for someone with diabetes regular exercise combined with a good diet can help control diabetes. Exercise not only burns calories, which can help with weight reduction, but it also can improve the body's response to the hormone insulin. As a result, following a regular exercise program can make oral diabetes medications and insulin more effective and can help control blood glucose levels.

Exercise also reduces some risk factors for heart disease. For example, exercise can lower fat and cholesterol levels in blood, which increase heart disease risk. It also can lower blood pressure and increase production of a cholesterol, called HDL, that protects against heart disease.

EXERCISING SAFELY

Infrequent, strenuous exercise can strain muscles and the circulatory system and can increase the risk of a heart attack during exercise. A doctor can decide how much exercise is safe for an individual. The doctor will consider how well controlled a person's diabetes is, the condition of the heart and circulatory system, and whether complications require that the person avoid certain types of activity.

The purpose of a good exercise program is to find an enjoyable activity and do it regularly. Doing strenuous exercise for six months and then stopping isn't as effective.

Walking is great exercise, especially for an inactive person, and it's easy to do. A person can start off walking for 15 to 20 minutes, three or four times a week, and gradually increase the speed or distance of the walks.

Precautions You May Need To Take

People taking oral drugs or insulin need to remember that strenuous exercise can cause dangerously low blood glucose and they should carry a food or drink high in sugar for medical emergencies. Signs of hypoglycemia include hunger, nervousness, shakiness, weakness, sweating, headache, and blurred vision. As a precaution, a person with diabetes should wear an identification bracelet or necklace to alert a stranger that the wearer has diabetes and may need special medical help in an emergency.

A doctor may advise someone with high blood pressure or other complications to avoid exercises that raise blood pressure. For example, lifting heavy objects and exercises that strain the upper body raise blood pressure.

continues

continued

People with diabetes who have lost sensitivity in their feet also can enjoy exercise. They should choose shoes carefully and check their feet regularly for breaks in skin that could lead to infection. Swimming or bicycling can be easier on the feet than running.

POINTS TO REMEMBER

- Exercise has three major benefits: it burns calories, improves the body's response to insulin, and reduces risk factors for heart disease.
- An exercise program should be started slowly and with the advice of a doctor.

NOTES:

Source: "Noninsulin-Dependent Diabetes," National Institutes of Health, NIH Publication No. 95–241, September 1992.

Why Is Exercise Important?

Exercise is an important part of diabetes care. Exercise will be part of the rehabilitation program. It is important to continue exercising after going home. Exercise will keep the body healthy by helping to:

- Keep blood sugar in the normal range (70 to 130 mg/dL)
- Use the insulin that is in the body
- Lower the level of fat in the blood
- Lose weight if needed
- Lower stress
- Increase energy levels

WHAT STEPS SHOULD BE FOLLOWED WHEN EXERCISING?

- Warm up before exercising
- Exercise at the same time each day
- Exercise for 30 minutes
- Exercise at least four times per week
- Start slowly and build up the exercise program

REMEMBER

It is important to know that exercise will lower blood sugar. Always have some sugar nearby. If low blood sugar signs occur (shakes, sweats, headache), take sugar RIGHT AWAY. If taking insulin or diabetes pills, check the blood sugar before starting the exercise. If the blood sugar is low, have a snack before beginning the exercise.

NOTES:

Source: St. Joseph Rehabilitation Hospital and Outpatient Center, *Patient Education and Discharge Planning Manual for Rehabilitation,* Aspen Publishers, Inc., © 1995.

Checking Blood Glucose Levels

When a person's body is operating normally, it automatically checks the level of glucose in blood. If the level is too high or too low, the body will adjust the sugar level to return it to normal. This system operates in much the same way that cruise control adjusts the speed of a car. With diabetes, the body doesn't do the job of controlling blood glucose automatically. To make up for this, someone with diabetes has to check blood sugar regularly and adjust treatment accordingly.

A doctor can measure blood glucose during an office visit. However, levels change from hour to hour and someone who visits the doctor only every few weeks won't know what his or her blood glucose is daily. Do-it-yourself tests enable people with diabetes to check their blood sugar daily.

URINE TESTING AT HOME

The easiest test you can do at home is a urine test. When the level of glucose in blood rises above normal, the kidneys eliminate the excess glucose in urine. Glucose in urine, therefore, reflects an excess of glucose in blood.

Urine testing is easy. Tablets or paper strips are dipped in urine. The color change that occurs indicates whether blood glucose is too high. However, urine testing is not completely accurate because the reading reflects the level of blood glucose a few hours earlier. In addition, not everyone's kidneys are the same. Even when the amount of glucose in two people's urine is the same, their sugar levels may be different. Certain drugs and vitamin C also can affect the accuracy of urine tests.

TESTING BLOOD GLUCOSE AT HOME

It's more accurate to measure blood glucose directly. Kits are available that allow people with diabetes to test their blood glucose at home. The test involves pricking a finger to draw a drop of blood. A spring-operated "lancet" does this automatically. The drop of blood is placed on a strip of specially coated plastic or into a small machine that "reads" how much glucose is in the blood. A doctor may suggest that you test your blood glucose several times a day. Monitoring your own blood glucose can show you how your body responds to meals, exercise, stress, and diabetes treatment.

A TEST YOUR DOCTOR CAN DO

Another test that measures the effectiveness of treatment is a "glycosylated hemoglobin" test. It measures the glucose that has become attached to hemoglobin, the molecule in red blood cells

continues

continued

that gives blood its red color. Over time, hemoglobin absorbs glucose, according to its concentration in blood. Once glucose is absorbed by hemoglobin it remains there until the blood cells die and new ones replace them. With the "glycosylated hemoglobin" test, a doctor can tell whether blood glucose has been very high over the last few months.

REMEMBER

Testing blood glucose levels regularly can show whether treatment is working.

NOTES:

Source: "Noninsulin-Dependent Diabetes," National Institutes of Health, NIH Publication No. 95–241, September 1992.

Keep Daily Records

ACTION STEPS

- **If you use insulin,** keep a daily record of:

    —When you gave yourself an insulin shot.

    —How much and what kind of insulin you gave in each shot.

    —If you tested your urine and found ketones.

- **Write down the results of your blood tests every day in a record book.** You can use a small notebook or ask your doctor for a blood testing record book. You may also want to write down what you eat, how you feel, and how much you have exercised.

- By keeping daily records of your blood and urine tests, you can tell how well you are taking care of your diabetes. Show your book to your doctor. The doctor can use your records to see if you need to make changes in your insulin shots or diabetes pills, or in your eating plan. Ask your doctor or nurse if you don't know what your test results mean.

- Things to write down every day in your notebook are:

    —if you had very low blood sugar

    —if you ate more or less food than you usually do

    —if you felt sick or very tired

    —what kind of exercise you did and for how long

continues

continued

Sample of a Noninsulin User Record Book

Daily Log   SAMPLE   **Week Starting** May 15, 1999

	Breakfast		Lunch		Dinner		Bedtime		Other		Notes
	Dose	Blood Sugar	Dose	Blood Sugar	Dose	Blood Sugar	Dose	Blood Sugar	Dose	Blood Sugar	
Mon		109		117		122		115			
Tues		111		106				★ 152			★ Missed evening walk. Start back tomorrow!
Wed		126		121		131		120			
Thurs		113		128		179		★ 241			★ Sick w/flu. Drinking diet soda ketones negative.
Fri		159		147		136		130			Feeling better today
Sat		127				124		★ 152		130 11 pm	★ Extra juice made sugar go up.
Sun		119		120		★ 166		130			★ Lunch at picnic.

Source: Do Your Level Best, NIH Publication No. 95-4016, The National Diabetes Outreach Program of the National Institute of Diabetes and Digestive and Kidney Diseases, National Institutes of Health, September 1995.

Diabetes To Do List

Do Every Day:	Sun	Mon	Tues	Wed	Thurs	Fri	Sat
check my glucose level							
inspect my feet							
brush and floss my teeth							
eat 5 servings of vegetables or fruit							
take diabetes medicine as prescribed							
spend at least 20 minutes _____, (e.g., exercise, stretch, walk) which relaxes me							

Do Every Day:	Sun	Mon	Tues	Wed	Thurs	Fri	Sat
check my glucose level							
inspect my feet							
brush and floss my teeth							
eat 5 servings of vegetables or fruit							
take diabetes medicine as prescribed							
spend at least 20 minutes _____, (e.g., exercise, stretch, walk) which relaxes me							

American Association of Diabetes Educators
Call 1-800-TEAMUP4 to find a diabetes educator near you.

Source: *Do Your Level Best,* NIH Publication No. 95-4016, The National Diabetes Outreach Program of the National Institute of Diabetes and Digestive and Kidney Diseases, National Institutes of Health, September 1995.

Sample Record for Each Physician Evaluation

EACH VISIT

Have your health care provider do these tests and set goals with you.
(Record dates and results in the boxes below.)

Tests and Goals	Dates and Results					
Blood Glucose (mg/dL)	2/1/96 145	6/11/96 118	9/28/96 180	1/5/97 105	4/3/97 110	
Hemoglobin A1c Test/Goal (%)	9.0% / 8.0%	8.9% / 8.0%	8.4% / 7.5%	not done	8.2% / 7.5%	
Weight/Goal (pounds)	180 / 170	175 / 165	172 / 165	170 / 165	165 / 160	
Blood Pressure (goal: ___/___ mm Hg)	140/90	140/86	138/84	136/82	124/80	
Foot Check	✓	✓	✓	✓	✓	

Source: Centers for Disease Control and Prevention. *Take Charge of Your Diabetes, 2nd Edition.* Atlanta: U.S. Department of Health and Human Services, 1997.

Record for Each Physician Evaluation

EACH VISIT

Have your health care provider do these tests and set goals with you.
(Record dates and results in the boxes below.)

Tests and Goals	Dates and Results					
Blood Glucose (mg/dL)						
Hemoglobin A1c Test/Goal (%)						
Weight/Goal (pounds)						
Blood Pressure (goal: ____/____ mm Hg)						
Foot Check						

Source: Centers for Disease Control and Prevention. *Take Charge of Your Diabetes, 2nd Edition.* Atlanta: U.S. Department of Health and Human Services, 1997.

Things To Do At Least Once a Year

- Get a flu shot (October to mid-November)

- Get a pneumonia shot (if you've never had one).

- Get a dilated eye exam.

- Get a foot exam (including check of circulation and nerves).

- Get a kidney test:
  —Have your urine tested for albumin.
  —Have your blood creatinine measured.
  —Get a 24-hour urine test (if your doctor advises).

- Get your blood fats checked for:
  —Total cholesterol
  —High-density lipoprotein (HDL)
  —Low-density lipoprotein (LDL)
  —Triglycerides

- Get a dental exam (at least twice a year)

- Talk with your health care team about:
  —How well you can tell when you have low blood glucose
  —How you are treating high blood glucose
  —Tobacco use (cigarettes, cigars, pipes, smokeless tobacco)
  —Your feelings about having diabetes
  —Your plans for pregnancy (if a woman)
  —Other_____

Source: Centers for Disease Control and Prevention, *Take Charge of Your Diabetes, 2nd edition.* Atlanta: U.S. Department of Health and Human Services, 1997.

Sample Record for Annual Test Results

AT LEAST ONCE A YEAR

*Have your health care provider do these tests and other services for you.
You may want to set some goals for these.
(Record the dates and results in the boxes below.)*

Tests and Other Services	Dates and Results						
Flu Shot	10/2/95	10/20/96	11/1/97				
Urine Protein or Albumin (mg)	10/2/95 40	10/20/96 50	11/1/97 55				
Blood Creatinine (mg/dL)	1.0	1.2	1.1				
Total Cholesterol (mg/dL)	190	180	175				
HDL Cholesterol (mg/dL)	30	35	40				
LDL Cholesterol (mg/dL)	150	140	135				
Triglycerides (mg/dL)	338	300	250				
Tobacco Use	5 cigars a day	2 cigars	0				
Eye Exam (dilated)	8/11/95	10/1/96	10/20/97				
Foot Exam	10/2/95	10/20/96	11/1/97				

Source: Centers for Disease Control and Prevention. *Take Charge of Your Diabetes, 2nd edition.* Atlanta: U.S. Department of Health and Human Services, 1997.

Record for Annual Test Results

AT LEAST ONCE A YEAR

Have your health care provider do these tests and other services for you.
You may want to set some goals for these.
(Record the dates and results in the boxes below.)

Tests and Other Services	Dates and Results						
Flu Shot							
Urine Protein or Albumin (mg)							
Blood Creatinine (mg/dL)							
Total Cholesterol (mg/dL)							
HDL Cholesterol (mg/dL)							
LDL Cholesterol (mg/dL)							
Triglycerides (mg/dL)							
Tobacco Use							
Eye Exam (dilated)							
Foot Exam							

Source: Centers for Disease Control and Prevention. *Take Charge of Your Diabetes, 2nd edition.* Atlanta: U.S. Department of Health and Human Services, 1997.

Questions To Ask Your Doctor about Blood Sugar Control

The Diabetes Control and Complications Trial (DCCT) showed that people with insulin-dependent diabetes who keep blood sugar levels as close to normal as possible can reduce their risk of eye, kidney, and nerve diseases.

Ask your doctor how you can improve blood sugar control. Questions you may want to ask include:

- How often and under what conditions should I test my blood sugar?

  _____
  _____
  _____

- What should I do with the results?

  _____
  _____
  _____

- What patterns should I try to achieve?

  _____
  _____
  _____

- What was my average blood sugar over the last 2 to 3 months (glycosylated hemoglobin)?

  _____

- What is a normal glycosylated hemoglobin?

  _____

- How can I get my glycosylated hemoglobin in the normal range?

  _____
  _____
  _____

- What changes should we make in my program as a result of the findings of the Diabetes Control and Complications Trial (DCCT)?

  _____
  _____
  _____
  _____

continues

continued

- What effect has diabetes had on my eyes?

  _____
  _____

- How often should I have a pupil exam?

  _____

- What effect has diabetes had on my kidneys?

  _____
  _____
  _____
  _____

- Do I have albumin in my urine, a sign of early diabetic kidney disease (microalubuminuria)?

  _____

- How should I take care of my feet?

  _____
  _____
  _____

- When should I get together with a dietitian to review what I eat?

  _____

- What exercises are best for me?

  _____
  _____
  _____

- What adjustments to my food or insulin should I make if I plan to exercise?

  _____
  _____
  _____
  _____

- What should my family and friends do if my blood sugar falls so low that I need their help (hypoglycemia)?

  _____
  _____
  _____
  _____

continues

continued

- (For women) What should I do about taking care of my diabetes if I plan to become pregnant?
  _____
  _____
  _____
  _____
  _____

- Are there any diabetes groups I could attend in our area?
  _____
  _____
  _____

NOTES:

Source: *Do Your Level Best,* The National Diabetes Outreach Program, National Institute of Diabetes and Digestive and Kidney Diseases, National Institutes of Health.

Managing Hypoglycemia

Glucose, a form of sugar, is the body's main fuel. Hypoglycemia, or low blood sugar, occurs when blood levels of glucose drop too low to fuel the body's activity.

Carbohydrates (sugars and starches) are the body's main dietary sources of glucose. During digestion, the glucose is absorbed into the blood stream (hence the term "blood sugar"), which carries it to every cell in the body. Unused glucose is stored in the liver as glycogen.

Hypoglycemia can occur as a complication of diabetes, as a condition in itself, or in association with other disorders.

Blood Sugar Range

The normal range for blood sugar is about 60 mg/dl (milligrams of glucose per deciliter of blood) to 120 mg/dl, depending on when a person last ate. In the fasting state, blood sugar can occasionally fall below 60 mg/dl and even to below 50 mg/dl and not indicate a serious abnormality or disease. This can be seen in healthy women, particularly after prolonged fasting. Blood sugar levels below 45 mg/dl are almost always associated with a serious abnormality.

HOW DOES THE BODY CONTROL GLUCOSE?

The amount of glucose in the blood is controlled mainly by the hormones insulin and glucagon. Too much or too little of these hormones can cause blood sugar levels to fall too low (hypoglycemia) or rise too high (hyperglycemia). Other hormones that influence blood sugar levels are cortisol, growth hormone, and catecholamines (epinephrine and norepinephrine).

The pancreas, a gland in the upper abdomen, produces insulin and glucagon. The pancreas is dotted with hormone-producing tissue called the islets of Langerhans, which contain alpha and beta cells. When blood sugar rises after a meal, the beta cells release insulin. The insulin helps glucose enter body cells, lowering blood levels of glucose to the normal range. When blood sugar drops too low, the alpha cells secrete glucagon. This signals the liver to release stored glycogen and change it back to glucose, raising blood sugar levels to the normal range. Muscles also store glycogen that can be converted to glucose.

WHAT ARE THE SYMPTOMS OF HYPOGLYCEMIA?

A person with hypoglycemia may feel weak, drowsy, confused, hungry, and dizzy. Paleness, headache, irritability, trembling, sweating, rapid heart beat, and a cold, clammy feeling are also signs of low blood sugar. In severe cases, a person can lose consciousness and even lapse into a coma.

continues

continued

The symptoms associated with hypoglycemia are sometimes mistaken for symptoms caused by conditions not related to blood sugar. For example, unusual stress and anxiety can cause excess production of catecholamines, resulting in symptoms similar to those caused by hypoglycemia but having no relation to blood sugar levels.

HYPOGLYCEMIA IN DIABETES

The most common cause of hypoglycemia is as a complication of diabetes. Diabetes occurs when the body cannot use glucose for fuel because either the pancreas is not able to make enough insulin or the insulin that is available is not effective. As a result, glucose builds up in the blood instead of getting into body cells.

The aim of treatment in diabetes is to lower high blood sugar levels. To do this, people with diabetes may use insulin or oral drugs, depending on the type of diabetes they have or the severity of their condition. Hypoglycemia occurs most often in people who use insulin to lower their blood sugar. All people with insulin-dependent diabetes (IDDM or Type I) and some people with noninsulin-dependent diabetes (NIDDM or Type II) use insulin. People with Type II diabetes who take oral drugs called sulfonylureas are also vulnerable to low blood sugar episodes.

Conditions that can lead to hypoglycemia in people with diabetes include taking too much medication, missing or delaying a meal, eating too little food for the amount of insulin taken, exercising too strenuously, drinking too much alcohol, or any combination of these factors. People who have diabetes often refer to hypoglycemia as an "insulin reaction."

Managing Hypoglycemia in Diabetes

People with diabetes should consult their health care providers for individual guidelines on target blood sugar ranges that are best for them. The lowest safe blood sugar level for an individual varies, depending on the person's age, medical condition, and ability to sense hypoglycemic symptoms. A target range that is safe for a young adult with no diabetes complications, for example, may be too low for a young child or an older person who may have other medical problems.

Because they are attuned to the symptoms, people with diabetes can usually recognize when their blood sugar levels are dropping too low. They can treat the condition quickly by eating or drinking something with sugar in it such as candy, juice, or non diet soda. Taking glucose tablets or gels (available in drug stores) is another convenient and quick way to treat hypoglycemia.

People with IDDM are most vulnerable to severe insulin reactions, which can cause loss of consciousness. A few patients with long-standing insulin-dependent diabetes may develop a

continues

continued

condition known as hypoglycemia unawareness, in which they have difficulty recognizing the symptoms of low blood sugar. For emergency use in patients with IDDM, physicians often prescribe an injectable form of the hormone glucagon. A glucagon injection (given by another person) quickly eases the symptoms of low blood sugar, releasing a burst of glucose into the blood.

Emergency medical help may be needed if the person does not recover in a few minutes after treatment for hypoglycemia. A person suffering a severe insulin reaction may be admitted to the hospital so that blood sugar can be stabilized.

People with diabetes can reduce or prevent episodes of hypoglycemia by monitoring their blood sugar levels frequently and learning to recognize the symptoms of low blood sugar and the situations that may trigger it. They should consult their health care providers for advice about the best way to treat low blood sugar. Friends and relatives should know about the symptoms of hypoglycemia and how to treat it in case of emergency.

Episodes of hypoglycemia in people with IDDM may become more common now that research has shown that carefully controlled blood sugar helps prevent the complications of diabetes. Keeping blood sugar in a close-to-normal range requires multiple injections of insulin each day or use of an insulin pump, frequent testing of blood glucose, a diet and exercise plan, and guidance from health care professionals.

OTHER CAUSES OF HYPOGLYCEMIA

Hypoglycemia in people who do not have diabetes is far less common than once believed. However, it can occur in some people under certain conditions such as early pregnancy, prolonged fasting, and long periods of strenuous exercise. People on beta blocker medications who exercise are at higher risk of hypoglycemia, and aspirin can induce hypoglycemia in some children. Drinking alcohol can cause blood sugar to drop in some sensitive individuals, and hypoglycemia has been well documented in chronic alcoholics and binge drinkers. Eating unripe ackee fruit from Jamaica is a rare cause of low blood sugar.

Diagnosis

To diagnose hypoglycemia in people who do not have diabetes, the doctor looks for the following three conditions:

- The patient complains of symptoms of hypoglycemia.
- Blood glucose levels are measured while the person is experiencing those symptoms and found to be 45 mg/dl or less in a woman or 55 mg/dl or less in a man.
- The symptoms are promptly relieved upon ingestion of sugar.

continues

continued

For many years, the oral glucose tolerance test (OGTT) was used to diagnose hypoglycemia. Experts now realize that the OGTT can actually trigger hypoglycemic symptoms in people with no signs of the disorder. For a more accurate diagnosis, experts now recommend that blood sugar be tested at the same time a person is experiencing hypoglycemic symptoms.

The doctor will also check the patient for health conditions such as diabetes, obtain a medication history, and assess the degree and severity of the patient's symptoms. Laboratory tests to measure insulin production and levels of C-peptide (a substance that the pancreas releases into the bloodstream in equal amounts to insulin) may be performed.

Reactive Hypoglycemia

A diagnosis of reactive hypoglycemia is considered only after other possible causes of low blood sugar have been ruled out. Reactive hypoglycemia with no known cause is a condition in which the symptoms of low blood sugar appear 2 to 5 hours after eating foods high in glucose.

Ten to 20 years ago, hypoglycemia was a popular diagnosis. However, studies now show that this condition is actually quite rare. In these studies, most patients who experienced the symptoms of hypoglycemia after eating glucose-rich foods consistently had normal levels of blood sugar—above 60 mg/dl. Some researchers have suggested that some people may be extra sensitive to the body's normal release of the hormone epinephrine after a meal.

People with symptoms of reactive hypoglycemia unrelated to other medical conditions or problems are usually advised to follow a healthy eating plan. The doctor or dietitian may suggest that such a person avoid foods high in carbohydrates; eat small, frequent meals and snacks throughout the day; exercise regularly; and eat a variety of foods, including whole grains, vegetables, and fruits.

Rare Causes of Hypoglycemia

Fasting hypoglycemia occurs when the stomach is empty. It usually develops in the early morning when a person awakens. As with other forms of hypoglycemia, the symptoms include headache, lack of energy, and an inability to concentrate. Fasting hypoglycemia may be caused by a variety of conditions such as hereditary enzyme or hormone deficiencies, liver disease, and insulin-producing tumors.

In hereditary fructose intolerance, a disorder usually seen in children, the body is unable to metabolize the natural sugar fructose. Attacks of hypoglycemia, marked by seizures, vomiting, and unconsciousness, are treated by giving glucose and eliminating fructose from the diet.

Galactosemia, a rare genetic disorder, hampers the body's ability to process the sugar galactose. An infant with this disorder may appear normal at birth, but after a few days or weeks of drinking

continues

continued

milk (which contains galactose), the child may begin to vomit, lose weight, and develop cataracts. The liver may fail to release stored glycogen into the blood, triggering hypoglycemia. Removing milk from the diet is the usual treatment.

A deficiency of growth hormone causes increased sensitivity to insulin. This sensitivity occurs because growth hormone opposes the action of insulin on muscle and fat cells. For this reason, children with growth hormone deficiency sometimes suffer from hypoglycemia, which goes away after treatment.

People with insulin-producing tumors, which arise in the islet cells of the pancreas, suffer from severe episodes of hypoglycemia.

To diagnose these tumors, called insulinomas, a doctor will put the patient on a 24- to 72-hour fast while measuring blood levels of glucose, insulin, and proinsulin. High levels of insulin and proinsulin in the presence of low levels of glucose strongly suggest an insulin-producing tumor. These tumors are usually benign and can be surgically removed.

In rare cases, some cancers such as breast cancer and adrenal cancer may cause hypoglycemia through secretion of a hormone called insulin-like growth factor II. The treatment is removal of the tumor, if possible.

NOTES:

Source: "Hypoglycemia," NIH Publication No. 95-3926, National Institutes of Health, May 1995.

How Is Hypoglycemia Treated?

It is important to treat an insulin reaction or low blood sugar RIGHT AWAY. Be careful not to overtreat.

HYPOGLYCEMIA: TREATMENT

1. Eat/drink any **ONE** of the following:

   - 4 oz of orange juice or other juice
   - 4 oz of Coke or other soda containing sugar
   - Two or three glucose tablets
   - Five to eight Life Savers

2. Wait 15 minutes. Repeat above if not feeling better.

3. Within 30 minutes of feeling better, eat a sandwich and a glass of milk. If it is mealtime, eat the meal instead of this snack.

4. After the insulin reaction, check to see why the reaction happened. Try to fix the problem. For example:

   - Eat meals on time and eat entire meal.
   - With more exercise or activity, have a snack.
   - Make sure the right dose of insulin was taken. TALK TO THE DOCTOR ABOUT THE RIGHT DOSE OF INSULIN.

Source: St. Joseph Rehabilitation Hospital and Outpatient Center, *Patient Education and Discharge Planning Manual for Rehabilitation,* Aspen Publishers, Inc., © 1995.

Guidelines for Sick Days

Keep a daily record of your sick days by following the guidelines below. If you feel too sick to follow any of these guidelines, ask a family member or a friend to help you. By following these instructions and by keeping a diary, you can work with your health care provider to feel better.

Health care provider's name: _____

Health care provider's telephone number: _____

1. If you feel too sick to eat normally, call your health care provider right away. Describe in detail how you feel.
2. Keep taking insulin when you feel sick. Don't stop taking insulin even if you can't eat. Your health care provider may change your insulin dose or may tell you to drink liquids that have sugar in them.
3. Weigh yourself every day and write down your weight.
4. Take your temperature every morning and evening. Write down the readings. (For small children or for someone who is breathing through the mouth, use a rectal thermometer.) If your temperature is above normal (99°F), drink extra liquids.
5. If you weigh 80 pounds or more, try to drink at least 12 eight-ounce glasses of liquid per day. Write down how much you drink. If you throw up, call your health care provider right away. You may need to go to the hospital or have special medical treatment.
6. Every 4 hours or before every meal, measure the glucose level in your blood. Write down the results. If the level is less than 60 mg/dL or consistently higher than 240 mg/dL, call your health care provider. Every 4 hours or each time you pass urine, test your urine for ketones and write down the results.
7. If you start to have trouble breathing, call your health care provider (or have someone do it for you) or go to a nearby emergency room.
8. Every 4 to 6 hours, write down whether you feel awake or sleepy. If you feel very sleepy or can't concentrate, have someone call your health care provider right away.
9. If your health care provider asks you to, call every day to describe your daily record (see "Record for Sick Days" below). Your health care provider may adjust your daily insulin dosage.

continues

continued

RECORD FOR SICK DAYS

How often	Question	Answer	
Every day	How much do you weigh today?	_____ pounds	
Every evening	How much did you drink today?	_____ glasses	
Every morning and every evening	What is your temperature?	AM _____ PM _____	

Every 4 hours or before every meal	How much medication did you take?	Time	Dose
		_____	_____
		_____	_____
		_____	_____
		_____	_____
		_____	_____

Every 4 hours or before every meal	What is the level of glucose in your blood?	Time	Level
		_____	_____
		_____	_____
		_____	_____
		_____	_____

Every 4 hours or each time you pass urine	What is the level of ketones in your urine?	Time	Level
		_____	_____
		_____	_____
		_____	_____
		_____	_____

Every 4 to 6 hours	How are you breathing?	Time	Condition
		_____	_____
		_____	_____
		_____	_____
		_____	_____

If you feel unusually sleepy or can't concentrate, have someone call your health care provider or take you to an emergency room.

Source: *The Prevention and Treatment of Complications of Diabetes Mellitus: A Guide for Primary Care Practitioners*, Department of Health and Human Services, Public Health Service, Centers for Disease Control, National Center for Chronic Disease Prevention and Health Promotion, Division of Diabetes Translation, January 1, 1991. Adapted from Take Charge of Your Diabetes: A Guide for Care, Centers for Disease Control and Prevention.

Diabetic Emergencies

HIGH BLOOD GLUCOSE

Signs

Very high blood glucose levels cause symptoms that are hard to ignore: frequent urination and excessive thirst. However, in someone who is elderly or in poor health these symptoms may go unnoticed. Without treatment, a person with high blood glucose or hyperglycemia can lose fluids, become weak, confused, and even unconscious. Breathing will be shallow and the pulse rapid. The person's lips and tongue will be dry, and his or her hands and feet will be cool.

What To Do

A doctor should be called immediately.

LOW BLOOD GLUCOSE

The opposite of high blood glucose, very low blood glucose or hypoglycemia, is also dangerous.

Causes

Hypoglycemia can occur when someone hasn't eaten enough to balance the effects of insulin or oral medicine. Prolonged, strenuous exercise in someone taking oral diabetes drugs or insulin also can cause hypoglycemia, as can alcohol.

Signs

Someone whose blood glucose has become too low may feel nervous, shaky, and weak. The person may sweat, feel hungry, and have a headache. Severe hypoglycemia can cause loss of consciousness.

What To Do

A person with hypoglycemia who begins to feel weak and shaky should eat or drink something with sugar in it immediately, like orange juice. If the person is unconscious, he or she should be taken to a hospital emergency room right away. An identification bracelet or necklace that states that the wearer has diabetes will let friends know that these symptoms are a warning of illness that requires urgent medical help.

Source: "Noninsulin-Dependent Diabetes," National Institutes of Health, NIH Publication No. 95–241, September 1992.

Surgery and Diabetes

SURGERY AND BLOOD GLUCOSE LEVELS

Surgery is stressful, both physically and mentally. It can raise blood glucose levels even in someone who is careful about control. To make sure that surgery and recovery are successful for someone with diabetes, a doctor will test blood glucose and keep it under careful control, usually with insulin. Careful control makes it possible for someone with diabetes to have surgery with little risk, or no more risk than someone without diabetes.

TELL YOUR SURGEON YOU HAVE DIABETES

To plan a safe and successful surgery, the surgeon and attending physicians must know that the person they're treating has diabetes. While tests done before surgery can detect diabetes, you should inform the doctor of your condition. A surgical team also will evaluate the possible effect of complications of diabetes, such as heart or kidney problems.

NOTES:

Source: "Noninsulin-Dependent Diabetes," National Institutes of Health, NIH Publication No. 95–241, September 1992.

Pregnancy and Diabetes

Having a baby places extra demands on a woman's body. Diabetes makes it more difficult for her body to adjust to these demands and it can cause problems for both mother and baby.

GESTATIONAL DIABETES

Some women may develop a form of diabetes during pregnancy called gestational diabetes. Gestational diabetes develops most frequently in the middle and later months of pregnancy, after the time of greatest risk for birth defects. Although this kind of diabetes often disappears after the baby's birth, treatment is necessary during pregnancy to make sure the diabetes doesn't harm the mother or fetus.

BEFORE YOU ARE PREGNANT

If you have diabetes, you should keep your condition under control before you become pregnant, so that your diabetes won't increase the risk of birth defects. A woman whose diabetes isn't well-controlled may have an unusually large baby. Diabetes also increases the risk of premature birth and problems in the baby, such as breathing difficulties, low blood sugar, and occasionally, death.

WHILE YOU ARE PREGNANT

Blood glucose monitoring and treatment with insulin can ensure that a baby will be healthy. Oral diabetes drugs aren't given during pregnancy because the effects of these drugs on the unborn baby aren't known. By following the advice of a doctor trained to treat gestational diabetes, you can make sure your blood glucose is normal and your baby is well nourished.

AFTER YOUR BABY IS BORN

About half of women with gestational diabetes will no longer have abnormal blood glucose tests shortly after giving birth. But many women with gestational diabetes will develop noninsulin-dependent diabetes later in their lives. Regular checkups can ensure that if a woman does develop diabetes later, it will be diagnosed and treated early.

Source: "Noninsulin-Dependent Diabetes," National Institutes of Health, NIH Publication No. 95–241, September 1992.

Pregnancy, Diabetes, and Women's Health

BECOMING PREGNANT WHEN YOU HAVE DIABETES

Women with diabetes can have healthy babies, but it takes planning ahead and effort. Pregnancy can make both **high** and **low blood glucose** levels happen more often. It can make **diabetic eye disease** and **diabetic kidney disease** worse. High glucose levels during pregnancy are dangerous for the baby, too.

If you don't want to become pregnant, talk with your health care provider about birth control.

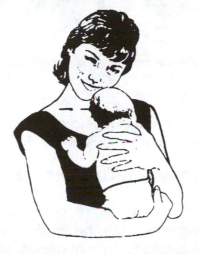

You can protect you and your baby
by controlling your blood glucose
before and during pregnancy.

PROTECTING YOUR BABY AND YOURSELF

Keeping your glucose levels near normal before and during pregnancy can help protect you and your baby. That's why it's so important to plan your pregnancies ahead of time.

If you want to have a baby, discuss it with your health care provider. Work with your diabetes care team to get and keep your blood glucose in the normal or near-normal range before you become pregnant. Your glucose records and your hemoglobin A1c test results will show when you have maintained a safe range for a period of time.

You may need to change your meal plan and your usual physical activity, and you may need to take more frequent insulin shots. Testing your glucose several times a day will help you see how well you're balancing things. Record the test results in your logbook or on a log sheet.

continues

continued

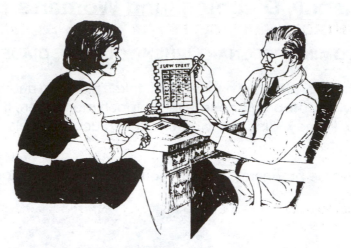

Your blood glucose and hemoglobin A1c records will help you and your health care team know when your glucose range is safe for pregnancy.

Get a complete check of your eyes and kidneys before you try to become pregnant. Don't smoke, drink alcohol, or use drugs—doing these things can harm you and your baby.

HAVING DIABETES DURING PREGNANCY

Some women have diabetes only when they're pregnant. This condition, which is called gestational diabetes, can be controlled just like other kinds of diabetes. Glucose control is the key. Your health care team can help you take charge of gestational diabetes.

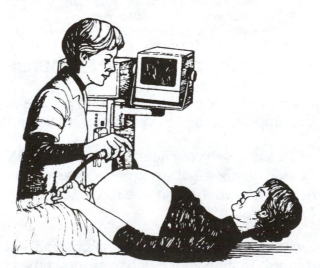

If you learn you have diabetes when you're pregnant, work closely with your health care team.

continues

continued

CONTROLLING DIABETES FOR WOMEN'S HEALTH

Some women with diabetes may have special problems, such as bladder infections. If you have an infection, it needs to be treated right away. Call your doctor.

Some women get yeast infections in their vagina, especially when their blood glucose is high. A sign of a yeast infection may be itching in the vagina. If you notice vaginal itching, tell your health care provider. You may learn about medicines you can buy at the drugstore and about how to prevent yeast infections.

Some women with diabetes may have trouble with sexual function. Discomfort caused by vaginal itching or dryness can be treated.

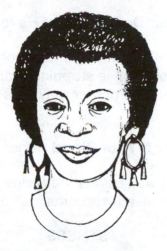

Getting Pap smears and mammograms is important to every woman's health.

Ask your doctor how often you should get a Pap smear and a mammogram (breast X-ray). Regular Pap smears and mammograms help detect cervical and breast cancer early. All women—whether or not they have diabetes—need to keep up with these tests.

Source: Centers for Disease Control and Prevention. *Take Charge of Your Diabetes, 2nd edition.* Atlanta: U.S. Department of Health and Human Services, 1997.

Stress and Illness and Diabetes

One way the body responds to stress is to increase the level of blood glucose. In a person with diabetes, stress may increase the need for treatment to lower blood glucose levels.

ILLNESS

Illnesses such as colds and flu are forms of physical stress that a doctor can treat.

Drink Plenty of Fluids

Your doctor will advise you to drink plenty of fluids. When blood glucose is high, your body gets rid of glucose through urine, and this fluid needs to be replaced.

Tell Your Doctor If You Have Nausea

If nausea makes eating or taking oral diabetes drugs a problem, call your doctor. Not eating can increase the risk of low blood glucose, while stopping oral medications or insulin during illness can lead to very high blood glucose. Your doctor may prescribe insulin temporarily if you cannot take medicine by mouth.

Call Your Doctor If Your Blood Sugar Is Out of Control

Great thirst, rapid weight loss, high fever, or very high urine or blood glucose are signs that blood sugar is out of control. If you have these symptoms, call a doctor immediately.

STRESS

Like illness, stress that results from losses or conflicts at home or on the job can affect diabetes control. Urine and blood glucose checks can be clues to the effects of stress. If stress is making diabetes control difficult for you, a doctor can advise treatment and suggest sources of help.

POINTS TO REMEMBER

- Special situations such as stress and illness call for extra careful diabetes control.
- Special control may require the use of insulin, even in people who don't normally use insulin.

Source: "Noninsulin-Dependent Diabetes," National Institutes of Health, NIH Publication No. 95–241, September 1992.

Dealing with Diabetes

Good diabetes care requires a daily effort to follow a diet, stay active, and take medicine when necessary. Talking to people who have diabetes or who treat diabetes may be helpful for someone who needs emotional support. It's very important for people with diabetes to understand how to stay healthy, follow a proper diet, exercise, and be aware of changes in their bodies. People with diabetes can live long, healthy lives if they take care of themselves.

POINTS TO REMEMBER

- Good diabetes care is a daily responsibility.
- Local diabetes organizations offer programs so people with diabetes can share experiences and support.
- The good health care urged for people with diabetes is beneficial to anyone who wishes to stay healthy.

FINDING HELP

A person with diabetes is responsible for his or her daily care and a doctor is the best source of information on that care. A doctor in family practice or internal medicine can diagnose and treat diabetes, and may refer the patient to a doctor who specializes in treating diabetes.

Specialists

"Endocrinologists" and "diabetologists" are doctors with advanced training and experience in diabetes treatment. The local chapters of the American Diabetes Association or the Juvenile Diabetes Foundation have lists of doctors who specialize in diabetes. Another alternative is to contact a university-based medical center. These centers may have special diabetes clinics or may be able to suggest diabetes doctors who practice in the community.

REMEMBER

Medical guidance is available from a variety of sources such as diabetes groups, local medical societies and hospitals, and diabetes clinics.

Source: "Noninsulin-Dependent Diabetes," National Institutes of Health, NIH Publication No. 95–241, September 1992.

Traveling with Diabetes

PREPARING AND PACKING

Preparing for travel, especially international travel, begins weeks ahead of your departure. For starters, you will want to call your insurance company to find out if there are any limitations to your health insurance in different states or different countries. If so, you may want to get supplemental travel insurance to cover emergencies. Be aware, too, that Medicare does not cover treatment outside the United States.

For international travel you need to determine whether you need inoculations. Those who plan to travel to countries that have a high rate of hepatitis A virus, for example, should receive the hepatitis A vaccine or immune globulin. The infectious disease division of many university hospitals can provide you with more information about inoculations through their travel centers. Your local public health department should also have this information (check in your phone book). You may also want to obtain a list of English-speaking foreign doctors from the International Association for Medical Assistance to Travelers by calling (716) 754-4883.

Make sure you have adequate medical identification before you leave. You will want to carry it with you at all times during your travels, along with a summary of your health history and a letter from your doctor describing your usual care, including your need for needles and syringes, if applicable. In addition, ask your doctor for prescriptions for any medicines you take. Make sure the generic names of drugs and the dosage you take are indicated. You cannot fill prescriptions outside the state where they were written, but the information will be helpful should you need to see a doctor while traveling.

To be on the safe side, plan to carry twice as much medicine as you think you will need. Since checked luggage can go astray, always pack diabetes supplies, tablets or foods to treat hypoglycemia, and medications in your carry-on luggage. If you are traveling with a companion, have that person carry half of your supplies. If you take insulin, pack a glucagon emergency kit and make sure your travel companion knows how to use it.

The problems associated with the unpredictability of travel are best managed when you know your blood sugar level, so by all means, bring your glucose meter. All of the glucose meters currently available can safely pass through airport detection systems. Pack extra batteries and more strips than you'll ever need.

Pack your diabetes supplies and other drugs first before you get involved in deciding which clothes to bring and whether or not you'll need a swimsuit. Include the following in your traveling medicine chest: antidiarrhea medication (such as Imodium AD tablets or Sugar-Free Kaopectate), laxatives (such as Sugar-Free Metamucil), sugar-free cough syrup, and motion sickness medicine.

continues

continued

TRAVELING WITH INSULIN

Taking insulin on the road requires some special preparations, especially if you'll be traveling through different time zones. If that's the case, make an appointment with your health care provider to discuss your travel plans and how to adjust your insulin schedule. Here are some other things to keep in mind:

Temperature control. Since the potency of insulin can be affected by improper storage, it's a good idea to store it according to the manufacturer's recommendations. Ideally, insulin should be refrigerated at 36°F to 46°F. Opened vials of Lilly insulin can be kept for 32 days when refrigerated. Opened vials of Novo Nordisk insulin can be kept for 90 days when refrigerated. Unopened vials of either brand can be refrigerated until the expiration date.

Insulin can be stored at a controlled room temperature of less than 86°F if the entire vial's contents will be used in 30 days. This is a popular option when traveling for a few weeks. Some people just discard the unrefrigerated insulin after a month and use a new refrigerated vial when they return home. Insulin can also be kept cool by using an insulated carrying case.

Storage guidelines differ for Humulin cartridges and Novo Nordisk PenFill and disposable pen (Prefilled). Humulin R (Regular) cartridges, Humalog (lispro) cartridges, Novolin R PenFill (Regular) cartridges, and Novolin R Prefilled syringes can be stored at room temperature for 30 days after puncture. Humulin N and 70/30 cartridges and Novolin PenFill, Prefilled 70/30, and NPH can be stored at room temperature for seven days after puncture.

Pens and pumps. Insulin pen devices are useful for travel. They are more portable and convenient to use when you're away from home than the conventional syringe and insulin vial (see "Insulin Pens," below). Insulin pumps offer another convenience to travelers; changing the clock in the pump eases dosage adjustment across time zones.

Disposal. Most travelers bring home all syringes, pen needles, pump supplies, and lancets for proper disposal.

Injecting at high altitude. If you will need to give yourself an injection during an airplane flight, you need to know that the cabin pressure becomes lower as you go higher. You may have noticed that those little bags of potato chips you are sometimes served appear puffed up at altitude. That's because the air pressure inside the bag is higher than the cabin pressure. The same thing can happen to your insulin vial. To get around this, carry a used syringe with the plunger removed and, with the vial upright, push the syringe through the cap on the vial. This will allow any excess air to escape, and the air pressure in the vial will then be equal to the cabin pressure.

Then you can use a regular syringe to inject air and withdraw the insulin you need. Many people forget to inject air into the vial before withdrawing insulin, but it's an important step, especially if you mix two types of insulin in one syringe.

continues

continued

INSULIN PENS

Insulin pens can be especially convenient for travel. They are lightweight, compact, and portable. The insulin is packaged in a cartridge that fits into the pen, and a needle is attached to the end of the pen. You dial in your dose of insulin, inject the needle into your skin, and press a button to inject the insulin. You cannot mix two types of insulin using a pen, but both Lilly and Novo Nordisk manufacture cartridges of 70/30 insulin. Here are some of the options:

Autopen

The Autopen by Owen Mumford is available in two models, each designed for use with either Lilly of Novo Nordisk 1.5-ml insulin cartridges. The AN 3100 model delivers insulin in one-unit increments with a maximum dose of 16 units. The AN 3000 model delivers doses in two-unit increments with a maximum dose of 32 units. (This means you can't inject a dose of 5 units; you would have to inject either 4 or 6 units.)

B-D Pen

The B-D pen is designed for use with cartridges of Lilly or Novo Nordisk insulin. Each cartridge contains 150 units. The B-D pen delivers a maximum dose of 30 units per injection in one-unit increments. You can use either 30-gauge, 8-mm (short) B-D Ultra-Fine pen needles or 29-gauge, 12.7-mm (standard) B-D Ultra-Fine pen needles.

Novolin Prefilled Syringes

This syringe already contains the insulin so there is no cartridge to insert. You just dial in the dose and inject. The Novolin Prefilled syringe contains 150 units of either Novolin N, Novolin R, or Novolin 70/30. The maximum dose is 58 units per injection, and the insulin is delivered in two-unit increments. The Novolin Prefilled syringe uses 30-gauge, 8-mm NovoFine pen needles.

NovoPen 1.5

The NovoPen 1.5 is designed to fit cartridges of Novolin insulin. Each Novolin Penfill contains 150 units of insulin. The maximum dose that the pen can deliver is 40 unit per injection in one-unit increments. It uses 30-gauge, 8-mm NovoFine pen needles.

When you get back on the ground, the air pressure in the vial will be lower than the outside air pressure, so before you withdraw insulin, push the no-plunger syringe through the cap on the vial again to equalize the pressure.

Time zones. There is no single set of rules for insulin adjustment across time zones. The guiding principle is to try to avoid hypoglycemia. Slight elevations in blood sugar are not a concern, but

continues

continued

low blood sugar can interfere with safety. Don't be fooled by formulas that give a simplified approach to changing insulin doses across times zones. No single set of rules could apply to flights of six hours or twelve hours leaving day or night.

In general, eastbound flights lead to a shorter day, and your health care provider may advise you to shorten the time between injections and/or reduce the insulin dose of one or more injections. Westbound flights will lengthen your day, meaning you may have an extra mealtime; your health care provider may suggest an extra dose of Regular insulin or Humalog to cover this. You will not need to adjust insulin doses when flying directly north or south, but you still need to consider the potential for flight delays.

One method of adjusting to the altered eating and sleeping schedules that are part of travel (especially across time zones) is to keep your wristwatch set to the same time as your city of departure for the day of travel and make your insulin and meal decisions based on that time. Your travel companion can change his or her watch to local time (or you can carry another timepiece with you) so that you do not miss connecting flights.

Individual needs. Seek individualized advice based on your travel plans, the nature of your trip, your injection regimen, and your unique needs. For example, the time and dose of your injection may differ depending on whether you plan to join a tour group after arrival of rent a car and navigate the roads yourself in a foreign country. Dose adjustment will differ based on whether you take three injections per day or one injection at bedtime. Different recommendations will also be given if you have hypoglycemia unawareness, a tendency toward motion sickness, if you plan to travel alone, or if you'll be traveling with small children.

Adjusting for activity. The type of activities you plan to do during your trip will also affect whether and how you adjust your insulin dosage. A business trip to London involving meetings and minimal sightseeing greatly differs from a ski trip to Switzerland or a walking tour of Italy.

Without preparation, vigorous activity can lead to *postexercise, late-onset hypoglycemia*. After vigorous exercise, your body tries to replace the stored sugar in your muscles (glycogen) that was used as fuel during exercise, and it takes the sugar from your blood and puts it back into your muscles for up to the next 24 hours. This can lead to an unexpected drop in blood sugar. If your trip involves vigorous activity, you can eat snacks before and after exercise based on frequent blood glucose monitoring to prevent this.

BUSINESS TRIPS

Traveling for business is in many ways different from taking a traveling vacation. For one thing, someone else often makes your travel arrangements. While that spares you some hassle, you may

continues

continued

find that your secretary or your company's travel office doesn't make your health needs a priority. You may be expected to take long flights and perform upon arrival without a break for a nap or a snack.

If your work demands that you travel frequently, ask to have a role in planning your itinerary. If a trip will last for more than a day or two, ask to stay at a hotel with a gym or workout room so you can get some exercise. Always save room in your carry-on luggage for snacks. And try to avoid the extremes of low and high blood sugar.

STAYING HEALTHY ON THE ROAD

Even the most wonderful vacation can feel like an ordeal when you're sick or just under the weather. Planning ahead raises your chances of staying healthy.

Eating well on the road is challenging because the timing of meals can vary, and dining out typically involves higher-calorie, higher-fat food choices. You may drink more alcohol than you would at home, especially if certain alcoholic beverages are part of the dinner culture where you are visiting. The same tips for dining out at home apply to travel: Try to choose low-fat foods, and try to moderate the portions. Most restaurants serve large portions of food. You might choose to avoid "all-you-can-eat" buffets because of the temptation to overeat.

Traveler's diarrhea is a common malady that can be prevented by avoiding tap water and ice cubes in countries where the water isn't purified. Most hotels provide information about the safety of their drinking water. To be safe, drink bottled water from a well-known company.

Constipation commonly occurs when you are away from home and not following your usual schedule. To prevent constipation, be sure to drink plenty of fluids, including exercise in your plans, and arrange time for privacy. Hurried bathroom stops will only add to the problem.

If you plan to travel to developing countries or countries with questionable sanitation, there are special precautions to investigate, including the country's rate of hepatitis A virus. Since hepatitis A is transmitted by sewage-contaminated water and food, avoid buying food from street vendors and be careful when eating in restaurants that cater to local people instead of tourists.

It is always wise to stay away from animals whenever you travel, and remember to pack insect repellent.

Vacation often means spending more time outdoors than usual, and that means more exposure to the sun. Before you leave home, ask your doctor if any of the drugs you're taking causes *photosensitivity*, or increased sensitivity to sunlight. Drug-induced photosensitivity can cause symptoms that mimic sunburn, rashes, and allergic reactions. If you are taking such a drug, ask

continues

continued

your doctor what you can do to avoid a reaction (using sunscreen doesn't always help). Sulfonylurea pills (glyburide, glipizide, glimepiride) are among the drugs that can cause photosensitivity. Even if you are not taking drugs, protect your skin by limiting your exposure to the sun at the hottest parts of the day and by wearing sunscreen, a wide-brimmed hat, and clothes that cover your arms and legs.

Care of your feet is another part of diabetes self-care that cannot be neglected when traveling. Reserve your high heels for special evenings out, and wear comfortable walking shoes when exploring a new city or strolling through museums. Water shoes offer foot protection when swimming; hiking boots will support your feet on rougher terrain. Always bring at least one spare pair of shoes in case you get caught in rain; wet shoes take a long time to dry and make for miserable feet.

AIRLINE TRAVEL

Even though it's usually the fastest way to travel, flying can feel like the slowest when you think about the time it takes to get to and from the airport, wait for your luggage, and sit through the seemingly inevitable delays. For people who require insulin to treat diabetes, consistent timing of meals and injections contributes to better blood sugar control. To make sure delays don't ruin your timing, plan on them happening. Prepare an itinerary that allows for traffic on the way to the airport, delayed or canceled flights, and late or lost luggage.

You may be able to minimize delays by taking nonstop flights (one take-off and one landing) or direct flights (which include a layover but no change of planes). However, there are fewer nonstop flights these days, and the cost of flying nonstop can be prohibitive). When you are stuck with layovers and plane changes, your preparations (and a good book) can make a difference.

Meals in flight. The safest approach to meal planning during air travel is not to rely on airline meals or meal schedules. For one thing, meals are served when it is convenient for the airplane staff, not when the passengers are hungry. For another, many airlines have cut back drastically on their meal service, offering only peanuts or pretzels and a beverage instead of lunch or dinner. Make sure your food needs are met by carrying nonperishable items such as peanut butter, crackers, sandwiches, fruit, boxed juices, and sugar substitute, in case you are served just coffee or tea. (Carrying your own food is sage advice for all travel, whatever your method of transportation.)

If your flight does include a meal, you may want to order a special diabetic meal. The special meal order must be made ahead of time and should be verified with the airline 36 hours before the flight. Some airlines also offer vegetarian, low-cholesterol, or kosher meals.

Staying hydrated. Dehydration is common on long flights because of the very low humidity in pressurized airline cabins. Dehydration aggravates fatigue and causes dryness of the eyes, nose,

continues

continued

throat, and skin. You can prevent dehydration by drinking calorie-free liquids, and you can keep your skin moist with moisturizing lotions. Since the beverage cart may come by only once or twice during a long flight, many experienced travelers carry a liter or two of bottled water with them when flying.

Dehydration is also common with a change in climate (hot or cold) and can be made worse by diuretics, some high blood pressure medicines, antidepressants, and antihistamines. Because of the way metformin (Glucophage) works in the body, severe dehydration is especially dangerous if you take this drug to treat diabetes.

Move around. The prolonged sitting that comes with travel by plane, bus, car, or train can interfere with circulation. It doesn't help that most airlines have cut back on both legroom and seat cushioning in recent years. For most of us this is an annoyance, but for people with circulation problems, sitting still for hours on end can be dangerous.

To keep your blood moving on an airplane, try to get an aisle seat so you can walk up and down the aisle periodically. Flexing your ankles and stretching as much as possible within the confines of your seat can also minimize muscle stiffness and improve circulation. Business class seats tend to be wider and hence less punishing. If possible, consider upgrading your seat (frequent flyer miles can be used for this purpose).

Jet lag. After a very long flight that crosses several time zones, you may find yourself feeling dazed, lightheaded, restless, and irritable. If so, you are probably suffering from jet lag. The symptoms of jet lag can mimic hypoglycemia, however, so make sure you test your blood sugar if you experience these symptoms.

Rapidly crossing several time zones upsets the body's *circadian rhythm*, its normal, 24-hour cycle of sleeping, waking, and other bodily functions. The most important factor contributing to jet lag is the disturbance of sleep. It is helpful to adjust to the sleep schedule of your destination as soon as possible. For morning arrivals, try to stay awake instead of napping when you arrive. Avoid stimulants such as coffee and cola drinks or alcohol before going to bed.

CAR TRAVEL

Hopping in the car is second nature to most Americans, and driving can be a great way to visit some of the beautiful places close to your home. Before you set out on a journey, however, take a minute to test your blood sugar level and pack some snacks in a bag or cooler. Knowing your blood sugar level before you get behind the wheel will help you avoid hypoglycemia and help you make decisions about when and where to stop next for food.

While highway rest stops are great for using the bathroom and fueling the car, the food they offer tends to be high-fat, high-sodium fast food. Having snack foods readily available is one of the

continues

continued

benefits of car travel. Most of the time you don't have to be concerned with limiting your luggage, so you can bring a cooler full of healthy snacks and beverages. Even if a special restaurant is your destination, bring some snacks just in case—like any other type of travel, car trips can be unpredictable.

For some people, traveling by car is seen as something to endure until they reach their destination. Stopping periodically for breaks will not only interrupt the monotony but will help prevent highway hypnosis, which makes you less alert. Even if driving doesn't bore you, sitting for long periods of time can interfere with your circulation; getting out of the car to stretch and take a brief walk every couple of hours will help prevent serious problems.

Having a cellular phone in the car can be a real help if you need to secure roadside assistance or call for help. It can also provide a sense of security, especially for people who travel alone. (Just don't chat on the phone and drive at the same time!)

OTHER WAYS OF GETTING THERE

Airplanes and cars may be the most popular modes of transportation, but they're not the only ones. Some people prefer trains, buses, or ships. And some even go for such adventurous options as bicycles, horses, or their own two feet.

Cruises. If a cruise is your type of adventure and you tend to get motion sickness, you may want to investigate the variety of preparations on the market for motion sickness; they include tablets, ear patches, and wristbands. Some are available over the counter, while others require a doctor's prescription.

Overeating can be a problem on cruises, considering there can be as many as eight meals a day, including midnight buffets. To avoid coming home heavier than when you left, ask your waiter if there's a low-calorie menu or if you can be served half-portions of entrées or desserts. With buffet-style meals, walk around the whole buffet first to see what you want before putting food on your plate.

Tours. Organized tours offer the benefit of a scheduled itinerary. You know in advance the time and place of your next meal and can make decisions based on that information. When choosing a tour, consider a trip that allows free time and time for rest.

To be sure that your travel stories are tales of fun, relaxation, and adventure, not inconvenience or illness, planning is the key. And don't forget the postcards!

Source: Virginia Peragallo-Dittko, RN, MA, CDE, "Planes, Trains, and Diabetes: A Guide to Safe Travel," U.S. Department of Health and Human Services, National Institutes of Health.

Oral Medications for Diabetes

Oral diabetes medicines, or oral hypoglycemics, can lower blood glucose in people who have diabetes, but who are able to make some insulin. They are an option if diet and exercise don't work. Oral diabetes medications are not insulin and are not a substitute for diet and exercise.

Although experts don't understand exactly how each oral medicine works, they know that these medicines increase insulin production and affect how insulin lowers blood glucose.

Oral medications are most effective in people who developed diabetes after age 40, have had diabetes less than 5 years, are normal weight, and have never received insulin or have taken only 40 units or less of insulin a day.

WHO SHOULD NOT TAKE ORAL MEDICATIONS FOR DIABETES?

Pregnant and nursing women shouldn't take oral medications because their effect on the fetus and newborn is unknown, and because insulin provides better control of diabetes during pregnancy.

There is also some question about whether oral diabetes medications increase the risk of a heart attack. Experts disagree on this point and many people with noninsulin-dependent diabetes use oral medicines safely and effectively. The Food and Drug Administration (FDA), the agency of the federal government that approves medications for use in this country, requires that oral diabetes medicines carry a warning concerning the increased risk of heart attack. Whether someone uses a medication depends on its benefits and risks, something a doctor can help the patient decide.

WHAT ORAL MEDICATIONS ARE AVAILABLE?

Six FDA-approved oral diabetes medications are now on the market. Their generic names are tolbutamide, chlorpropamide, tolazamide, acetohexamide, glyburide, and glipizide. The generic name refers to the chemical that gives each medicine its particular effect. Some of these medications are made by more than one pharmaceutical company and have more than one brand name. All six are different types of one class of medication, called sulfonylureas, but each affects metabolism differently. A doctor will choose a patient's medication based on the person's general health, the amount his or her blood glucose needs to be lowered, the person's eating habits, and the medicine's side effects.

TAKING ORAL MEDICATIONS

The purpose of oral medications is to lower blood glucose. Therefore, the person taking them must eat regular meals and engage in only light to moderate exercise, to prevent blood glucose

continues

continued

from dipping too low. Medications taken for other health problems, including illness, also can lower blood sugar and may react with the diabetes medicine. Therefore, a doctor needs to know all the medications a person is taking to prevent a harmful interaction. Lowering blood sugar too much can cause hypoglycemia, with symptoms such as headache, weakness, shakiness, and if the condition is severe enough, collapse.

POSSIBLE SIDE EFFECTS

Oral diabetes medications usually don't cause side effects. However, a few people do experience nausea, skin rashes, headache, either water retention or diuresis (increased urination), and sensitivity to direct sunlight. These effects should gradually subside, but a person should see a doctor if they persist. For reasons that aren't always clear, sometimes oral diabetes medications don't help the person for whom they're prescribed. Investigations are under way to learn why this happens.

POINTS TO REMEMBER

- Oral diabetes medications may be used when diet and exercise alone don't control diabetes.
- Oral diabetes medicines aren't a substitute for diet and exercise.

NOTES:

Source: "Noninsulin-Dependent Diabetes," National Institutes of Health, NIH Publication No. 95–241, September 1992.

Oral Hypoglycemic Agents

WHAT THEY ARE

Oral hypoglycemic agents are medications that your doctor may prescribe to help control your blood sugar levels. You may also hear them referred to as "sulfonylureas."

Oral hypoglycemic agents are not "oral insulin" or "insulin pills." Insulin is destroyed by the digestive system and therefore is not effective if taken by mouth. Since you have what is called "Type II or noninsulin-dependent diabetes," your pancreas is still making insulin. However, it is not making enough, or the cells in your body are not able to use it effectively.

Oral hypoglycemic agents help to control diabetes in a variety of ways. Some help your pancreas to produce more insulin. Others help the cells to use insulin more effectively. Some of these medications also slow down the production of sugar by the liver, thus lowering your blood glucose.

TREATMENT PLAN

It is important for you to take these medications exactly as prescribed. Do not take more or fewer pills without consulting your doctor.

Oral agents are a supplement, not a substitute, for your diabetes regimen. It is still very important for you to follow your diet carefully, exercise regularly, and maintain a normal weight. It is also helpful to check your blood sugar regularly to make sure your diabetes is under control. Your diabetes educator can help you plan a schedule of blood sugar testing.

SIDE EFFECTS

Some side effects may occur when you start taking the medication and will go away after a few weeks. Others may mean your dosage needs to be changed or the medication should be discontinued. If any of the following symptoms occur, **call your doctor:**

- nausea/stomachache
- skin rash
- hives
- acne
- vomiting
- dizziness

It is also important to watch for symptoms of low blood sugar—such as feeling weak, shaky, sweaty, or irritable. Low blood sugar (less than 60 mg) can last many hours with oral hypoglycemic agents; therefore, treat with food or sugar, and notify your doctor if these symptoms occur.

continues

continued

DRUG INTERACTIONS

Certain medications may increase or decrease the effect of oral hypoglycemic agents, including aspirin (salicylate) and alcohol. Consult your doctor about using aspirin or alcohol while taking oral agents. If another doctor prescribes medication for you, be sure that the doctor is aware that you take an oral hypoglycemic agent.

You should not take oral hypoglycemic agents if you become pregnant or are breastfeeding. Your doctor will prescribe alternative means of controlling your blood sugar. Birth defects can occur in pregnancies of women with diabetes if their blood sugars are not in excellent control.

NOTES:

Source: Adapted from materials developed by Deborah Hinnen, RN, MN, CDE, Diabetes Treatment Center at St. Joseph's Medical Center, Wichita, Kansas, and Diane Guthrie, RN, PhD, CDE, University of Kansas School of Medicine, Wichita, Kansas. © 1987 by the American Association of Diabetes Educators.

What Are Diabetes Pills?

Diabetes pills, also known as oral hypoglycemic agents, help control diabetes in two ways. They help:

- the pancreas make more insulin
- the body's cells use the insulin the right way

NOTE: DIABETES PILLS ARE NOT INSULIN.

In order for diabetes pills to work:

- Follow a low-sugar, low-fat diet.
- Exercise.
- Lose weight, if needed.

When Are These Pills Used?

If blood sugar remains high, even with diet and exercise, diabetes pills may be needed.

Precautions When Taking Diabetes Pills

- When first taking diabetes pills, watch for
  1. an upset stomach
  2. rash
  3. loss of appetite

Call the doctor right away if any of the above symptoms occur.

- Take the pills exactly as the doctor ordered.
- Do not skip meals. If a meal is skipped, blood sugar could become too low.
- Watch exercise.
  1. Extra exercise may make blood sugar too low.
  2. An extra snack may be needed.
- Do not drink alcohol if a headache and red face develop.
- Tell the doctor about any other medications taken. Some medicines stop diabetes pills from working right (example: aspirin).

continues

continued

ORAL HYPOGLYCEMIC AGENTS (DIABETES PILLS)

Medication	Generic Name	When It Starts To Work	How Long It Works	Normal Doses
Diabeta Micronase	Glyburide	4 hours after taking	16–24 hours	1.25–20 mg/day
Glucotrol	Glipizide*	1–3 hour after taking	12–24 hours	5–40 mg/day
Orinase	Tolbutamide*	3–5 hours after taking	6–12 hours	500–3000 mg/day
Diabinese	Chlorpropamide	2–4 hours after taking	60 hours	100–500 mg/day
Tolinase	Tolazamide	4–6 hours after taking	12–24 hours	100 mg/day
Dymelor	Acetohexamide*	3–6 hours after taking	12–18 hours	250–1500 mg/day

*Take 1/2 hour before meals. All others may be taken with meals.

Source: St. Joseph Rehabilitation Hospital and Outpatient Center, *Patient Education and Discharge Planning Manual for Rehabilitation,* Aspen Publishers, Inc., © 1995.

Insulin

Like oral diabetes medications, insulin is an alternative for some people with noninsulin-dependent diabetes who can't control their blood glucose levels with diet and exercise. In special situations, such as surgery and pregnancy, insulin is a temporary but important means of controlling blood glucose.

WHEN IS INSULIN NEEDED?

Sometimes it's unclear whether insulin or oral medications are more effective in controlling blood glucose; therefore, a doctor will consider a person's weight, age, and the severity of the diabetes before prescribing a medicine. Experts do know that weight control is essential for insulin to be effective. A doctor is likely to prescribe insulin if diet, exercise, or oral medications don't work, or if someone has a bad reaction to oral medicines. A person also may have to take insulin if his or her blood glucose fluctuates a great deal and is difficult to control.

USING INSULIN

A doctor will instruct a person with diabetes on how to purchase, mix, and inject insulin. Various types of insulin are available that differ in purity, concentration, and how quickly they work. They also are made differently. In the past, all commercially available insulin came from the pancreas glands of cows and pigs. Today, human insulin is available in two forms: one uses genetic engineering and the other involves chemically changing pork insulin into human insulin. The best sources of information on insulin are the company that makes it and a doctor.

POINTS TO REMEMBER

- Insulin may be used when diet, exercise, or oral medications don't control diabetes.
- Weight control is important when taking insulin.
- Insulin is taken in special situations such as surgery and pregnancy.

Source: "Noninsulin-Dependent Diabetes," National Institutes of Health, NIH Publication No. 95–241, September 1992.

What Is Insulin?

WHAT IS INSULIN?

Insulin is a hormone (chemical) made in the body. It is made by cells in the pancreas called the islets of Langerhans. If these cells do not make enough insulin, then insulin must be injected into the body. Insulin cannot be taken in pill form because stomach juices destroy insulin.

WHAT ARE THE DIFFERENT TYPES OF INSULIN?

Insulin comes in three main types and one mixture.

1. Short-acting insulin (regular).
2. Intermediate-acting insulin (NPH [Neutral Protamine Hagedorn], or Lente)
3. Long-acting insulin (Ultralente)
4. Humulin 70/30 insulin mixture

1. **Short-Acting Insulin (Clear, Regular, R)**
   Short-acting insulin begins working (onset) within 15 to 30 minutes after injection. It works hardest (peaks) 1 to 3 hours after injection and is out of the body (duration) in 6 to 12 hours.

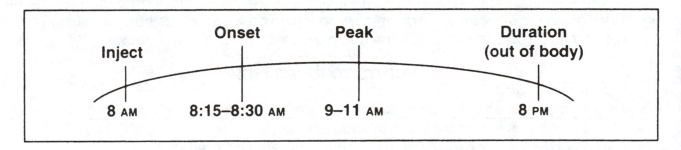

Regular (R) is the most common type of short-acting insulin. Regular insulin is a clear solution.

continues

continued

2. Intermediate-Acting Insulin (Cloudy, NPH, Lente, N, L)

Intermediate-acting insulin begins to work in 1 to 3 hours after injection. It works hardest (peaks) 8 to 12 hours after injection. It is out of the body 18 to 24 hours later.

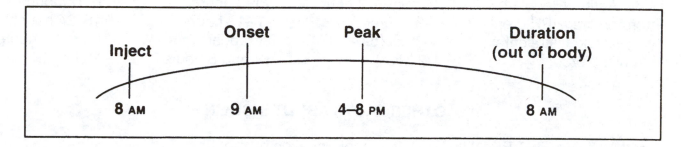

NPH and **Lente** are the most common types of intermediate insulins. These insulins look cloudy.

3. Long-Acting Insulin (Cloudy, Ultralente, U)

Long-acting insulin begins to work 1 to 3 hours after injection. It does not peak as the other insulins do. It keeps working for up to 36 hours.

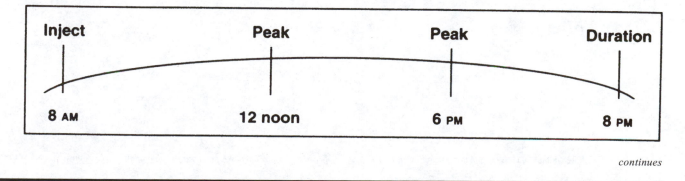

4. Humulin 70/30 Insulin

This insulin is a mixture of regular and NPH : 70% of the insulin is NPH, and 30% of the insulin is regular. It will follow the patterns of both regular and NPH.

continues

continued

Summary: Insulin

Chart	Onset	Peak	Duration
Short-Acting (Regular)	15 min.–1/2 hour	1–3 hours	6–12 hours
Intermediate (NPH, Lente)	1–3 hours	8–12 hours	18–24 hours
Long-Acting (Ultralente)	1–3 hours	gradual	up to 36 hours
Humulin (70/30)	1/2 hour	4 and 6 hours	12 hours

OTHER FACTS ABOUT INSULIN

- INSULIN MUST BE INJECTED. It cannot be taken by mouth.

- Insulin is measured in units (like height is measured in inches).

- Insulin is made in different strengths. Most people use a strength called U-100.

- Use a U-100 syringe with U-100 insulin.

- Do not change brands of insulin without talking to a doctor.

- Eat 30 minutes after taking insulin.

- Always take insulin—do not skip it.

NOTES:

Source: St. Joseph Rehabilitation Hospital and Outpatient Center, *Patient Education and Discharge Planning Manual for Rehabilitation*, Aspen Publishers, Inc., © 1995.

How To Give an Insulin Shot

1. After drawing up insulin, clean injection area with alcohol swab or water. ***The abdomen is the best place for insulin shots; insulin is absorbed faster and more evenly.***

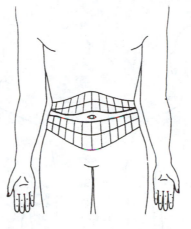

2. Pinch a large area of skin and hold it firmly. With the other hand, hold the syringe like a pencil. Push the needle straight into the skin. Be sure the needle is in all the way so it reaches the proper space between the skin and the muscle, into the subcutaneous tissue.

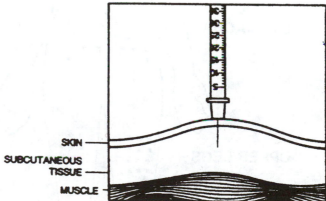

3. To inject the insulin, push the plunger all the way down, using less than five seconds to inject the dose.

4. Pull the needle straight out of the skin, and cover the injection site with a finger, or an alcohol swab or cotton ball and apply slight pressure for several seconds. DO NOT RUB. Rubbing may spread the insulin too quickly or irritate your skin.

5. Use a different site each time, at least 1 inch away from the last injection. Avoid injecting in the area 2 inches around the bellybutton and waistline. If on multiple injections a day, give all injections in the same body area. For example: if injection at breakfast given on the right side of the abdomen, then give all injections for that day on the right side.

Courtesy of Veterans Administration Medical Center, San Diego, California.

Where Is Insulin Injected?

Insulin can be injected into the arm, stomach, thigh, and buttocks. (See the dots below.) The stomach and upper legs are the best areas. Try not to inject into the same spot more than once a month.

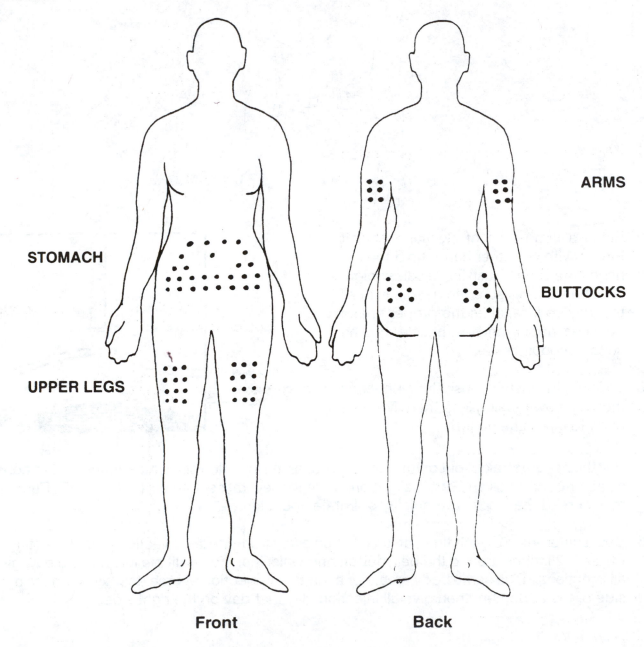

STOMACH

UPPER LEGS

ARMS

BUTTOCKS

Front   Back

Source: St. Joseph Rehabilitation Hospital and Outpatient Center, *Patient Education and Discharge Planning Manual for Rehabilitation,* Aspen Publishers, Inc., © 1995.

How To Draw Up and Inject Insulin

1. Roll bottle upside down and sideways between hands.

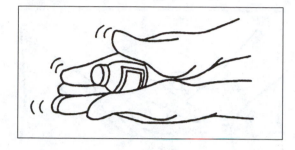

2. Wipe off top of bottle with alcohol swab (cotton and alcohol).

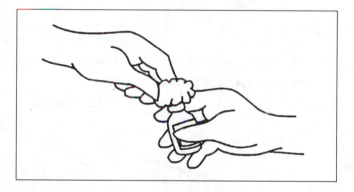

3. Pull plunger of syringe to number of units of insulin you should inject.

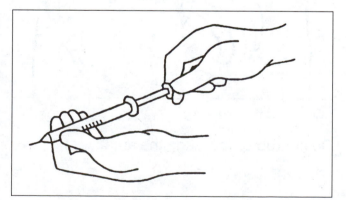

4. Put needle through top of insulin bottle and push plunger down. This puts air into the bottle of insulin.

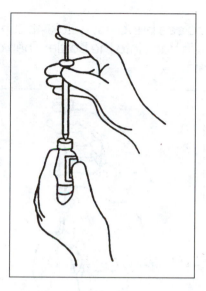

5. With needle still in bottle, turn bottle upside down.

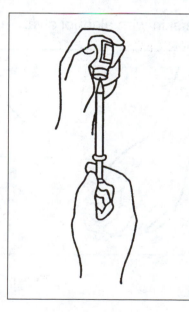

continues

continued

6. Pull plunger out to the number of units of insulin you should inject. Check insulin in syringe for bubbles. If you do not see bubbles, remove needle from bottle.

If you see bubbles, quickly push all of the insulin back into the bottle. Then do Step 6 again.

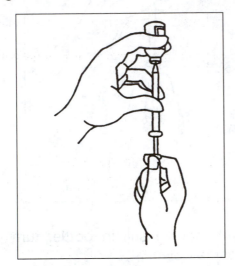

7. Wipe skin with alcohol swab.

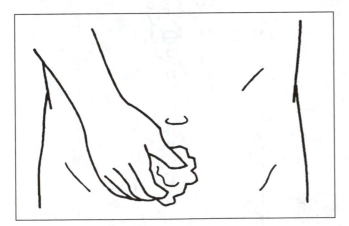

8. Pinch skin gently. Pick up syringe like a pencil and push needle straight into skin. Push plunger down.

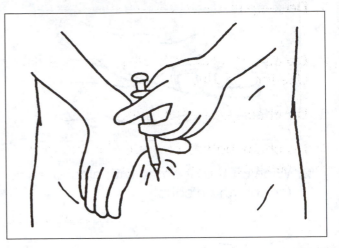

9. Pull needle out from skin. Press the skin with finger for a few seconds.

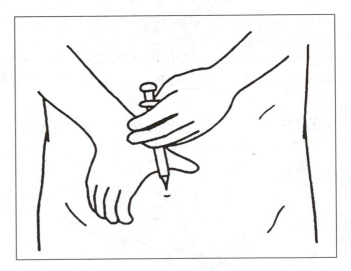

Do not rub or massage the area.

How To Care for Insulin

Do	Don't
1. **Do** keep insulin at room temperature.	1. **Do not** freeze insulin or leave it in direct sunlight.
2. **Do** date insulin bottle when first opened. Use for 1 month.	2. **Do not** use after 1 month.
3. **Do** check expiration date.	3. **Do not** use after expiration date.
4. **Do** check bottles of insulin for changes. (Does insulin look the same?)	4. **Do not** use insulin if it looks different.

How To Care for Syringes

Most people use plastic disposable syringes—use once and then throw away. If using the syringe more than once, do not wipe the needle with alcohol. Alcohol destroys the coating on the needle. Carefully replace the cap on the needle. Do not use the syringe more than two or three times.

Be sure to protect other people from being stuck with the used needles. Put used syringes (to be thrown away) in a coffee tin or some other heavy plastic or metal container. Keep the lid on at all times. Keep this tin away from children. **When the coffee tin is full, put tape across the top and throw it away. Do not put with recyclable garbage.**

NOTES:

Source: St. Joseph Rehabilitation Hospital and Outpatient Center, *Patient Education and Discharge Planning Manual for Rehabilitation,* Aspen Publishers, Inc., © 1995.

Alternative Therapies for Diabetes

Alternative therapies are treatments that are neither widely taught in medical schools nor widely practiced in hospitals. Alternative treatments that have been studied to manage diabetes include acupuncture, biofeedback, guided imagery, and vitamin and mineral supplementation. The success of some alternative treatments can be hard to measure. Many alternative treatments remain either untested or unproven through traditional scientific studies.

Acupuncture

Acupuncture is a procedure in which a practitioner inserts needles into designated points on the skin. Some Western scientists believe that acupuncture triggers the release of the body's natural painkillers. Acupuncture has been shown to offer relief from chronic pain. Acupuncture is sometimes used by people with neuropathy, the painful nerve damage of diabetes.

Biofeedback

Biofeedback is a technique which helps a person become more aware of and learn with the body's response to pain. This alternative therapy emphasizes relaxation and stress-reduction techniques. *Guided imagery* is a relaxation technique that some professionals who use biofeedback do. With guided imagery, a person thinks of peaceful mental images, such as ocean waves. A person may also include the images of controlling or curing a chronic disease, such as diabetes. People using this technique believe condition can be eased with these positive images.

Chromium

The benefit of added *chromium* for diabetes has been studied and debated for several years. Several studies report that chromium supplementation may improve diabetes control. Chromium is needed to make glucose tolerance factor, which helps insulin improve its action. Because of insufficient information on the use of chromium to treat diabetes, no recommendations for supplementation yet exist.

Magnesium

Although the relationship between *magnesium* and diabetes has been studied for decades, it is not yet fully understood. Studies suggest that a deficiency in magnesium may worsen the blood sugar control in Type II diabetes. Scientists believe that a deficiency of magnesium interrupts insulin secretion in the pancreas and increases insulin resistance in the body's tissues. Evidence suggests that a deficiency of magnesium may contribute to certain diabetes complications.

continues

continued

Vanadium

Vanadium is a compound found in tiny amounts in plants and animals. Early studies showed that vanadium normalized blood glucose levels in animals with Type I and Type II diabetes. A recent study found that when people with diabetes were given vanadium, they developed a modest increase in insulin sensitivity and were able to decrease their insulin requirements. Currently researchers want to understand how vanadium works in the body, discover potential side effects, and establish safe dosages.

To learn more about alternative therapies for diabetes treatment, contact the National Institutes of Health's Office of Alternative Medicines Clearinghouse at (888) 644-6226.

NOTES:

Source: "Alternative Therapies for Diabetes," National Institute of Diabetes and Digestive and Kidney Diseases," National Institutes of Health, March 1998.

Diabetes Mellitus Nutritional Goals

GUIDELINES

1. Maintain as near-normal blood-glucose levels as possible, considering diet, exercise, and medication.
2. Maintain optimal serum-lipid levels (cholesterol, triglycerides).
3. Ensure an adequate energy intake to attain/maintain a reasonable body weight or to recover from an illness.
4. Prevent and treat any acute and long-term complications of diabetes.
5. Improve your overall health with good nutrition.

Treatment for high blood sugar begins with diet. The effort and attention that you put into your food choices and meal plan can result in many health benefits. (However, if diabetes or high blood sugar is not treated, it can lead to heart disease, kidney failure, blindness, and vascular and nerve disease.)

The best choices for a health-promoting diet are foods that are low in fats, cholesterol, and sugar and high in fiber. Your planning should include

- reaching and maintaining a reasonable weight
- eating well-balanced meals at regular times
- not skipping meals
- selecting low-fat and fat-free foods
- limiting sugar and foods made with sugar
- limiting egg yolks to no more than four per week

- eating foods high in fiber daily (e.g., whole-grain bread and cereals, dry beans, fresh fruits, and vegetables)
- avoiding alcohol (discuss specifics with your physician)
- including a small, protein-rich bedtime snack if you are taking insulin
- using cooking methods that minimize added fats
- making grocery-shopping decisions that emphasize lean meats, more fish, and unprocessed foods (become an expert label reader)
- choosing noncaloric beverages to quench thirst
- making exercise an important part of your diabetes treatment plan (check with your health care provider for exercise tips and tolerance)

DIET SPECIFICS

1. Protein intake should be 10–20 percent of total daily calories. If neuropathy exists, the protein level for adults should be not more than the Recommended Daily Allowance of 0.8 g/kg/desirable body weight/day, approximately 10 percent of daily calories.
2. Fat intake should be less than 30 percent of total daily calories, less than 10 percent from saturated fat and less than 300 mg cholesterol per day. (If the patient has elevated LDL, low-density lipoproteins, saturated fat should be less than 7 percent of total calories and dietary cholesterol intake should be less than 200

continues

continued

mg/day.) Omega-3 fats, polyunsaturated fats found in fish, do not need to be limited.

3. Carbohydrate intake should be planned and based on individual nutrition assessment and treatment goals.

- Sucrose and sucrose-containing food can be used as part of the meal plan if substituted for other carbohydrates.
- Fructose has a more modulating affect on plasma glucose than does sucrose and many starchy carbohydrates, but large amounts (20 percent of calories) have adverse affects on serum cholesterol and LDL cholesterol.
- Nonnutritive sweeteners approved by the FDA, saccharin, aspartame, and acesulfame K, are considered safe to consume.

4. Fiber intake, especially soluble fiber, is recommended at a level of 20–35 g per day. Soluble fiber, if eaten in large amounts, helps to lower serum lipids, and all fiber reduces the risk for colon cancer and may help in the prevention or treatment of gastrointestinal disorders.

5. Sodium intake should not exceed 3,000 mg if you are normotensive. With mild to moderate hypertension, less than 2,400 mg per day is recommended. With hypertension and neuropathy, 2,000 mg of sodium per day, or less, is recommended.

6. Alcohol, if diabetes is well controlled and if not contraindicated by medications, may be consumed by people with insulin-dependent diabetes—if ingested with and in addition to the usual meal plan. (Alcohol should be avoided by people who have a history of alcohol abuse, during pregnancy, and if taking sulfonylureas. Alcohol intake is inadvisable for patients with pancreatitis, dyslipidemia, or neuropathy.) Calories from alcohol should be calculated as fat calories, with one alcoholic beverage equal to two fat exchanges.

NOTES:

Source: Barbara Stover Gingerich and Deborah Anne Ondeck, *Clinical Pathways for the Multidisciplinary Home Care Team,* Aspen Publishers, Inc., © 1996.

Noninsulin-Dependent Diabetes Mellitus and Diet

Noninsulin-dependent diabetes mellitus (NIDDM), also known as adult onset or Type II diabetes, often appears gradually when your body is unable to efficiently use the insulin it produces. Insulin helps sugar get into cells to maintain normal blood-sugar (glucose) levels. Type II is the most common form of diabetes. It frequently begins after age 40, however, it can occur at any age.

Sugar can only move into the cells through special entrances, but there is a problem with these entrances in people with Type I diabetes. As a result, little or no sugar moves into the cells even though insulin is present, and sugar builds up in the blood causing hyperglycemia (hyper = high; glycemia = sugar in the blood).

The symptoms of Type II diabetes appear gradually and may not be recognized as diabetes easily.

Symptoms of Type II diabetes may include the following:

- Frequent urination
- Blurred eyesight
- Slow healing cuts or sores
- Problems with sexual function
- Numbness/tingling in hands and feet
- Increased thirst
- Feeling tired
- Increased hunger
- Frequent infections
- Dry, itchy skin

Treatment for Type II diabetes includes **meal planning, weight loss if indicated, exercise (as tolerated), and medications (pills or insulin).** People who maintain a healthy body weight are better able to control their blood glucose levels. So, if you are overweight, it's important to follow a meal plan designed to help you lose weight. Once you've reaching your desired weight, you'll need to follow a meal plan to maintain your healthier body weight.

Many people with Type II diabetes take pills to lower their blood sugar levels. These pills are not insulin. Diabetes pills:

- lower the level of sugar in the blood
- prevent the body from releasing additional sugar into the blood
- help the body use insulin efficiently
- help the body release more of its own insulin into the bloodstream
- work with meals and exercise to keep blood sugar in the target range

Some people with Type II diabetes sometimes also take insulin.
The meal plan you should follow is the same as what is recommended for all Americans.

- Eat more starches, fiber, and naturally occurring sugars. These are found in bread and pasta, rice, fruits, and vegetables. Limit foods rich in refined sugars such as cake, candy, and regular soft drinks.

continues

continued

- Eat a variety of foods to help ensure that you're getting the right balance of nutrients. Use the food pyramid recommendations as a guide.
- Schedule eating times and maintain the schedule as closely as possible. Eating meals at regular times helps your body regulate its blood-glucose levels.
- Avoid eating large meals because they will raise your blood-glucose levels.

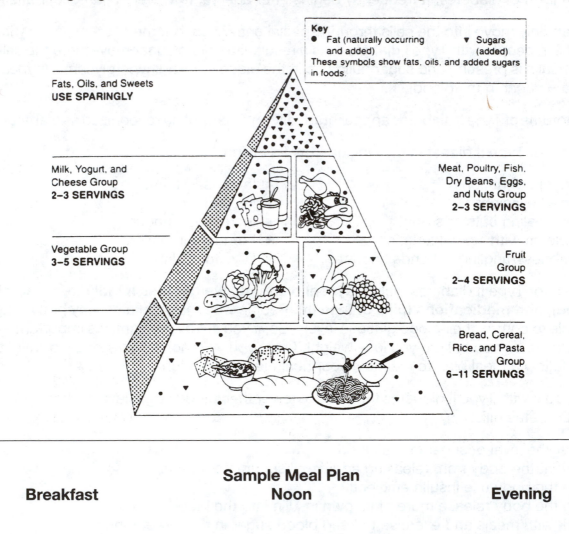

Key
● Fat (naturally occurring and added)   ▼ Sugars (added)
These symbols show fats, oils, and added sugars in foods.

Fats, Oils, and Sweets
USE SPARINGLY

Milk, Yogurt, and
Cheese Group
2–3 SERVINGS

Meat, Poultry, Fish,
Dry Beans, Eggs,
and Nuts Group
2–3 SERVINGS

Vegetable Group
3–5 SERVINGS

Fruit
Group
2–4 SERVINGS

Bread, Cereal,
Rice, and Pasta
Group
6–11 SERVINGS

	Sample Meal Plan	
Breakfast	**Noon**	**Evening**
Snacks		**Snacks**

Insulin-Dependent Diabetes Mellitus and Diet

Insulin-dependent diabetes mellitus (IDDM), also known as juvenile onset or Type I diabetes, often begins very suddenly in childhood when the pancreas stops producing insulin. Insulin lowers the level of blood sugar by helping sugar leave the bloodstream and enter the cells. Because there is no insulin, sugar cannot enter cells to be used for energy and blood sugars remain elevated.

Symptoms of Type I diabetes may include the following:

- Frequent urination to rid the body of excess glucose
- Increased thirst due to fluid lost in urination
- Sudden weight loss when the body uses its fat cells for energy
- Increased fatigue
- Increased hunger

With Type I diabetes, you need insulin shots every day to live. Insulin helps the body in many ways by:

- lowering the level of sugar in the blood
- allowing the body to use energy from food
- allowing sugar from the blood to enter muscle and fat cells
- keeping the body from sending extra sugar into the blood when you are sick or under other kinds of stress
- allowing the body to use energy and protein for growth; this being especially important in children and during pregnancy
- working with meal planning and exercise to keep blood-sugar levels in the target range

Once insulin is injected into your body, it begins to lower blood-glucose levels regardless of food intake and exercise pattern. Therefore, it is very important to coordinate the timing of your meals and your insulin injections. Monitoring your diet and coordinating food intake and exercise helps to keep your blood-glucose levels near normal.

To coordinate your insulin needs, meal plan and exercise, you'll need to do the following:

- Take your insulin.
- Eat well-balanced meals.
- Schedule meal times consistently and maintain that schedule as closely as possible every day. Eating meals and snacks at regular times will help your body to balance your insulin and food intake.
- Eat enough of the right foods to provide sufficient calories to maintain your recommended body weight. Controlling your weight helps control your blood glucose levels.
- Coordinate exercise activity with your insulin schedule and mealtimes so that you do not develop hypoglycemia (low blood-sugar levels).

continues

continued

DIABETES AND MEAL PLANNING

The food guide pyramid is the best place to start for people with diabetes. The pyramid shows the kinds of foods everyone needs to be healthy. The best food choices for the person with diabetes are also the best food choices for the whole family. It is important to eat foods from all of the food groups. You should choose more of the foods at the base of the pyramid and less of those at the peak.

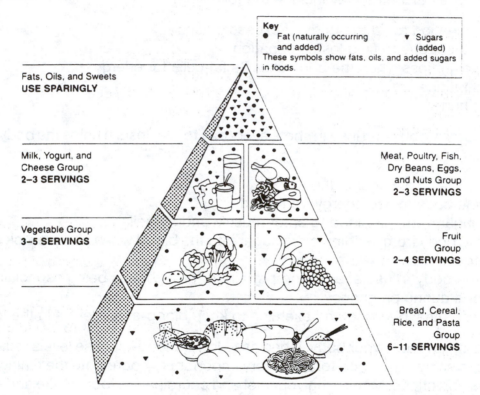

Key
● Fat (naturally occurring and added)   ▼ Sugars (added)
These symbols show fats, oils, and added sugars in foods.

Fats, Oils, and Sweets
USE SPARINGLY

Milk, Yogurt, and Cheese Group
2–3 SERVINGS

Meat, Poultry, Fish, Dry Beans, Eggs, and Nuts Group
2–3 SERVINGS

Vegetable Group
3–5 SERVINGS

Fruit Group
2–4 SERVINGS

Bread, Cereal, Rice, and Pasta Group
6–11 SERVINGS

The food pyramid will help you do the following:

- Eat a variety of foods.
- Maintain a healthy weight.
- Choose a diet low in fat, saturated fat, and cholesterol.
- Choose a diet with plenty of vegetables, fruits, and grains.
- Use sugar in moderation.

Your meal plan should be modified according to your diabetes medication, exercise, and any other health concerns you may have. You and your dietitian will discuss the kinds of foods you like, when you eat, and how you prepare food to design a meal plan for your individual lifestyle.

How Can I Find Out How Much To Eat Each Day?

Ask yourself these questions:

- Am I a small woman who exercises?
  Yes or **No** (circle one)
- Am I a small woman who wants to lose weight?
  Yes or **No** (circle one)
- Am I a medium woman who wants to lose weight?
  Yes or **No** (circle one)
- Am I a medium woman who does not exercise much?
  Yes or **No** (circle one)

If your answer to every question is **No**, go to the next section. If you answered **Yes** to any of these questions, eat between 1,200 and 1,600 calories a day.

Eat these numbers of servings to eat 1,200 to 1,600 calories a day:

6 starches
3 vegetables
2 fruits
2 milk and yogurt
2 protein foods
4–6 fats
0–1 sugary foods

Ask yourself these questions:

- Am I a large woman who needs to lose weight?
  Yes or **No** (circle one)
- Am I a small man at a healthy weight?
  Yes or **No** (circle one)
- Am I a medium man who needs to lose weight?
  Yes or **No** (circle one)
- Am I a medium man who does not exercise much?
  Yes or **No** (circle one)

If your answer to every question is **No**, go to the next section. If you answered **Yes** to any of these questions, eat between 1,600 and 2,000 calories a day.

Eat these numbers of servings from these food groups to eat 1,600 to 2,000 calories a day:

8 starches
4 vegetables
3 fruits
2 milk and yogurt
2 protein foods
6–8 fats
0–1 sugary foods

continues

continued

Ask yourself these questions:

- Am I a large man who does not need to lose weight?
  Yes or **No** (circle one)
- Am I a large man who needs to lose weight?
  Yes or **No** (circle one)
- Am I a medium to large man who does a lot of exercise or has an active job?
  Yes or **No** (circle one)
- Am I a large woman who does a lot of exercise or has an active job?
  Yes or **No** (circle one)

If you answer **Yes** to any of these questions, eat between 2,000 and 2,400 calories a day.

Eat these numbers of servings from these food groups to eat 2,000 to 2,400 calories a day:

10 starches
4 vegetables
3 fruits
2 milk and yogurt
2 protein foods
8–10 fats
0–1 sugary foods

NOTES:

Source: *I Have Diabetes: How Much Should I Eat?* NIH Pub. No. 98-4243, National Institute of Diabetes and Digestive and Kidney Diseases, National Institutes of Health, Public Health Service, U.S. Department of Health and Human Services, 1997.

Make Your Own Food Pyramid

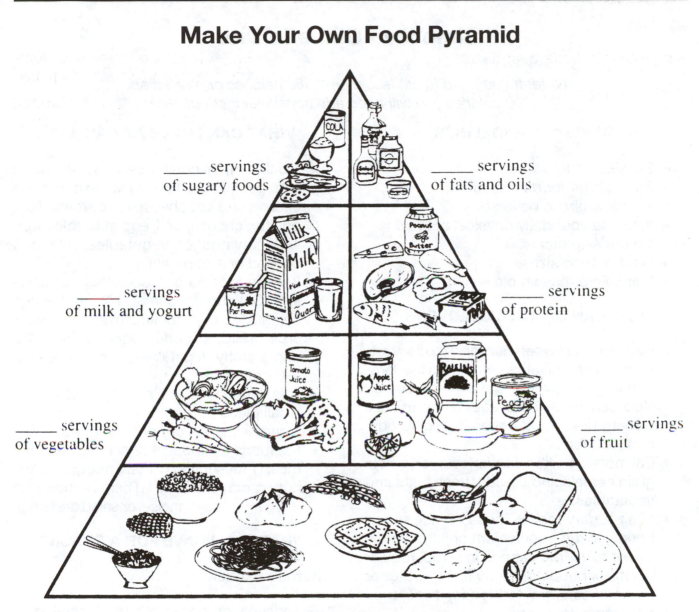

_____ servings of sugary foods

_____ servings of fats and oils

_____ servings of milk and yogurt

_____ servings of protein

_____ servings of vegetables

_____ servings of fruit

_____ servings of starches

Source: _I Have Diabetes: How Much Should I Eat?_ NIH Pub. No. 98-4243, National Institute of Diabetes and Digestive and Kidney Diseases, National Institutes of Health, Public Health Service, U.S. Department of Health and Human Services, 1997.

Simplified Diabetic Diet

Note: If you need to eat less than 1,500 calories or more than 1,900 calories you will need additional diet instructions.

GENERAL GUIDELINES

- Eat sweets less often.
- Eat high-fat foods less often.
- Avoid alcoholic beverages.
- Increase your daily physical activity.
- Do not skip meals.
- Limit portion sizes.
- Maintain a reasonable weight.

YOU CAN DO THE FOLLOWING

- Use artificial sweeteners and food sweetened with artificial sweeteners in moderation (e.g., sugar-free gelatin or pudding). You can drink beverages with artificial sweeteners in moderation (e.g., diet soda, diet iced tea).
- Eat more high-fiber foods: legumes, whole grain cereals and breads, fresh fruits and vegetables.
- Limit sugary foods: These include sugar, honey, syrup, regular jam or jelly, candy, sweet rolls, fruit canned in syrup, regular gelatin or pudding, cake with icing, pies or other sweets, frosted foods, sweetened beverages (e.g., soda).
- Limit high-fat foods: These include fried foods, foods with cream, cheese or butter sauce, cold cuts, bacon, sausage, hot dogs, nuts, seeds, salad dressing, lard, gravy, solid shortening, and whole milk dairy products. Trim meat of fat and remove skin from poultry.
- Limit fruit servings to 3–4 per day

WHAT CAN I HAVE AT A MEAL?

- Meat, fish, or poultry servings limited to 3 oz. per meal, 3/4 cup tuna fish or cottage cheese or 3 oz. cheese (1 oz. meat, fish, poultry, cheese, or 1 egg at breakfast).
- 1–2 servings of vegetables (1/2 cup cooked or 1 cup raw).
- 2 servings of starchy foods (1 starch serving = 3/4 cup dry cereal, 1/2 cup cooked cereal, 1/2 cup cooked pasta or rice, 1 slice bread, 1/2 cup cooked beans, 1/2 cup starchy vegetables, 1 small potato, 4–6 crackers).
- 1 fruit or fruit juice serving (1/2 cup, 1 small piece of fruit).
- 1 cup skim milk or nonfat yogurt.
- Fat foods limited to 1–2 servings at each meal (1 fat serving = 1 tsp. margarine, oil, butter, mayonnaise, 1 Tbsp. reduced-fat margarine, mayonnaise, or salad dressing).

WHAT CAN I HAVE FOR A SNACK?

Afternoon snack:

1–2 servings of starch foods (1 serving of starch = 4–6 crackers, 3/4 cup dry cereal, 3/4 oz. pretzels, 2 rice cakes, 1 slice bread, 8 animal crackers, 3 graham cracker squares).

Evening snack (avoid late snacking):

1–2 servings of starch foods and 1 oz. meat, fish, poultry, or cheese or 1 cup skim milk or nonfat yogurt.

Courtesy of Anna M. Sousa, MS, RD.

No Concentrated Sweets

The following guidelines are for individuals who need to avoid sugar and foods containing large amounts of sugar. These foods are referred to as *concentrated sweets.* Limiting concentrated sweets in your diet can help to control blood sugar levels.

IMPORTANT POINTS TO REMEMBER

- Eat at least three meals, evenly spaced throughout the day. Avoid long periods without food.
- Try to achieve and maintain your desirable weight.
- Eat a balanced diet by including foods from each food group: fruits and vegetables; bread and cereal; meat, fish, or poultry; dairy products; and fats.
- Artificial sweeteners and artificially sweetened foods are available. Use should be discussed with the dietitian.
- The following foods are sources of concentrated sweets and should be limited:
  —Sugar, honey, jam, jelly, molasses
  —Syrups (maple, corn, pancake syrup)
  —Candy, regular chewing gum
  —Regular gelatin, pudding, custard
  —Sherbet, water ice, ice cream
  —Cakes, cookies, pastry, pies, sweet rolls, sweet breads, doughnuts
  —Beverages that contain sugar or corn syrup, regular soda pop, milkshakes
  —Chocolate or flavored milk, eggnog, fruited or flavored yogurt
  —Condensed milk
  —Fruits canned in syrup

NOTES:

Courtesy of Youville Lifecare, Cambridge, Massachusetts.

How To Calculate Total Available Glucose

Total available glucose (TAG) is calculated as follows:

TAG = Carbohydrate (CHO) (grams) + [Animal Protein (PRO) (grams) × .58]

	CHO	+ Animal PRO (.58)	= TAG
1 Fruit exchange	= 15 g	+ 0	= 15
1 Meat exchange	= 0	+ 7 g (.58)	= 4
1 Milk exchange	= 12 g	+ 8 g (.58)	= 17
1 Bread exchange	= 15 g	+ 0	= 15
1 Vegetable exchange	= 5 g	+ 0	= 5

The number that results from this formula can be used to determine what each of your meals might include.

Counting total available glucose is a way to ensure consistency in diet from day to day. Carbohydrate is counted because it tends to raise blood sugars. Animal proteins also raise blood sugar levels because they are eventually converted to carbohydrate by the body. Fat does not raise blood sugar levels because very little of it is converted to carbohydrate. You should try to keep your fat intake low enough to prevent increases in weight. You also should consider the type of fat you eat to be sure it is optimum for possible prevention of coronary heart disease.

NOTES:

Courtesy of Linda G. Snetselaar.

Examples of Foods To Add for Exercise

Food	Amount
Chewy granola bars	½ bar
Dried fruit	¼ cup
Fig bars	1 bar
Fruit/cereal bars	½ bar
Fruit rolls	1
Fruit snacks	½ pouch
Grapes	15
Raisins	2 Tbs. or 1 small box

Beverages

Juice	4 oz
Regular soft drinks	4 oz
Sports drink (e.g., Gatorade)	8 oz

Note: Each food in the serving size listed provides 10 to 15 grams of carbohydrate.

NOTES:

Source: Lea Ann Holzmeister, "Children and Adolescents," in *Handbook of Diabetes Medical Nutrition Therapy,* Margaret A. Powers, ed., Aspen Publishers, Inc., © 1996.

Carbohydrate Content of Foods Appropriate for Sick-Day Use

	Carbohydrate Content (g)			Carbohydrate Content (g)
Starch Exchanges			**Fruit Exchanges**	
1 slice bread	15		½ twin Popsicle	10
½ cup hot cereal	15		Fruit juices (unsweetened):	
6 saltine crackers (2-in. squares	15		⅓ cup cranberry, grape	15
4 soda crackers (2½-in. squares)	15		⅓ cup prune juice	15
			½ cup apple, pineapple	15
3 graham crackers (2½-in. squares)	15		½ cup apricot	15
			½ cup cherry, grapefruit, orange, or peach juice	15
½ cup ice cream	15			
1 cup soup, broth	15		**Milk Exchanges**	
1 cup soup, cream				
(reconstituted with water)	15		1 cup milk	12
(reconstituted with milk)	25		1 cup yogurt	12
			¼ cup plain pudding	12
Meat Exchanges				
			Other Carbohydrates	
¼ cup low-fat cottage cheese	0			
1 oz. American or Swiss cheese	0		½ cup ice milk	15
			½ cup regular gelatin	15
1 poached or soft-boiled egg	0		¼ cup sherbet	15
			4 oz. regular carbonated beverage, cola-type	15
Vegetable Exchanges				
½ cup tomato juice	5			
½ cup vegetable juice	5			

Source: Karmeen D. Kulkarni, "Adjusting Nutrition Therapy for Special Situations," in *Handbook of Diabetes Medical Nutrition Therapy,* Margaret A. Powers, ed., Aspen Publishers, Inc., © 1996.

Diabetic Toddler Feeding Guidelines

1. **If your child wants to drink more fruit juice** than the 4-oz serving allowed:
   - Dilute the juice with water or diet soda pop.
   - Offer a piece of fruit instead, which takes longer to eat and is more filling.
2. **If your child doesn't like milk:**
   - Flavor the milk with sugar-free Nestle's Quik.
   - Offer other high-calcium foods such as cheese, plain or sugar-free pudding, or sugar-free frozen fudge pop.
3. **If your child won't eat vegetables,** don't make an issue of it. Vegetables are so low in carbohydrates that they have minimal effect on blood glucose levels. Similar nutrients are found in fruit, juice, or vitamin and mineral supplements.
4. **If your child won't eat fruit:**
   - Offer fruit juice (limit to one 4-oz serving per day).
   - Use vitamin and mineral supplements.
5. **If your child won't finish his or her meal or snack,** don't force the issue:
   - Offer beverages (milk provides both carbohydrates and proteins).
   - Serve child-size portions.
6. **If your child wants more food,** offer "free" foods such as sugar-free Popsicle, Kool-Aid, Jell-O, and nonstarchy vegetables. Foods containing less than 20 calories and 5 g carbohydrates per serving can generally be eaten freely.
7. **If your child goes on a food jag** (requesting one food often), don't object because boredom will eventually lead to change.
8. **If your child takes a long time to eat:**
   - Offer child-size portions (your expectations of how much your child can eat may be too high).
   - Ask your health care provider for guidance.
9. **If your child doesn't like eating breakfast:**
   - Vary food offered (e.g., different cereals, bagels, English muffins, frozen waffles).
   - Mix sugar-free Carnation Instant Breakfast in milk for a meal in itself.
   - Try nontraditional breakfast foods (e.g., sandwiches, pizza, leftovers).

Source: Lea Ann Holzmeister, "Children and Adolescents," in *Handbook of Diabetes Medical Nutrition Therapy,* Margaret A. Powers, ed., Aspen Publishers, Inc., © 1996.

Exchange Lists for Meal Planning for Vegetarian Diabetics

STARCHY FOODS

A starch exchange provides approximately 15 grams of carbohydrate, 3 grams of protein, a trace of fat, and 80 calories.

Breads

½ bagel
½ hamburger bun
½ English muffin
½ 6-in. pita

1 6-in. poori (Indian bread)
1 dinner roll
1 slice whole grain bread
1 6-in. corn or flour tortilla

Cereals/Grains

⅓ cup bran cereal
½ cup bran, corn, or other flakes
½ cup shredded wheat
1 shredded wheat biscuit
3 Tbsp. Grapenuts
1½ cups puffed rice or wheat
½ cup cooked cereal (oatmeal, 7-grain, oat bran, bear mush, farina, Wheatena, etc.)
½ cup cooked grits
⅓ cup cooked rice (white or brown)
½ cup cooked bulgur

⅓ cup cooked couscous
⅓ cup cooked millet
⅓ cup cooked quinoa
½ cup cooked pasta
¾ cup mung bean (cellophane) noodles
⅓ cup polenta
⅓ cup cooked wheat berries
3 cups air-popped popcorn
3 Tbsp. wheat germ
5 Tbsp. bran

Starchy Vegetables

½ cup corn
1 6-in. corn on the cob
½ cup lima beans
⅔ cup parsnips
½ cup green peas
½ cup plantain

1 3-oz. potato
½ cup mashed potatoes
1 cup winter squash
⅓ cup sweet potatoes or yams
¼ cup chestnuts

continues

continued

Crackers/Cookies

4 Rye Krisps
3 graham crackers
5 oblong melba toasts
2 rice cakes
¾ oz. matzo
8 animal crackers

2 thin breadsticks
2 Fig Newtons
3 ginger snaps
2 oatmeal cookies
6 vanilla wafers

Dried Beans

½ cup vegetarian baked beans, cooked
   beans, peas, or lentils*
3 Tbsp. miso

Other†

¼ cup bread dressing
1 2½-in. biscuit
1 2-in. square corn bread
¼ cup granola
1 4-in. pancake
2 4-in. crisp taco shells
½ cup chow mein noodles

*Count as one exchange of starch plus one exchange of protein.
†Count each as one exchange of starch plus one exchange of fat.

VEGETABLES

An exchange provides approximately 5 grams of carbohydrate, 2 grams of protein, no fat, and 25 calories. One exchange of vegetables is equal to ½ cup of cooked or 1 cup of raw vegetables (any of the following). Note that starchy vegetables such as potatoes and winter squash are included on the starchy foods exchange list.

Alfalfa sprouts
Artichoke
Asparagus
Bamboo shoots
Beans (green, wax, Italian)
Beets
Bok choy
Brussels sprouts

Cabbage
Carrots
Cauliflower
Eggplant
Greens (kale, collards, mustard,
   turnip greens, beet, Swiss chard)
Jicama
Kohlrabi

continues

continued

Leeks
Mushrooms
Okra
Onions
Pea pods
Pepper
Radicchio
Rutabaga

Sauerkraut
Sea vegetables
Spinach
Summer squash and zucchini
Tomatoes
Tomato or vegetable juice
Turnips
Water chestnuts

FRUITS AND JUICES

One exchange of fruit provides approximately 15 grams of carbohydrate, no protein or fat, and about 60 calories.

Fresh Fruits

1 apple
½ cup unsweetened applesauce
4 apricots
½ banana
¾ cup blackberries
¾ cup blueberries
1 cup cantaloupe chunks
12 cherries
½ grapefruit
15 grapes
⅜ honeydew melon or 1 cup honeydew cubes
1 kiwi fruit

½ mango
1 nectarine
1 orange
1 cup papaya or ½ papaya
1 peach
1 pear
¾ cup pineapple
2 plums
1 cup raspberries
1¼ cup strawberries
2 tangerines
1¼ cup watermelon cubes

Dried Fruits

7 apricot halves
2½ dates
1½ figs

3 prunes
2 Tbsp. raisins

continues

continued

Juices

½ cup apple juice or cider
⅓ cup cranberry juice cocktail
½ cup grapefruit juice
⅓ cup grape juice

½ cup orange juice
½ cup pineapple juice
⅓ cup prune juice

PROTEIN FOODS

One protein exchange provides 7 grams of protein and 3 grams of fat.

½ cup tofu
1 tofu hotdog
¼ cup tempeh
1 oz. seitan
¼ cup roasted soynuts

¼ cup prepared textured soy protein
2 Tbsp. Parmesan cheese
3 egg whites
1 whole egg
¼ cup egg substitute

Count as one protein exchange plus one starch exchange:

½ cup cooked dried beans

Count as one protein exchange plus one fat exchange:

1 oz. soy cheese
1 oz. dairy cheese
1 veggieburger

Count as one protein exchange plus two fat exchanges:

½ Tbsp. peanut butter, tahini, almond butter, or other nut or seed butter
2 Tbsp. nuts
1 Tbsp. seeds

MILKS

One milk exchange provides approximately 12 grams of carbohydrate, 8 grams of protein, between 0 and 2 grams of fat, and about 90 calories.

continues

continued

1 cup "light" soymilk
1 cup Vegelicious
1 cup Rice Dream
1 cup skimmed cow's milk

1 cup buttermilk
½ cup skimmed milk cottage cheese
¾ cup nonfat plain yogurt

Count as one milk exchange plus one fat exchange:

1 cup 2% cow's milk

Count as one milk exchange plus two fat exchanges:

1 cup whole cow's milk

Count as one milk exchange plus one fat exchange:

1 cup regular soymilk

Count as one milk exchange plus one fruit exchange:

¾ cup fruit-flavored, nonfat yogurt

FATS

One fat exchange provides approximately 5 grams of fat and about 45 calories.

⅛ avocado
1 tsp. mayonnaise
1 Tbsp. reduced-calorie mayonnaise
1½ Tbsp. tofu mayonnaiuse (Nayonnaise)
1 tsp. vegetable oil
10 small or 5 large olives
2 tsp. mayonnaise type salad dressing
2 Tbsp. low-fat salad dressing
1 tsp. margarine

1 tsp. butter
1 Tbsp. reduced-calorie margarine
1 Tbsp. cream cheese
1 Tbsp. tofu cream cheese
2 Tbsp. sour cream
2 Tbsp. shredded coconut
1 Tbsp. coconut cream
1 Tbsp. coconut milk

Source: Mark Messina and Virginia Messina, *The Dietitian's Guide to Vegetarian Diets*, Aspen Publishers, Inc., © 1996.

Sample Diet Plan Handout for Low Literacy Client with Diabetes

Task: What can I eat for lunch? Use the numbers written in the squares for each of the 6 food groups to determine how many servings you should have from each food group. Then use the food groups to select the foods for lunch.

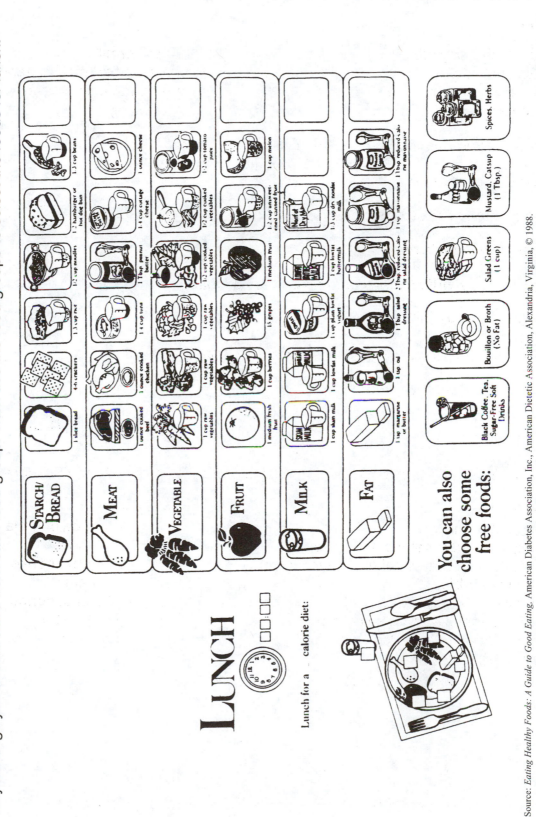

Source: *Eating Healthy Foods: A Guide to Good Eating,* American Diabetes Association, Inc., American Dietetic Association, Alexandria, Virginia, © 1988.

Diabetes Complications

WHAT PROBLEMS CAN DIABETES CAUSE?

A key goal of diabetes treatment is to prevent complications because, over time, diabetes can damage the heart, blood vessels, eyes, kidneys, and nerves, although the person may not know damage is taking place. It's important to diagnose and treat diabetes early, because it can cause damage even before it makes someone feel ill.

HOW DOES DIABETES CAUSE PROBLEMS?

How diabetes causes long-term problems is unclear. However, changes in the small blood vessels and nerves are common. These changes may be the first step toward many problems that diabetes causes.

WHO WILL DEVELOP PROBLEMS?

Scientists can't predict who among people with diabetes will develop complications, but complications are most likely to occur in someone who has had diabetes for many years. However, because a person can have diabetes without knowing it, a complication may be the first sign.

POINTS TO REMEMBER

- Diabetes can cause long-term complications such as heart, kidney, eye, and nerve disease.
- Careful treatment of diabetes and checking for signs of complications can lower the chances that someone will be troubled by these conditions.
- An identification bracelet or necklace stating that the wearer has diabetes can help ensure that friends or strangers won't ignore symptoms that signal a medical emergency.

Source: "Noninsulin-Dependent Diabetes," National Institutes of Health, NIH Publication No. 95–241, September 1992.

What Are Possible Complications of Diabetes?

High blood sugar may damage the eyes, heart, blood vessels, nerves, feet, and kidneys. The best way to lower chances of having these problems is to KEEP THE BLOOD SUGAR WITHIN NORMAL LEVEL. Other suggestions:

Complications	Suggestions
1. Eyes (Retinopathy)	• Have eyes tested at least once a year by an eye doctor (ophthalmologist) • Keep blood pressure at a normal level.
2. Kidney Damage (Nephropathy)	Test urine for protein from time to time.
3. Nerve Damage (Neuropathy)	Tell the doctor about any pain or loss of feeling in legs, feet, or hands.
4. Foot Problems	Follow daily foot care.

5. Heart and Blood Vessel Problems (Cardiovascular)	• Keep a healthy body weight.
	• Eat less fat, especially red meat and fatty meats.
	• DO NOT SMOKE.
	• Keep blood pressure at a normal level.
	• Tell the doctor if there is:
	—Pain in:
	  • Chest
	  • Neck
	  • Arms
	—Trouble breathing

6. Sexual Problems	• **Men** Men with diabetes may be unable to get and keep an erection because of nerve damage caused by high blood sugars. This comes on slowly. There are medications and devices to help. • **Women** Women are less likely to have sexual problems. Increased blood sugar may cause vaginal infections. There may be a decrease in the amount of lubrication during intercourse. If this happens, K-Y jelly or other vaginal lubrication jelly can help. Do not use petroleum jelly. Talk about any questions or concerns with the doctor or nurse.

REMEMBER: KEEP NORMAL BLOOD SUGAR (GLUCOSE) LEVEL (70 TO 130 mg/dL) TO HELP PREVENT PROBLEMS.

Source: St. Joseph Rehabilitation Hospital and Outpatient Center, *Patient Education and Discharge Planning Manual for Rehabilitation*, Aspen Publishers, Inc., © 1995.

Managing Complications

Whether you have insulin-dependent (type I) or noninsulin-dependent (type II) diabetes, you may someday face one or more diabetes complications. Complications are medical problems that occur more often in people with diabetes. Over time, diabetes can cause changes in blood vessels or nerves. These changes can lead to medical problems. You may have diabetes for decades before complications show up, if they ever do.

If they do occur, these complications can affect many different parts of the body. Large blood vessels may become narrow. When a blood flow is slowed, you run a risk of heart disease or stroke. Small blood vessels often get damaged, too. Damage to vessels in the eyes (retinopathy) can threaten your vision. The damage can lead to blindness if not treated early. The small blood vessels in the kidney may also be injured, leading to kidney disease, or nephropathy.

Nerve damage, or neuropathy, is another common complication of diabetes. Neuropathy can numb parts of the body, especially the feet and legs, or cause feelings of tingling or burning. It can also impair the function of internal organs such as the stomach and bladder.

The combination of neuropathy and blood vessel disease can lead to amputation. If you lose feeling in your feet, you may not feel blisters or small sores. Diabetes raises the chances that these wounds will become infected. If they do, blood vessel damage can make infections hard to heal. An out-of-control infection could require amputation to save the rest of the limb.

WARNING SIGNS

Complications don't come out of nowhere. Some complications, such as kidney disease, do not cause symptoms early on. But they can be detected through special screening tests by your health-care team, so regular checkups are important.

Other complications, such as nerve damage, may be spotted because of physical symptoms. If you notice a change in your health, take action. Do not ignore small warning signs that point to a complication. You may be able to slow things down and avoid more serious trouble. If you have any of the following symptoms, tell your doctor:

- blurry or spotty vision
- tiredness
- pale skin color (could indicate poor blood flow)
- obesity (defined as 20 percent or more over your ideal body weight)
- numbness or tingling in hands or feet
- chest pain
- infections that occur often or cuts that heal slowly
- constant headaches (may signal high blood pressure).

continues

continued

Any other changes in your health that feel "wrong" should be brought to the attention of your doctor.

New treatments exist for many complications. Laser surgery can repair damage to the eyes. Many quick surgical techniques have made it easier to treat the blockage of arteries. Kidney transplantation has grown more successful for people with kidney disease. New methods of treating blocked blood vessels and wounds may help prevent amputation. In most cases, the faster and earlier you spot the problem, the better the outcome.

FACING TROUBLE

Some people work hard to control their blood glucose level and care for themselves. Yet they may still face the shock of learning they have a complication.

News of a complication is not a signal to stop caring for your diabetes. Yes, it is bad news. You may feel angry or hopeless. You may think "I've done so much to take care of myself, and how this happens. What was the point?"

The point was this: the care you took may have delayed the complication for years. In fact, the problem may be milder because you took such good care of yourself. Keep it up, because a healthy body is better able to fight back.

Paying attention to your health will also help you cope mentally. You will know that you are doing everything you can to live well with the complication.

- Do not smoke.
- Keep your blood glucose levels close to normal.
- Eat a healthy, balanced diet.
- Get regular exercise (with your doctor's okay).
- See your doctor (dentist and eye doctor, too) regularly, even if you feel great.
- Check your feet each day for small cuts or blisters. Your doctor should check your feet at each visit.
- Keep your weight under control.
- Keep your blood pressure and blood fat levels in the normal range.

When you are diagnosed with a complication, you take on a new job: learning to cope with this change. An action plan can help. Here are some suggestions:

- **Keep a positive attitude.** Staying hopeful and upbeat can improve and possibly lengthen your life. A negative attitude makes living with the complication harder, not only on you, but on your family and friends.

continues

continued

- **Be an active member of your health care team.** Speak up. If you don't think something will work for you, explain your feelings. Make suggestions. Ask about other treatments.
- **Learn about your complication.** Chances are, the better you understand your complication, the less out of control you will feel.

  Groups that focus on your complications may be good resources. Your local American Diabetes Association chapter can refer you to organizations such as the National Kidney Foundation or the Foundation for the Blind. Such organizations often know about the latest medical advances. They may supply names of leading doctors in the field and medical centers doing the latest research. They may even have information about insurance or government reimbursement.
- **Think about seeing a specialist** (a doctor with special training) who works with your complication. Don't worry about making your primary care doctor angry. Any doctor who wants the best for you will be glad you want to see a specialist. In fact, your doctor may refer you to a specialist when your complication is diagnosed.
- **Try to get a second opinion.** Any time you face a major change in your health or diabetes care, it is a good idea to get a second opinion. Before you go, check your health insurance. It may pay for the second opinion or even require it.
- **Ask questions of any health care professional who examines you.** What are the likely side effects of this treatment? How often will I need the treatment? Will I need new medications? How many patients with this problem have you treated? What were the results?
- **Be a wise medical consumer.** Don't be afraid to discuss money with your doctor. Some treatments cost more than others, but the most costly option may not be the best choice for you. What are the alternatives? Know what your insurance will pay for. If your insurance doesn't cover a treatment, you can try an appeal to the insurance company.
- **Build a support system.** You will probably feel better if you can open up, at least to one or two people.

  Make your family and friends part of that system. Let them know what it's like to live with your complication. Tell them about problems and choices you might face. When you don't talk about your feelings and needs, its hard for others to know how to help.

  If you find it hard to talk with family or friends, you may want to get help from a social worker or psychologist. Short-term counseling can help you through a time of high stress and change. Social workers may be able to help you find other resources that would help.

  Ask your doctor or American Diabetes Association chapter to put you in touch with others who have dealt with the same complication. Talking with someone who has been there is a good way to get moral support. It may also give you leads on treatment options or doctors.

LIVING WELL WITH COMPLICATIONS

Coping with a complication may mean making some changes in your lifestyle. But with work, you can often continue doing the same activities that you have always enjoyed. To stay active, you

continues

continued

will need the support of others. You will also need to rely strongly on yourself. There are many ways you can manage your own treatment and your own rehabilitation—retraining yourself to do tasks such as walking, preparing food, and exercising.

Vision Loss

If eye disease has left you with serious vision loss or blindness, many resources can help you. First, you may want to contact local agencies that work with the blind (you can get names from the American Diabetes Association). Large print books and books on cassette can give you access to written material. Low-vision aids, such as telescopes or magnifiers placed on glasses, can help you see objects far and near.

You can also regain certain skills through rehabilitation. You can learn to walk along using a cane or a guide dog. You can learn to pour coffee and even to inject your own insulin with the help of devices that indicate when you have measured the right amount. Counseling can teach you to function in your job, housekeeping, and child care. You can sharpen your other senses: hearing, small, touch, and the sense of your body's movement in space.

Amputation

An amputation is a scary prospect. But be confident that surgeons will always try to save as much of your leg or foot as possible. They just need to make sure that the part they leave will be able to heal. If you are having an amputation, you will want to work with a health-care team that includes a physician, a physical therapist, a prosthetist (someone who makes artificial limbs), a social worker, and a psychologist.

Physical therapy will start a day or two after surgery. You will work with your physical therapist on balance by using parallel bars. Later, you will move up to a walker or crutches. The therapist can show you how to fall and get up safely.

About four to eight weeks after surgery, the prosthetist will fit you with an artificial foot or leg. New designs permit easier walking and even running using prosthetic feet.

Losing a limb can often cause feelings of grief. It may help to talk to peer counselors who have also had amputations or to see a psychologist or social worker.

Dialysis

Dialysis is a common treatment for kidney disease. It replaces the function of the kidney by cleaning the blood. Depending on the type of dialysis, you will get treatment every day or three

continues

continued

times a week. A team of people will help you decide how to carry out dialysis: a nephrologist (a kidney specialist), a nephrology nurse who may also be a trained dialysis nurse, a kidney transplant surgeon and coordinator, a social worker, a psychologist, a renal dietitian, and a physical therapist.

The two types of dialysis are hemodialysis and peritoneal dialysis. Hemodialysis cleans the blood by filtering it through a machine outside the body. If you choose hemodialysis, you will probably get treated at a dialysis center three times a week. Each session will take about three to five hours. You may be able to get training with a partner so that the two of you can perform hemodialysis at home.

Unlike hemodialysis, peritoneal dialysis cleans the blood using a solution poured into the abdomen through a tube called a catheter. You can learn to perform this type of dialysis on your own at home. It is usually done daily.

Nerve Damage

The best way to handle nerve damage is to prevent injuries and additional complications. For example, when you lose feeling in your feet and toes, as in distinal neuropathy, it is easy to injure your foot without ever feeling it. For this reason, you should check your feet every day. Also check your shoes to make sure they contain no stones, staples, rough spots, or other sharp or lumpy objects that could hurt your feet.

Loss of feeling is why electric blankets and heating pads carry warning labels that say people with diabetes should not use them without talking to their doctors first. You can be seriously burned by an electric blanket or heating pad because you cannot feel how hot it really is.

Be on the alert for urinary infections. These tend to happen again and again when your bladder is affected by nerve damage known as autonomic neuropathy. Tell your doctor if you have cloudy or bloody urine, painful urination, low back pain, and fever. One way to help prevent these infections is to urinate every three to four hours when you are awake, even if you don't feel as if you need to.

There are drugs that can treat faintness, stomach trouble, or diarrhea caused by autonomic neuropathy.

WHAT EXERCISE CAN DO

Staying active in your health-care is a key aspect of coping well. Staying physically active is equally important for most people. When diabetes seems to be dealing you hard blows, exercise may be the last things you want to think about. After all, isn't it out of the question for someone

continues

continued

in your condition? No. In fact, regular exercise is a good idea for almost everyone. When you live with a diabetes complication, you may need exercise more than ever. Here's why.

When a physical problem, like vision loss or surgery, keeps you from being active, your whole body suffers. That's because parts of your body are not getting used enough. Muscles need to be regularly exercised to stay strong. If they aren't, they become too weak to do even easy tasks like taking out the trash or making the bed.

You can make your muscles stronger and more effective by regular exercise. This doesn't mean you have to lift weights, go to the gym, or make drastic changes. Regular exercise can be very modest. In fact, if you haven't done much for a long time, or are adjusting to limited mobility, you must start slowly. Of course, you need to talk about exercise with your doctor. Never start an exercise program without your doctor's okay. Very high blood glucose levels may make exercise dangerous. If you are over 35 years of age, be sure to have a heart evaluation before starting an exercise program.

Below are some common complications and exercises that might be good choices for each. Discuss these with your doctor. Ask your doctor to help you find an exercise physiologist who has worked with people with your complication. You, your doctor, and the exercise specialist can plan a safe exercise program for you.

Nerve Damage in the Limbs

If you have nerve damage to the hands, legs, or feet, you may feel pain, tingling, or numbness in those areas. Exercise won't cure the problem, but it can help. Regular exercise can help you keep your strength, flexibility, and blood flow to those damaged areas. If you combine regular exercise with good blood glucose control, you may be able to relieve some of the pain. This may take some time, however.

Good choices for people with nerve damage in the legs or feet are activities that don't put a lot of stress on the legs, feet, or nearby joints. These might include bicycling or easy rowing on a rowing machine. If pushing with your feet doesn't feel good or is not safe, you can try a special machine you pedal with your arms.

Swimming and aqua aerobics are also good choices for almost anyone. Be sure to take care of your feet. Wear shoes such as water socks while you are in the water on walking around the pool and locker room area. If you have an open wound, do not use the pool until it heals.

Autonomic Neuropathy

Avoid activities that require quick changes in body position. You may have problems with low blood pressure, which can make you faint. Aerobics or sports such as baseball, basketball, or tennis are not good choices for you. Do not exercise at high intensity.

continues

continued

Good exercise choices include: recumbent stationary cycling (using a special kind of bike that you allows you to stretch your legs out in front of pedal) and aqua aerobics.

Retinopathy and Vision Loss

If you have proliferative retinopathy (serious damage to the small blood vessels of the eye), exercise can hurt your vision. First, get treatment. After treatment, when your retinopathy is stable, you will probably be able to exercise. Make sure your eye doctor and your primary care doctor say your eyes are ready.

When you have retinopathy or vision loss from diabetes, you may be told not to do exercises when you put your head below your waist. You may also be told not to play contact sports like basketball or football.

If your vision is mildly impaired, you can still enjoy aerobic exercise. Here are some choices: ride a stationary bike, take a brisk walk on a treadmill, row at an easy pace on a rowing machine, dance with a partner who can guide you, or ride on the back of bicycle built for two.

Water exercises are great for people with low or partial vision. You can swim laps, guiding yourself by touching the pool's lane ropes. You can do aqua aerobics in the pool's shallow end.

Kidney Disease and High Blood Pressure

You need to take care when you exercise. Get your doctor's okay on your exercise plans. Avoid activities that are high intensity. They will increase your blood pressure. If your workout feels too hard, it probably is. Do not do competitive weight lifting. You can use light weights to build muscle strength and mass.

If you do endurance aerobic sports—like running for 45 minutes—it is important to drink fluids before, during, and after the workout.

Blood Vessel Damage

Has your doctor told you have intermittent claudication? Do you get an aching pain in your legs when you walk? This happens because the blood vessels in your legs sometimes close up so that your working muscles can't get as much blood as they need. Talk to your doctor about types of exercise that might help increase blood flow in the legs. Talk to your doctor about interval walking. You alternate resting and walking short distances to avoid pain and fatigue. Ask your doctor if any of your medications will make it hard to exercise.

continues

continued

Heart Disease and High Blood Pressure

If you have heart disease or high blood pressure, you can still benefit from regular exercise. But you must work out a program with your doctor and exercise specialist. Your doctor may refer you to a cardiac rehabilitation program. This is a medically supervised program that tests your fitness level and makes specific exercise suggestions for you. When you start to exercise in such a program, you can build your confidence and abilities in a safe environment.

After Transplantation

Why is exercise a key part of your recovery from kidney, pancreas, or kidney/pancreas transplantation? First, organ transplantation usually leads to weight gain for people with diabetes. This happens because you can eat more foods than you could before transplantation, and you have to take the drug prednisone. Prednisone helps your body accept the new organ, but it also causes weight gain.

Prednisone also causes muscles to waste and weaken. Regular aerobic exercise and strength training are the best ways to keep these side effects under control. You need to go slowly, however. Discuss your exercise program with your health-care team and exercise specialist.

Amputation and Limited Mobility

If you have limited mobility from diabetes or other health problems (such as arthritis), some good exercise choices might be water exercise or chair aerobics. Often, there are special classes available. Staying with regular exercise can help you keep the mobility you have.

You may have trouble with balance or standing on your feet. Or you may have had a foot or leg amputation. If your feet can't hold your body weight, you can try riding a stationary bike, chair exercise, or some form of adapted water exercise. You will be surprised how much exercise can help improve your strength and flexibility. Discuss your options with your doctor and exercise specialist.

A FINAL WORD

It's important to know that whatever diabetes complication you have, there are resources to help you cope. Talk to your health-care team, American Diabetes Association chapter, trained counselor, or other people in the same situation. You do not have to face a complication alone.

Source: "Diabetes Day-By-Day 40," *Coping with Complications,* © American Diabetes Association, Alexandria, Virginia.

Heart Disease and Diabetes

Heart disease is the most common life-threatening disease linked to diabetes. Experts say diabetes doubles a person's risk of developing heart disease.

WHAT IS HEART DISEASE?

In heart disease, deposits of fat and cholesterol build up in the arteries that supply the heart with blood. If this buildup blocks blood from getting to the heart, a potentially fatal heart attack can occur.

RISK FACTORS

Besides diabetes, other risk factors include

- high blood pressure
- being overweight
- high amounts of fats and cholesterol in blood
- cigarette smoking

Eliminating these risk factors, along with treating diabetes, can reduce the risk of heart disease. The American Heart Association has literature that explains what heart disease is and how to prevent it.

NOTES:

Source: "Noninsulin-Dependent Diabetes," National Institutes of Health, NIH Publication No. 95–241, September 1992.

Women with Diabetes: Risk Factor for Heart Disease

Diabetes, or high blood sugar, is not only a serious disorder but also an independent risk factor for coronary heart disease. More than 80 percent of people who have diabetes die of some form of cardiovascular disease, usually heart attack. The risk of death from coronary heart disease is doubled in women with diabetes. Many diabetic women also have higher blood pressure and blood cholesterol levels than nondiabetic women.

In addition to coronary heart disease, untreated diabetes can contribute to the development of kidney disease, blindness, problems in pregnancy and childbirth, nerve and blood vessel damage, and a reduced ability to fight infection.

Diabetes is often called a "woman's disease" because, after age 45, about twice as many women as men develop the disease. This maturity-inset diabetes is generally noninsulin-dependent diabetes mellitus (NIDDM). In NIDDM, the most common form of diabetes, the pancreas produces insulin but the body is unable to use it effectively. For reasons not entirely clear, the risks of heart disease and heart-related death are higher for diabetic women than for diabetic men.

Although there is no cure for diabetes, there are steps one can take to control it. About 85 percent of NIDDM patients are at least 20 percent overweight. Obesity and aging seem to promote the development of diabetes in those who are susceptible to the disease.

Weight reduction and increased physical activity appear to help postpone or even prevent diabetes. For effective and lasting weight loss, exercise should be accompanied by an appropriate diet. Regular, brisk exercise will help one to maintain a healthy weight. Attaining normal weight is also important for those who have diabetes. It helps them to achieve better metabolic balance and improved health, as well as reducing the risk of coronary heart disease.

Source: *The Healthy Heart Handbook for Women,* Publication No. 89-2720, U.S. Department of Health and Human Services, National Heart, Lung, and Blood Institute, 1989.

Kidney Disease and Diabetes

The kidneys filter waste products from the blood and excrete them in the form of urine, maintaining proper fluid balance in the body. While people can live without one kidney, those without both must have special treatment, called dialysis.

People with diabetes are more likely to develop kidney disease than other people. Most people with diabetes will never develop kidney disease, but proper diabetes treatment can further reduce the risk.

High blood pressure also can add to the risk of kidney disease. Therefore, regular blood pressure checks and early treatment of the disorder can help prevent kidney disease.

URINARY TRACT INFECTIONS

Urinary tract infections are also a cause of kidney problems. Diabetes can affect the nerves that control the bladder, making it difficult for a person to empty his or her bladder completely. Bacteria can form in the unemptied bladder and the tubes leading from it, eventually causing infection.

The symptoms of a urinary tract infection include frequent, painful urination, blood in the urine, and pain in the lower abdomen and back.

Without prompt examination and treatment by a doctor, the infection can reach the kidneys, causing pain, fever, and possibly kidney damage. A doctor may prescribe antibiotics to treat the infection and may suggest that the person drink large amounts of water.

OTHER KIDNEY PROBLEMS

Kidney problems are one cause of water retention, or edema, a condition in which fluid collects in the body, causing swelling, often in the legs and hands. A doctor can decide if swelling or water retention relates to kidney function.

A nephrologist, a doctor specially trained to diagnose and treat kidney problems, can identify the cause of problems and recommend ways to reduce the risk of kidney disease.

Source: "Noninsulin-Dependent Diabetes," National Institutes of Health, NIH Publication No. 95–241, September 1992.

Diabetes and Your Kidneys

Some people with diabetes will develop kidney problems. These problems are serious because the kidneys remove waste materials from your body. Doctors feel there are two main reasons that influence whether people with diabetes will develop kidney problems:

1. contracting diabetes at a young age

2. having diabetes for a long time

You can take steps to decrease the possibility that you will have kidney problems. Studies have shown that people with diabetes are less likely to develop kidney problems if they do not have high blood sugar levels. Therefore, maintain a level of blood sugar as nearly normal as possible.

High blood pressure also increases your risk of developing kidney problems. Your blood pressure should be checked each time you see your doctor. The earlier the doctor discovers high blood pressure, the sooner it can be treated. If your doctor finds that you have high blood pressure, he or she may prescribe a drug to treat it.

Eating a lot of salt can increase your chances of getting high blood pressure. It is a good idea to cut down on the amount of salt you eat.

- Leave the salt shaker off the dinner table.

- Cook with unsalted water.

- Avoid buying canned soups and foods with a high salt content. (Some grocery stores have special shelves for low-salt foods.)

People with diabetes are more likely to have kidney infections. If you have a kidney infection, you may feel as if you have to urinate all the time. You may also have a burning feeling when you urinate. If you have either of these feelings, see your doctor immediately. He or she will want to collect a urine sample to detect the infection. The doctor may prescribe a drug to help your body fight infection.

Your doctor may want to test your urine and take blood samples regularly. These steps will allow the doctor to detect a developing kidney problem early. If you do develop kidney disease, your doctor may refer you to a special medical center.

Source: *The Prevention and Treatment of Five Complications of Diabetes: A Guide for Primary Care Practitioners.* National Diabetes Advisory Board, U.S. Department of Health and Human Services, Public Health Service, Centers for Disease Control, Atlanta, Georgia, 1983.

Kidney Disease: Options for Prevention and Treatment

Kidneys are remarkable organs. Inside them are millions of tiny blood vessels that act as filters. Their job is to remove waste products from the blood.

But sometimes this filtering system breaks down. Failing kidneys lose their ability to filter out waste products. One cause of kidney failure is diabetes.

WHY DIABETES DAMAGES KIDNEYS

When our bodies digest the protein we eat, the process creates waste products that build up in the blood. In the kidneys, millions of tiny blood vessels (capillaries) with even tinier holes in them act as filters. As blood flows through the blood vessels, small molecules such as waste products squeeze through the holes. These waste products become part of the urine. Useful substances, such as protein and red blood cells, are too big to pass through the holes in the filter. They stay where they belong—in the blood.

Diabetes can damage this system. High levels of glucose make the kidneys filter too much blood. All this extra work is hard on the filters. After many years, they start to leak. Useful protein is lost in the urine. Having small amounts of protein in the urine is called microalbuminuria. Having larger amounts is called proteinuria or macroalbuminuria.

In time, the stress of overwork causes some filters to collapse. This collapse makes more work for the remaining filters and they, too, begin collapsing. As the capillaries lose their filtering ability, waste products start to build up in the blood.

Finally, the kidneys fail. This failure is called end-stage renal disease (ESRD). ESRD is very serious. A person with ESRD needs either to have a kidney transplant or to have the blood filtered by machine (dialysis).

WHO GETS KIDNEY DISEASE

Not everyone with diabetes develops kidney disease. Factors that can influence development include genetics, blood glucose control, and blood pressure.

The better a person keeps diabetes under control, the lower the chance of getting kidney disease. High blood pressure should also be kept under control. The healthier the blood pressure, the healthier the kidneys will be.

More than 30 percent of people with insulin-dependent (type I) diabetes will one day have kidney disease, compared with perhaps 10 percent of people with noninsulin-dependent (type II)

continues

continued

diabetes. People with type I diabetes have 15 times the risk of ESRD as those with type II diabetes. The longer a person has diabetes, the higher the risk of kidney disease—up to a point. After 40 years with diabetes, if a person does not yet have kidney disease, he or she probably never will.

Men are 50 percent more likely to get kidney disease than women. Native Americans are seven times more likely to have kidney disease than other white people. Other ethnic groups at greater risk are blacks (three to four times the risk of whites) and Mexican Americans.

Most people who get diabetic kidney disease also have diabetic eye problems.

SYMPTOMS AND DIAGNOSIS

The kidneys work so hard to make up for the failing capillaries that kidney disease produces no symptoms until almost all function is gone. Also, the symptoms are not specific. The first symptom is often fluid buildup. Others include loss of sleep, tiredness, poor appetite, upset stomach, vomiting, weakness, and difficulty concentrating.

It is vital to see a doctor regularly. The doctor can test the urine for protein, check whether blood pressure is high, and detect diabetic eye problems.

PREVENTION

Diabetic kidney disease can be prevented by tight blood glucose control. In the Diabetes Control and Complications Trial, tight control reduced the risk of microalbuminuria by a third. In people who already had microalbuminuria, the risk of progressing to proteinuria was about half in people on tight control. Other studies have suggested that tight control can reverse microalbuminuria.

TREATMENTS FOR KIDNEY DISEASE

When kidney disease is diagnosed early (during microalbuminuria), several treatments may keep it from getting worse. When kidney disease is caught later (during proteinuria), ESRD always follows. Treatment at this stage can only delay the inevitable.

One important treatment is tight blood glucose control.

Another important treatment is tight control of blood pressure. Blood pressure has a dramatic effect on the rate at which the disease progresses. Even a mild rise in blood pressure can quickly make the disease worsen. Three ways to bring blood pressure down are losing weight, eating less salt, and avoiding alcohol and tobacco.

When these methods fail, certain medicines may be able to lower blood pressure. There are several kinds of blood pressure drugs. Not all are equally good for people with diabetes to take.

continues

continued

Some raise blood glucose levels or mask some of the symptoms of low blood glucose. Those that doctors prefer for people with diabetes are called calcium-channel blockers, alpha blockers, and ACE inhibitors.

ACE inhibitors may turn out to be the best drug treatment. Recent studies suggest that these drugs—which include captopril and enalapril—slow kidney disease in addition to lowering blood pressure. In fact, these drugs are helpful even in people who do not have high blood pressure.

Another treatment some doctors use is a low-protein diet. Protein seems to increase how hard the kidneys must work. A low-protein diet can decrease protein loss in the urine and increase protein levels in the blood. Never start a low-protein diet without talking to your doctor first.

Once kidneys fail, these treatments are no longer useful. Dialysis is then necessary. The person must choose whether to continue with dialysis or to get a kidney transplant. This choice should be made as a team effort. The team should include the doctor and diabetes educator, a nephrologist (kidney doctor), a kidney transplant surgeon, a social worker, and a psychologist.

KIDNEY TRANSPLANTS

A kidney transplant, if successful, frees the person from dialysis. It makes the quality of life dramatically better.

The immune system's job is to protect the body from foreign substances. As a result, the immune system will reject any organ it perceives as foreign. To reduce the chance that the immune system will reject the donated kidney, doctors prefer donors whose immune systems are similar to those of the patients. The best donor is a healthy relative. To further lower the chance of rejection, people with kidney transplants must take powerful drugs to suppress their immune systems for the rest of their lives.

Having a kidney transplant is a serious matter. The operation is a major one, and the drugs are dangerous with many side effects. But people who get kidney transplants are more likely to be alive after 5 years than people who stay on dialysis.

DIALYSIS

Dialysis is a way of cleaning the blood with an artificial kidney. Dialysis is the more common form of kidney-replacement therapy. There are two types of dialysis: hemodialysis and peritoneal dialysis.

No matter which type is chosen, the person undergoing dialysis needs to work closely with the health care team to keep diabetes under control.

continues

continued

HEMODIALYSIS

In hemodialysis, an artificial kidney removes waste from the blood. To get the blood to the artificial kidney, there has to be access to the blood vessels. The place where blood is drawn is called the access connection site. Preparing this site—usually in the arm—requires surgery. The surgeon may connect a vein to an artery to make a large "vein" called a fistula or a loop. (A vein carries blood to the heart. An artery carries blood away from the heart.) Or the surgeon may implant a straight piece of tubing.

The more common name for the fistula is an access. Usually, this surgery is done 2 to 3 months before dialysis is to begin so that the body has time to heal. In most cases, the surgeon puts the access in the arm not used for writing.

To begin dialysis, two needles are placed in the access. One is for outgoing blood, and the other is for blood returning to the body. Blood is pumped from the arm to a dialysis machine. One compartment of this machine holds this incoming blood. A second compartment has a specially treated solution called dialysate. Separating the two compartments is a thin membrane with thousands of tiny holes.

This membrane acts like the filters in a healthy kidney. The waste products in the blood pass through the holes into the dialysate. Blood cells, protein, and other vital substances are too large to pass through the holes. They remain in the first compartment and are returned to the body. Blood is removed at the same time. Only a small amount is absent from the body at once. Dialysate flows constantly during dialysis. After it picks up waste products from the blood, it is discarded down a drain.

For home hemodialysis, a partner (such as a relative or technician) must help the person and stay during the procedure. Both the patient and the dialysis partner must take training at a certified facility. This training takes four to six weeks.

Hemodialysis is not perfect for everyone. Some people have health complications. These include progressive nerve damage, problems regulating insulin dosages, malnutrition, increased rates of infection, and increased problems accessing the blood vessels. Sometimes, these complications are the result of diabetes, not of hemodialysis.

Hemodialysis can cause other problems as well. These include high or low blood pressure, upset stomach or vomiting, anemia, and bone disease.

PERITONEAL DIALYSIS

Many doctors think peritoneal dialysis a better treatment than hemodialysis. There are a variety of methods. The two most common forms are continuous ambulatory peritoneal dialysis (CAPD)

continues

continued

and automated peritoneal dialysis (APD). APD is also called continuous cyclic peritoneal dialysis (CCPD).

The principles for peritoneal dialysis are similar to those for hemodialysis. But instead of blood being cleaned in an artificial kidney, the body itself is used as a filter. In peritoneal dialysis, wastes are filtered out of the blood through the peritoneum. The peritoneum is a thin membrane that lines the abdominal cavity.

A small catheter is placed surgically in the lower abdomen. This catheter remains in the person indefinitely. Usually, the catheter is changed if it doesn't work or if it becomes infected and the infection won't heal.

In peritoneal dialysis, a cleansing fluid (dialysate) is poured into the abdominal cavity through the catheter. Waste products pass from the blood vessels through the peritoneal membrane and into the dialysate. After a while the dialysate—with the waste products—is drained from the abdomen.

People can perform CAPD themselves by connecting a flexible plastic bag filled with dialysate to a piece of tubing attached to the catheter. Next, the bag is raised to shoulder height. Gravity makes the dialysate flow down into the abdominal cavity. After the bag is empty, it can be disconnected. Some people leave the bag there, but roll it up and place it under their clothing. When the dialysate is in the abdomen, wastes and excess water pass from the tiny blood vessels in the peritoneal membrane into the dialysate. The person can move around freely and perform most daily activities.

Afterward, the bag is again connected to the catheter and lowered below the abdomen. Gravity now makes the dialysate containing waste products drain out. Once the bag is full, it is discarded. Then a new container of dialysate is connected, and the process is repeated.

An exchange, which includes draining the solution and adding new dialysate, takes about 45 minutes. Usually the dialysate remains in the abdomen 4 to 6 hours before being exchanged. At night, the dialysate is left in for about 8 hours. The exchange of dialysis needs to be done three to five times a day.

CAPD has several advantages over hemodialysis. First, it prevents major changes in body chemistry and fluid levels. Preventing large fluid gains may reduce stress on the heart and blood vessels. Second, people using this treatment are not tied to a machine. They can eat a more liberal diet and are better able to hold a job, go to school, or travel. Third, they have better control of blood pressure levels and less anemia. Fourth, they can put insulin in the peritoneal cavity with the dialysate. Insulin taken this way better controls blood glucose.

The major problem with CAPD is infection, which can occur in the abdomen or at the catheter. A person using CAPD must keep the catheter area clean and follow all procedures carefully. Some people get lower back problems and weak abdominal wall muscles or a hernia.

continues

continued

CAPD is not for everyone. A person must see well and have good motor skills.

CCPD is similar to CAPD in that the exchange of dialysate and blood is done in the abdominal cavity. The difference is that in CCPD, the exchange is done automatically by a machine called a cycler.

A cycler delivers the dialysate and drains it. It does not need to be done so manually. The exchange of dialysate usually occurs at night during sleep. The cycler does three to five short exchanges during the night. When the person using it wakes up, he or she unhooks the cycler from the catheter. Before disconnecting, new dialysate is pumped into the abdomen. That solution dialyzes during the day and then is drained in the evening.

This type of peritoneal dialysis may be ideal for people unable or unwilling to do CAPD. It is also better for people who do not see well, those prone to low blood pressure, and those who have weak abdominal wall muscles.

The problems of CCPD are the same as with CAPD. Putting insulin into the peritoneal cavity is harder with CCPD.

THE BOTTOM LINE

All treatments for ESRD cost a lot of money. Dialysis, depending on the type, can cost $20,000 to $30,000 a year.

Costs of kidney transplants vary more widely, in part because the costs of removing, preparing, and transporting the donor's kidney vary a lot. But you can expect to pay tens of thousands of dollars for a transplant.

Most insurance plans, including Medicare, will help pay for the costs of dialysis and kidney transplantation. Check with your insurer about its policies.

Source: "Diabetes Day-by-Day 36," *Kidney Disease,* © American Diabetes Association, Alexandria, Virginia.

End-Stage Renal Disease and Hemodialysis

WHEN YOUR KIDNEYS FAIL

Healthy kidneys clean the blood by filtering out extra water and wastes. They also make hormones that keep your bones strong and blood healthy. When both of your kidneys fail, your body holds up fluid. Your blood pressure rises. Harmful wastes build up in your body. Your body doesn't make enough red blood cells. When this happens, you need treatment to replace the work of your failed kidneys.

HEMODIALYSIS

Purpose

Hemodialysis is a procedure that cleans and filters your blood. It rids your body of harmful wastes and extra salt and fluids. It also controls your blood pressure and helps your body keep the proper balance of chemicals such as potassium, sodium, and chloride.

How It Works

Hemodialysis uses a dialyzer, or special filter, to clean your blood. The dialyzer connects to a machine. During treatment, your blood travels through tubes into the dialyzer. The dialyzer filters out wastes and extra fluids. The newly cleaned blood flows through another set of tubes and back into your body.

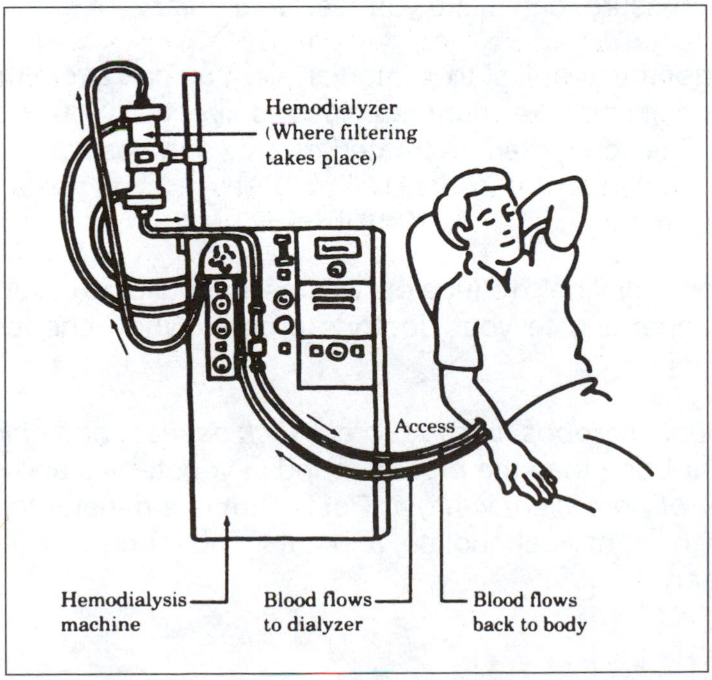

continues

continued

Getting Ready

Before your first treatment, an access to your bloodstream must be made. The access provides a way for blood to be carried from your body to the dialysis machine and then back into your body. The access can be internal (inside the body—usually under your skin) or external (outside the body).

Who Performs It?

Hemodialysis can be done at home or at a center. At a center, nurses or trained technicians perform the treatment. At home, you perform hemodialysis with the help of a partner, usually a family member or friend. If you decide to do home dialysis, you and your partner will receive special training.

The Time It Takes

Hemodialysis usually is done three times a week. Each treatment lasts from 2 to 4 hours. During treatment, you can read, write, sleep, talk, or watch TV.

Possible Complications

Side effects can be caused by rapid changes in your body's fluid and chemical balance during treatment. Muscle cramps and hypotension are two common side effects. Hypotension, a sudden drop in blood pressure, can make you feel weak, dizzy, or sick to your stomach.

It usually takes a few months to adjust to hemodialysis. You can avoid many of the side effects if you follow the proper diet and take your medicines as directed. You should always report side effects to your doctor. They can often be treated quickly and easily.

Your Diet

Hemodialysis and a proper diet help reduce the wastes that build up in your blood. A dietitian can help you plan meals according to your doctor's orders. When choosing foods, you should remember to:

- *Eat balanced amounts of foods high in protein such as meat and chicken.* Animal protein is better used by your body than the protein found in vegetables and grains.
- *Watch the amount of potassium you eat.* Potassium is a mineral found in salt substitutes, some fruits, vegetables, milk, chocolate, and nuts. Too much or too little potassium can be harmful to your heart.

continues

continued

- *Limit how much you drink.* Fluids build up quickly in your body when your kidneys aren't working. Too much fluid makes your tissues swell. It can also cause high blood pressure and heart trouble.
- *Avoid salt.* Salty foods make you thirsty and cause your body to hold water.
- *Limit foods such as milk, cheese, nuts, dried beans, and soft drinks.* These foods contain the mineral phosphorus. Too much phosphorus in your blood causes calcium to be pulled from your bones. Calcium helps keep bones strong and healthy. To prevent bone problems, your doctor may give you special medicines. You must take these medicines everyday as directed.

Pros and Cons

Each person responds differently to similar situations. What may be a negative factor for one person may be positive for another. However, in general, the following are pros and cons for each type of hemodialysis.

In-Center Hemodialysis

Pros	Cons
• You have trained professionals with you at all times. • You can get to know other patients.	• Treatments are scheduled by the center. • You must travel to the center for treatment.

Home Hemodialysis

Pros	Cons
• You can do it at the hours you choose. *(But you still must do it as often as your doctor orders.)* • You don't have to travel to a center. • You gain a sense of independence and control over your treatment.	• Helping with treatments may be stressful to your family. • You need training. • You need space for storing the machine and supplies at home.

Working with Your Health Care Team

Questions you may want to ask:

- Is hemodialysis the best treatment choice for me? Why or why not?
- If I am treated at a center, can I go to the center of my choice?
- What does hemodialysis feel like? Does it hurt?
- What is self-care dialysis?

continues

continued

- How long does it take to learn hemodialysis? Who will train my partner and me?
- What kind of blood access is best for me?
- As a hemodialysis patient, will I be able to keep working? Can I have treatment at night if I plan to keep working?
- How much should I exercise?
- Who will be on my health care team? How can they help me?
- Who can I talk with about sexuality, family problems, or money concerns?
- How/where can I talk to other people who have faced this decision?

NOTES:

Source: "End-Stage Renal Disease: Choosing a Treatment That's Right for You," NIH Publication No. 94-2412, National Institutes of Health, June 1994.

Hemodialysis—Know Your Number

WHAT IS THE NUMBER?

The **number** is a measure of a waste product in your blood, called urea. Dialysis acts like your kidneys by taking waste products out of your blood. The number tells you how much your urea has gone down after dialysis.

Two measures are used:

- Urea Reduction Ratio (URR)
- KT/V

WHY IS MY NUMBER IMPORTANT?

The number shows you how well your dialysis treatments are working.

If you have too much urea in your blood after dialysis, it can make you feel sick.

People with less urea in their blood feel better, are healthier, and live longer.

WHAT SHOULD MY NUMBER BE?

If your dialysis center uses URR, the urea in your blood should have gone down by 65 percent (0.65) or more after your dialysis treatment.

If your dialysis center uses KT/V, your number should be 1.2 or above after your dialysis treatment.

Your dialysis staff can give you more information about these measurements.

HOW CAN I FIND OUT WHAT MY NUMBER IS?

Your nurse, dietitian, or doctor at your dialysis center can give you your number. You may want to record your number on the URR or KT/V chart below.

Your number may change a little. But if your URR is less than 0.65 or your KT/V is less than 1.2, it is important for you and your doctor to talk about possible ways to improve your number.

ARE THERE OTHER NUMBERS I NEED TO KNOW ABOUT?

There are many tests done for you at the dialysis center. However, studies have shown that URR or KT/V results help show how well your dialysis is working.

continues

continued

WHAT CAN I DO TO HELP KEEP MY NUMBER UP?

- Always go to all of your scheduled dialysis treatments.
- Stay for the full treatment.
- Make sure you follow your diet.
- Follow the advice of your dialysis staff on caring for yourself.
- Talk to your doctor or nurse if your number is low.

Talk to your dialysis staff if you need help with transportation, meals, or other things.

At the end of this handout are two charts you can use to keep track of your URR or KT/V number.

Ask your dialysis nurse or your doctor for your number.

Keep a record of your number by putting an **X** in the box on the chart below. If your **X** falls below the dotted line, talk to your doctor, or nurse.

If your dialysis center is not collecting this information, discuss it with them or call the End-Stage Renal Disease Network in your area.

For Urea Reduction Ratio (URR)

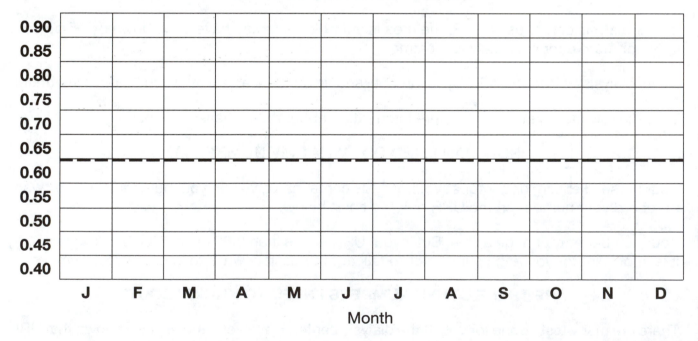

continues

continued

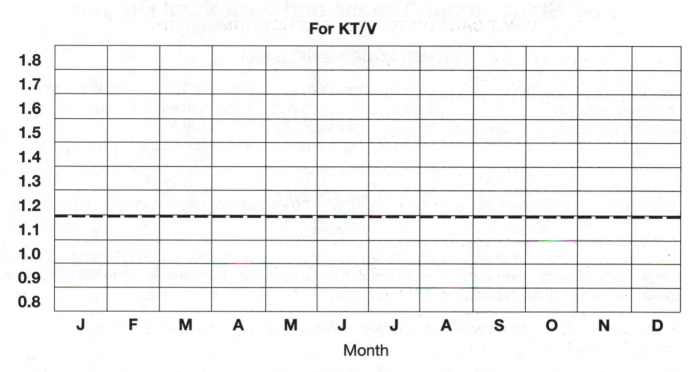

For KT/V

Source: "It's Your Life . . . Know Your Number. A Patient Guide to Two Important Measures That Show How Well Your Hemodialysis Is Working," U.S. Department of Health and Human Services, Health Care Financing Administration.

End-Stage Renal Disease and Peritoneal Dialysis

WHEN YOUR KIDNEYS FAIL

Healthy kidneys clean the blood by filtering out extra water and wastes. They also make hormones that keep your bones strong and blood healthy. When both of your kidneys fail, your body holds up fluid. Your blood pressure rises. Harmful wastes build up in your body. Your body doesn't make enough red blood cells. When this happens, you need treatment to replace the work of your failed kidneys.

Peritoneal Dialysis

Purpose

Peritoneal dialysis is another procedure that replaces the work of your kidneys. It removes extra water, wastes, and chemicals from your body. This type of dialysis uses the lining of your abdomen to filter your blood. This lining is called the peritoneal membrane.

How It Works

A cleansing solution, called dialysate, travels through a special tube into your abdomen. Fluid, wastes, and chemicals pass from tiny blood vessels in the peritoneal membrane into the dialysate. After several hours, the dialysate gets drained from your abdomen, taking the wastes from your blood with it. Then you fill your abdomen with fresh dialysate and the cleaning process begins again.

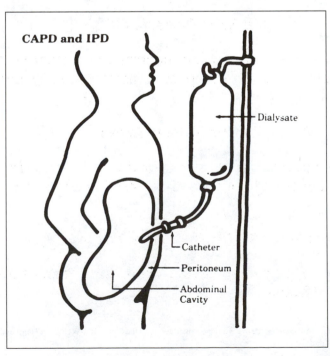

continues

continued

Getting Ready

Before your first treatment, a surgeon places a small, soft tube called a catheter into your abdomen. This catheter always stays there. It helps transport the dialysate to and from your peritoneal membrane.

Types of Personal Dialysis

There are three types of peritoneal dialysis:

1. Continuous Ambulatory Peritoneal Dialysis (CAPD)—With CAPD, your blood is always being cleaned. The dialysate passes from a plastic bag through the catheter and into your abdomen. The dialysate stays in your abdomen with the catheter sealed. After several hours, you drain the solution back into the bag. Then you refill your abdomen with fresh solution through the same catheter. Now the cleaning process begins again. While the solution is in your body, you may fold the empty plastic bag and hide it under your clothes, around your waist, or in a pocket.
2. Continuous Cyclic Peritoneal Dialysis (CCPD)—CCPD is like CAPD except that a machine, which connects to your catheter automatically fills and drains the dialysate from your abdomen. The machine does this at night while you sleep.
3. Intermittent Peritoneal Dialysis (IPD)—IPD uses the same type of machine as CCPD to add and drain the dialysate. IPD can be done at home, but it's usually done in the hospital. IPD treatments take longer than CCPD.

Who Performs It?

CAPD is a form of self-treatment. It needs no machine and no partner. However, with IPD and CCPD, you need a machine and the help of a partner (family member, friend, or health professional).

The Time It Takes

With CAPD, the dialysate stays in your abdomen for about 4 to 6 hours. The process of draining the dialysate and replacing fresh solution takes 30 to 40 minutes. Most people change the solution four times a day.

With CCPD, treatments last from 10 to 12 hours every night.

With IPD, treatments are done several times a week, for a total of 36 to 42 hours per week. Sessions may last up to 24 hours.

continues

continued

Possible Complications

Peritonitis, or infection of the peritoneum, can occur if the opening where the catheter enters your body gets infected. You can also get it if there is a problem connecting or disconnecting the catheter from the bags. Peritonitis can make you feel sick. It can cause fever and stomach pain.

To avoid peritonitis, you must be careful to follow the procedure exactly. You must know the early signs of peritonitis. Look for reddening or swelling around the catheter. You should also note if your dialysate looks cloudy. It is important to report these signs to your doctor so that the peritonitis can be treated quickly to avoid serious problems.

Your Diet

Diet for peritoneal dialysis is slightly different than diet for hemodialysis.

- You may be able to have more salt and fluids.
- You may eat more protein.
- You may have different potassium restrictions.
- You may need to cut back on the number of calories you eat. This limitation is because the sugar in the dialysate may cause you to gain weight.

Pros and Cons

There are pros and cons to each type of peritoneal dialysis.

Continuous Ambulatory Peritoneal Dialysis

Pros	Cons
• You can perform treatment alone. • You can do it at times you choose. • You can do it in many locations. • You don't need a machine.	• It disrupts your daily schedule.

Continuous Cyclic Peritoneal Dialysis

Pros	Cons
• You can do it at night, mainly while you sleep.	• You need a machine and help from a partner.

continues

continued

Intermittent Peritoneal Dialysis

Pros	Cons
• Health professionals usually perform treatments.	• You may need to go to a hospital. • It takes a lot of time. • You need a machine.

Working with Your Health Care Team

Questions you may want to ask:

- Is peritoneal dialysis the best treatment choice for me? Why or why not? Which type?
- How long will it take me to learn peritoneal dialysis?
- What does peritoneal dialysis feel like? Does it hurt?
- How will peritoneal dialysis affect my blood pressure?
- How do I know if I have peritonitis? How is peritonitis treated?
- As a peritoneal dialysis patient, will I be able to continue working?
- How much should I exercise?
- Who will be on my health care team? How can they help me?
- Who can I talk with about sexuality, finances, or family concerns?
- How/where can I talk to other people who have faced this decision?

Dialysis Is Not a Cure

Hemodialysis and peritoneal dialysis are treatments that try to replace your failed kidneys. These treatments help you feel better and live longer, but they are not cures for end-stage renal disease (ESRD). While patients with ESRD are now living longer than ever, ESRD can cause problems over the years. Some problems are bone disease, high blood pressure, nerve damage, and anemia (having too few red blood cells). Although these problems won't go away with dialysis, doctors now have new and better ways to treat or prevent them. You should discuss these treatments with your doctor.

Source: "End-Stage Renal Disease: Choosing a Treatment That's Right for You," NIH Publication No. 94-2412, National Institutes of Health, June 1994.

End-Stage Renal Disease and Kidney Transplantation

KIDNEY TRANSPLANTATION

Purpose

Kidney transplantation is a procedure that places a healthy kidney from another person into your body. This one new kidney does all the work that your two failed kidneys cannot do.

How It Works

A surgeon places the new kidney inside your body between your upper thigh and abdomen. The surgeon connects the artery and vein of the new kidney to your artery and vein. Your blood flows through the new kidney and makes urine, just like your own kidneys did when they were healthy. The new kidney may start working right away or may take up to a few weeks to make urine. Your own kidneys are left where they are, unless they are causing infection or high blood pressure.

Getting Ready

You may receive a kidney from a member of your family. This kind of donor is called a living-related donor. You may receive a kidney from a person who has recently died. This type of donor is called a cadaver donor. Sometimes a spouse or a very close friend may donate a kidney. This kind of donor is called a living-unrelated donor.

It is very important for the donor's blood and tissues to closely match yours. This match will help prevent your body's immune system from fighting off, or rejecting, the new kidney. A lab will do the special tests on blood cells to find out if your body will accept the new kidney.

The Time It Takes

The time it takes to get a kidney varies. There are not enough cadaver donors for every person who needs a transplant. Because of this, you must be placed on a waiting list to receive a cadaver donor kidney. However, if a relative gives you a kidney, the transplant operation can be done sooner.

The surgery takes from 3 to 6 hours. The usual hospital stay may last from 10 to 14 days. After you leave the hospital, you will go to the clinic for regular follow-up visits.

If a relative or friend gives you a kidney, he or she will probably stay in the hospital for one week or less.

continues

continued

Possible Complications

Transplantation is not a cure. There is always a chance that your body will reject your new kidney, no matter how good the match. The chance of your body accepting the new kidney depends on your age, race, and medical condition.

Normally, 75 to 80 percent of transplants from cadaver donors are working one year after surgery. However, transplants from living relatives often work better than transplants from cadaver donors. This fact is because they are usually a closer match.

Your doctor will give you special drugs to help prevent rejection. These are called immunosuppressants. You will need to take these drugs every day for the rest of your life. Sometimes these drugs cannot stop your body from rejecting the new kidney. If this happens, you will go back to some form of dialysis and possibly wait for another transplant.

Treatment with these drugs may cause side effects. The most serious is that they weaken your immune system, making it easier for you to get infections. Some drugs also cause changes in how you look. Your face may get fuller. You may gain weight or develop acne or facial hair. Not all patients have these problems, and makeup and diet can help.

Some of these drugs may cause problems such as cataracts, extra stomach acid, and hip disease. In a smaller number of patients, these drugs also may cause liver or kidney damage when used for a long period of time.

Your Diet

Diet for transplant patients is less limiting than it is for dialysis patients. You may still have to cut back on some foods, though. Your diet will probably change as your medicines, blood values, weight, and blood pressure change.

- You may need to count calories. Your medicine may give you a bigger appetite and cause you to gain weight.
- You may have to limit eating salty foods. Your medications may cause salt to be held in your body, leading to high blood pressure.
- You may need to eat less protein. Some medications cause a higher level of wastes to build up in your bloodstream.

Pros and Cons

There are pros and cons to kidney transplantation.

continues

continued

Kidney Transplantation

Pros	Cons
• It works like a normal kidney. • It helps you feel healthier. • You have fewer diet restrictions. • There's no need for dialysis.	• It requires major surgery. • You may need to wait for a donor. • One transplant may not last a lifetime. Your body may reject the new kidney. • You will have to take drugs for the rest of your life.

Working with Your Health Care Team

Questions you may want to ask:

- Is transplantation the best treatment choice for me? Why or why not?
- What are my chances of having a successful transplant?
- How do I find out if a family member or friend can donate?
- What are the risks to a family member or friend if he/she donates?
- If a family member or friend doesn't donate, how do I get placed on a waiting list for a kidney? How long will I have to wait?
- What are the symptoms of rejection?
- Who will be on my health care team? How will they help me?
- Who can I talk to about sexuality, finances, or family concerns?
- How/where can I talk to other people who have faced this decision?

CONCLUSION

It's not always easy to decide which type of treatment is best for you. Your decision depends on your medical condition, lifestyle, and personal likes and dislikes. Discuss the pros and cons of each with your health care team. If you start one form of treatment and decide you'd like to try another, talk it over with your doctor. The key is to learn as much as you can about your choices. With that knowledge, you and your doctor will choose a treatment that suits you best.

PAYING FOR TREATMENT

Treatment for end-stage renal disease (ESRD) is expensive, but the Federal government helps pay for much of the cost. Often, private insurance or state programs pay the rest.

Medicare

Medicare pays for 80 percent of the cost of your dialysis treatments or transplant, no matter how old you are. To qualify:

continues

continued

- you must have worked long enough to be insured under Social Security (or be the child of someone who has) or
- you already must be receiving Social Security benefits

You should apply for Medicare as soon as possible after beginning dialysis. Often a social worker at your hospital or dialysis center will help you apply.

Private Insurance

Private insurance often pays for the entire cost of a treatment. Or it may pay for the 20 percent that Medicare does not cover. Private insurance also may pay for your prescription drugs.

Medicaid

Medicaid is a state program. Your income must be below a certain level to receive Medicaid funds. Medicaid may pay for your treatments if you cannot receive Medicare. In some states, it also pays the 20 percent that Medicare does not cover. It also may pay for some of your medicines. To apply for Medicaid, talk with your social worker or contact your local health department.

Veterans Administration (VA) Benefits

If you are a veteran, the VA can help you pay for treatment. Contact your local VA office for more information.

Social Security Income (SSI) and Social Security Disability Income (SSDI)

These benefits are available from the Social Security Administration. They assist you with the costs of daily living. To find out if you qualify, talk to your social worker or call your local Social Security office.

Source: "End-Stage Renal Disease: Choosing a Treatment That's Right for You," NIH Publication No. 94-2412, National Institutes of Health, June 1994.

Eye Problems and Diabetes

Diabetes can affect the eyes in several ways. Frequently, the effects are temporary and can be corrected with better diabetes control. However, long-term diabetes can cause changes in the eyes that threaten vision. Stable blood glucose levels and yearly eye examinations can help reduce the risk of serious eye damage.

BLURRED VISION

Blurred vision is one effect diabetes can have on the eyes. The reason may be that changing levels of glucose in blood also can affect the balance of fluid in the lens of the eye, which works like a flexible camera lens to focus images. If the lens absorbs more water than normal and swells, its focusing power changes. Diabetes also may affect the function of nerves that control eyesight, causing blurred vision.

CATARACT AND GLAUCOMA

Cataract and glaucoma are eye diseases that occur more frequently in people with diabetes. Cataract is a clouding of the normally clear lens of the eye. Glaucoma is a condition in which pressure within the eye can damage the optic nerve that transmits visual images to the brain. Early diagnosis and treatment of cataract and glaucoma can reduce the severity of these disorders.

DIABETIC RETINOPATHY

Retinopathy, a disease of the retina, the light sensing tissue at the back of the eye, is a common concern among people with diabetes. Diabetic retinopathy damages the tiny vessels that supply the retina with blood. The blood vessels may swell and leak fluid. When retinopathy is more severe, new blood vessels may grow from the back of the eye and bleed into the clear gel that fills the eye, the vitreous.

While most people with diabetes may never develop serious eye problems, people who have had diabetes for 25 years or more are more likely to develop retinopathy. Experts think high blood pressure may contribute to diabetic retinopathy, and that smoking can cause the condition to worsen. If someone experiences blurred vision that lasts longer than a day or so, sudden loss of vision in either eye, or black spots, lines, or flashing lights in the field of vision, a doctor should be alerted right away.

Treatment for diabetic retinopathy can help prevent loss of vision and can sometimes restore vision lost because of the disease. A yearly eye examination with dilated pupils makes it possible for an ophthalmologist, an eye doctor, to notice changes before the illness becomes harder to treat. Scientists are testing new means of treating diabetic retinopathy.

Source: "Noninsulin-Dependent Diabetes," National Institutes of Health, NIH Publication No. 95–241, September 1992.

Diabetes and Your Eyes

DIABETIC RETINOPATHY

Diabetes is a major cause of blindness in the United States. Blindness from diabetes is caused by changes in the small blood vessels of the eye retina, the thin light-sensitive inner lining of the back of the eye. This disease is called **diabetic retinopathy.**

About half of all people with diabetes have some changes in the retina after they have had the disease for 10 years. After 15 years, almost all people with diabetes have some changes in the retina. These changes do not affect vision in most cases. But in a small group of people, the changes are serious enough to threaten eyesight. In general, scientists feel the following key points influence whether a person with diabetes will develop vision problems:

- how old the person was when he or she contracted diabetes
- the length of time the person has had diabetes

PREVENTION

Blood Sugar Control

There may be a link between how well blood sugar levels are controlled and whether eye problems develop later. Some studies suggest that retinopathy occurs only in patients who have blood sugars above 200. Therefore, many physicians now support efforts to maintain excellent control of blood sugar levels in people with diabetes. This control might help to prevent retinopathy. You should follow closely the treatment plan your physician designs for you. If you do not follow this treatment plan, you could be taking chances with your health and your eyesight. It is also important to keep your blood pressure in the normal range.

Early Detection

Your physician should dilate your pupils and examine the back of your eyes every one or two years. He or she may refer you to an ophthalmologist (eye specialist) who has experience in diagnosing eye changes caused by diabetes. If these changes develop, physicians can offer different kinds of treatment. Your physician may also refer you to an ophthalmologist for specific treatment.

TREATMENT

Treatments include **laser photocoagulation** and **vitrectomy**. In laser photocoagulation, a physician uses a laser (light) beam to eliminate abnormal small blood vessels from the retina. A

continues

continued

study conducted by the National Eye Institute showed this treatment to be effective in most patients who have medium to serious eye disease. In many cases, the best time for treatment is **before** any vision problem is noticed by the patient. Another treatment, vitrectomy, involves the removal by surgery of the vitreous, the clear fluid filling the eye, when it has become cloudy from bleeding. This operation is also sometimes used to remove scar tissue.

Frequent eye checkups are necessary, even though your vision may be normal. You should also stick carefully to the treatment plan your physician gives you.

NOTES:

Source: *The Prevention and Treatment of Five Complications of Diabetes: A Guide for Primary Care Practitioners*. National Diabetes Advisory Board, U.S. Department of Health and Human Services, Public Health Service, Centers for Disease Control, Atlanta, Georgia, 1983.

Diabetic Retinopathy

Diabetic retinopathy is a potentially blinding complication of diabetes that damages the eye's retina. It affects half of all Americans diagnosed with diabetes.

At first, you may notice no changes in your vision. But don't let diabetic retinopathy fool you. It could get worse over the years and threaten your good vision. With timely treatment, 90 percent of those with advanced diabetic retinopathy can be saved from going blind.

The National Eye Institute (NEI) is the Federal government's lead agency for vision research. The NEI urges all people with diabetes to have an eye examination through dilated pupils at least once a year.

WHAT IS THE RETINA?

The retina is a light-sensitive tissue at the back of the eye. When light enters the eye, the retina changes the light into nerve signals. The retina then sends these signals along the optic nerve to the brain. Without a retina, the eye cannot communicate with the brain, making vision impossible.

HOW DOES DIABETIC RETINOPATHY DAMAGE THE RETINA?

Diabetic retinopathy occurs when diabetes damages the tiny blood vessels in the retina. At this point, most people do not notice any changes in their vision.

Some people develop a condition called **macular edema**. It occurs when the damaged blood vessels leak fluid and lipids onto the macula, the part of the retina that lets us see detail. The fluid makes the macula swell, blurring vision.

As the disease progresses, it enters its advanced, or **proliferative**, stage. Fragile, new blood vessels grow along the retina and in the clear, gel-like vitreous that fills the inside of the eye. Without timely treatment, these new blood vessels can bleed, cloud vision, and destroy the retina.

WHO IS AT RISK FOR THIS DISEASE?

All people with diabetes are at risk—those with Type I diabetes (juvenile onset) and those with Type II diabetes (adult onset).

During pregnancy, diabetic retinopathy may also be a problem for women with diabetes. It is recommended that all pregnant women with diabetes have dilated eye examinations each trimester to protect their vision.

continues

continued

WHAT ARE ITS SYMPTOMS?

Diabetic retinopathy often has no warning signs. At some point, though, you may have macular edema. It blurs vision, making it hard to do things like read and drive. In some cases, your vision will get better or worse during the day.

As new blood vessels form at the back of the eye, they can bleed (hemorrhage) and blur vision. The first time this happens it may not be very severe. In most cases, it will leave just a few specks of blood, or spots, floating in your vision. They often go away after a few hours.

These spots are often followed within a few days or weeks by a much greater leakage of blood. The blood will blur your vision. In extreme cases, a person will only be able to tell light from dark in that eye. It may take the blood anywhere from a few days to months or even years to clear from inside of your eye. In some cases, the blood will not clear. You should be aware that large hemorrhages tend to happen more than once, often during sleep.

HOW IS IT DETECTED?

Diabetic retinopathy is detected during an examination that includes:

- **Visual acuity test:** This eye chart test measures how well you see at various distances.
- **Pupil dilation:** The eye care professional places drops into the eye to widen the pupil. This allows him or her to see more of the retina and look for signs of diabetic retinopathy. After the examination, close-up vision may remain blurred for several hours.
- **Ophthalmoscopy:** This is an examination of the retina in which the eye care professional: (1) looks through a device with a special magnifying lens that provides a narrow view of the retina, or (2) wearing a headset with a bright light, looks through a special magnifying glass and gains a wide view of the retina.
- **Tonometry:** A standard test that determines the fluid pressure inside the eye. Elevated pressure is a possible sign of glaucoma, another common eye problem in people with diabetes.

Your eye care professional will look at your retina for early signs of the disease, such as: (1) leaking blood vessels, (2) retinal swelling, such as macular edema, (3) pale, fatty deposits on the retina—signs of leaking blood vessels, (4) damaged nerve tissue, and (5) any changes in the blood vessels.

Should your doctor suspect that you need treatment for macular edema, he or she may ask you to have a test called **fluorescein angiography**.

In this test, a special dye is injected into your arm. Pictures are then taken as the dye passes through the blood vessels in the retina. This test allows your doctor to find the leaking blood vessels.

continues

continued

HOW IS IT TREATED?

There are two treatments for diabetic retinopathy. They are very effective in reducing vision loss from this disease. In fact, even people with advanced retinopathy have a 90 percent chance of keeping their vision when they get treatment before the retina is severely damaged.

These two treatments are laser surgery and vitrectomy. It is important to note that although these treatments are very successful, they do not cure diabetic retinopathy.

Laser Surgery

Laser surgery is performed in a doctor's office or eye clinic. Before the surgery, your ophthalmologist will: (1) dilate your pupil and (2) apply drops to numb the eye. In some cases, the doctor also may numb the area behind the eye to prevent any discomfort.

The lights in the office will be dim. As you sit facing the laser machine, your doctor will hold a special lens to your eye. During the procedure, you may see flashes of light. These flashes may eventually create a stinging sensation that makes you feel a little uncomfortable.

You may leave the office once the treatment is done, but you will need someone to drive you home. Because your pupils will remain dilated for a few hours, you also should bring a pair of sunglasses.

For the rest of the day, your vision will probably be a little blurry. If your eye hurts a bit, your eye care professional can suggest a way to control this.

Doctors will perform laser surgery to treat severe macular edema and proliferative retinopathy.

Macular Edema

Timely laser surgery can reduce vision loss from macular edema by half. But you may need to have laser surgery more than once to control the leaking fluid.

During the surgery, your doctor will aim a high-energy beam of light directly onto the damaged blood vessels. This is called **focal laser treatment**. This seals the vessels and stops them from leaking. Generally, laser surgery is used to stabilize vision, not necessarily to improve it.

Proliferative Retinopathy

In treating advanced diabetic retinopathy, doctors use the laser to destroy the abnormal blood vessels that form at the back of the eye.

continues

continued

Rather than focus the light on a single spot, your eye care professional will make hundreds of small laser burns away from the center of the retina. This is called **scatter laser treatment**. The treatment shrinks the abnormal blood vessels. You will lose some of your side vision after this surgery to save the rest of your sight. Laser surgery may also slightly reduce your color and night vision.

Once you have proliferative retinopathy, you will always be at risk for new bleeding. This means you may need treatment more than once to protect your sight.

Vitrectomy

Instead of laser surgery, you may need an eye operation called a vitrectomy to restore your sight. A vitrectomy is performed if you have a lot of blood in the vitreous. It involves removing the cloudy vitreous and replacing it with a salt solution. Because the vitreous is mostly water, you will notice no change between the salt solution and the normal vitreous.

Studies show that people who have a vitrectomy soon after a large hemorrhage are more likely to protect their vision than someone who waits to have the operation.

Early vitrectomy is especially effective in people with insulin-dependent diabetes, who may be at greater risk of blindness from a hemorrhage into the eye.

Vitrectomy is often done under local anesthesia. This means that you will be awake during the operation. The doctor makes a tiny incision in the sclera, or white of the eye. Next, a small instrument is placed into the eye. It removes the vitreous and inserts the salt solution into the eye.

You may be able to return home soon after the vitrectomy. Or, you may be asked to stay in the hospital overnight. Your eye will be red and sensitive. After the operation, you will need to wear an eyepatch for a few days or weeks to protect the eye. You will also need to use medicated eye drops to protect against infection.

WHAT RESEARCH IS BEING DONE?

The NEI is currently supporting a number of research studies in both the laboratory and with patients to learn more about the cause of diabetic retinopathy. This research should provide better ways to detect, treat, and prevent vision loss in people with diabetes.

For example, it is likely that in the coming years researchers will develop drugs that turn off enzyme activity that has been shown to cause diabetic retinopathy. Some day, these drugs will help people to control the disease and reduce the need for laser surgery.

continues

continued

WHAT CAN YOU DO TO PROTECT YOUR VISION?

The NEI urges all people with diabetes to have an eye examination through dilated pupils at least once a year. If you have more serious retinopathy, you may need to have a dilated eye examination more often.

A recent study, the Diabetes Control and Complications Trial (DCCT), showed that better control of blood sugar levels slows the onset and progression of retinopathy and lessens the need for laser surgery for severe retinopathy.

The study found that the group that tried to keep their blood sugar levels as close to normal as possible, had much less eye, kidney, and nerve disease. This level of blood sugar control may not be best for everyone, including some elderly patients, children under 13, or people with heart disease. So ask your doctor if this program is right for you.

NOTES:

Source: "Diabetic Retinopathy," NIH Publication No. 99-2171, National Eye Institute, National Institutes of Health, January 1999.

Leg and Foot Problems and Diabetes

Leg and foot problems can arise in people with diabetes due to changes in blood vessels and nerves in these areas.

PERIPHERAL VASCULAR DISEASE

Peripheral vascular disease is a condition in which blood vessels become narrowed by fatty deposits, reducing blood supply to the legs and feet.

PERIPHERAL NEUROPATHY

Diabetes also can dull the sensitivity of nerves. Someone with this condition, called peripheral neuropathy, might not notice a sore spot caused by tight shoes or pressure from walking. If ignored, the sore can become infected, and because blood circulation is poor, the area may take longer to heal.

Proper foot care and regular visits to a doctor can prevent foot and leg sores and ensure that any sores that do appear don't become infected and painful. Helpful measures include inspecting the feet daily for cuts or sore spots. Blisters and sore spots are not as likely when shoes fit well and socks or stockings aren't tight. A doctor also may suggest washing feet daily, with warm, not hot, water; filing thick calluses; and using lotions that keep the feet from getting too dry. Shoe inserts or special shoes can be used to prevent pressure on the foot.

DIABETIC NEUROPATHY

Diabetic neuropathy, or nerve disease, dulls the nerves and can be extremely painful. A person with neuropathy also may be depressed. Scientists aren't sure whether the depression is an effect of neuropathy, or if it's simply a response to pain. Treatment, aimed at relieving pain and depression, may include aspirin and other pain-killing drugs.

Any sore on the foot or leg, whether or not it's painful, requires a doctor's immediate attention. Treatment can help sores heal and prevent new ones from developing. Problems with the feet and legs can cause life-threatening problems that require amputation—surgical removal of limbs—if they are not treated early.

Other Effects of Diabetic Neuropathy

Nerves provide muscle tone and feeling and help control functions like digestion and blood pressure. Diabetes can cause changes in these nerves and the functions they control. These changes are most frequent in people who have had other complications of diabetes, like problems with their feet.

continues

continued

Someone who has had diabetes for some years, and has other complications, may find that spells of indigestion or diarrhea are common. A doctor may prescribe drugs to relieve these symptoms.

Diabetes also can affect the nerves that control penile erection in men, which can cause impotence that shows up gradually, without any loss of desire for sex. A doctor can find out whether impotence is the result of physical changes, such as diabetes, or emotional changes, and suggest treatment or counseling.

NOTES:

Source: "Noninsulin-Dependent Diabetes," National Institutes of Health, NIH Publication No. 95–241, September 1992.

For People with Diabetes—How To Care for Your Feet

- Wash your feet daily. Dry them carefully, especially between the toes. Don't soak your feet (unless instructed to do so by your health care provider). If your feet are dry, apply a very thin coat of lubricant (oil or cream) to them after bathing and drying them. Don't put oil or cream between your toes.
- Inspect your feet daily. Use an unbreakable mirror to help see the bottom of your feet.
- If your vision is impaired, ask someone to check your feet for you. Check for scratches, cuts, or blisters. Always check between your toes.
- Cut your toenails by following the contour of the nail. Smooth the corners with an emery board. Don't trim into the corners of your toenails or cut ingrown toenails. If redness appears around your toenails, see your health care provider immediately.
- Don't cut corns or calluses. Don't use corn plasters or chemicals for removing corns or calluses. Don't use strong antiseptic solutions or adhesive tape on your feet.
- Avoid extreme temperatures. Test water with your hand or elbow before bathing. Don't walk on hot surfaces, such as sand at the beach or cement around swimming pools. In winter, wear wool socks and protective foot gear, such as fleece-lined boots. Don't apply hot water bottles or heating pads to your feet. If your feet are cold at night, wear socks.
- Don't walk barefooted—even indoors. Don't wear sandals with thongs between your toes. Don't wear shoes without stockings or socks. Inspect the inside of your shoes every day for foreign objects, nail points, torn linings, and rough areas. Shoes should be comfortable at the time of purchase. Don't buy shoes that are too tight and depend on them to stretch out. Break in new shoes before wearing them regularly. Ask your health care provider or podiatrist about the types of shoes most appropriate for you.
- Don't wear tight clothing (such as leg garters). Avoid crossing your legs; doing so can cause pressure on the nerves and blood vessels in the legs.
- Don't smoke.
- Don't drink alcohol excessively.
- See your health care provider regularly and be sure your feet are examined at least four times a year.
- Tell your health care provider or podiatrist immediately if you develop a blister or sore on your foot. Be sure to tell your podiatrist that you have diabetes.

Source: *The Prevention and Treatment of Complications of Diabetes Mellitus: A Guide for Primary Care Practitioners*, Department of Health and Human Services, Public Health Service, Centers for Disease Control, National Center for Chronic Disease Prevention and Health Promotion, Division of Diabetes Translation, January 1, 1991. Adapted from Take Charge of Your Diabetes: A Guide for Care, Centers for Disease Control and Prevention.

How To Take Care of Your Feet

Nerve damage, circulation problems, and infections can cause serious foot problems for people with diabetes.

Nerve damage can cause you to lose feeling in your feet. Sometimes nerve damage can deform or misshape your feet, causing pressure points that can turn into blisters, sores, or ulcers.

Poor circulation can make these injuries slow to heal. There may be changes in the color and temperature of your feet. Some people lose hair on their toes, feet, and lower legs.

The skin on your feet may be dry and cracked. Toenails may turn thick and yellow. Fungus infections can grow between your toes.

There is a lot you can do to prevent problems with your feet. Controlling your blood glucose and not smoking or using tobacco can help protect your feet. You can also keep small problems from getting out of control by following these recommendations.

INSPECTING YOUR FEET

You may have serious foot problems yet feel no pain. Look at your feet *every day* to see if you have scratches, cracks, cuts, or blisters, changes in color or temperature, or swelling.

Always check between your toes and on the bottoms of your feet. If you can't bend over to see the bottoms of your feet, use an unbreakable mirror. If you can't see well, ask a family member to help you. Call your doctor at once if you have a sore on your foot.

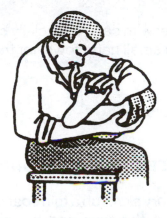

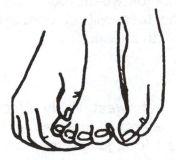

continues

continued

BATHING

Wash your feet every day. Don't soak your feet—it can dry out your skin, and dry skin can lead to infections.

DRYING

Dry your feet with care, especially between the toes. Use a small hand towel for this purpose.

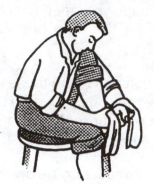

KEEPING FEET IN GOOD CONDITION

If you have *dry skin,* rub a thin coat of oil, lotion, or cream on the tops and bottoms of your feet—but not between your toes. Moisture between the toes will let germs grow that could cause an infection.

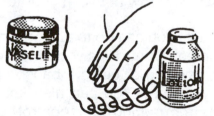

When your feet sweat, apply a foot powder, such as cornstarch. If fungus infection develops (athlete's foot, jungle rot), talk with your doctor right away to start treatment.

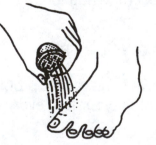

continues

continued

TOENAILS

Trim your toenails after you've washed and dried your feet—the nails will be softer and easier to trim.

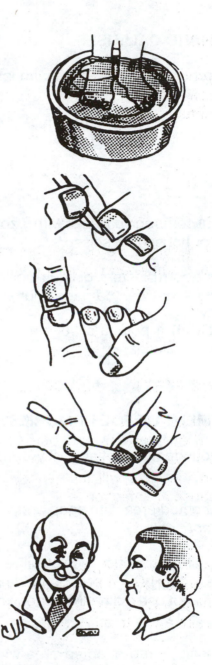

Use a wooden orange stick to clean under the toenails.

Trim your toenails straight across with toenail clippers or special toenail scissors. Leave 1/8" of nail showing.

Smooth your toenails with a file or emery board. Don't cut into the corners.

Don't trim your own nails if:

1. You can't see well.
2. You have hard, thick nails that are too hard to cut.
3. You have poor circulation or numbness in toes.
4. You have ingrown toenails.

Get them trimmed by a podiatrist (foot doctor) or another health care provider.

continues

continued

CORNS AND CALLUSES

Keep corns and calluses soft with lotion.

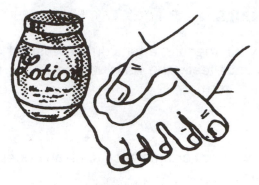

Never cut corns and calluses with razor blades, knives, or household scissors.

Never use corn plasters, or liquid corn or callus removers—they can damage your skin.

Consult with a podiatrist for proper care of corns and calluses.

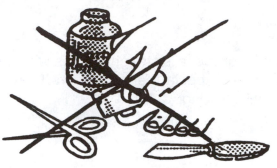

TREATMENT OF FOOT INJURIES

Notify your doctor right away if you injure your feet!

Wash affected area with soap and warm water. *Do not soak.*

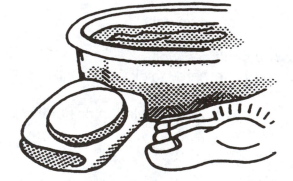

Apply a mild antiseptic, such as diluted hydrogen peroxide (H_2O_2): 1 part peroxide to 1 part water. Do not use iodine. Neosporin ointment is acceptable.

If necessary, wrap affected area with sterile gauze or Band-Aid to keep the wound clean.

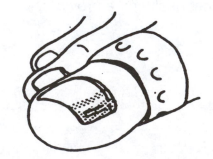

Stay off the foot as much as possible to allow it a chance to heal. If the area becomes red, painful, or swollen, it is likely to be infected. Consult with your doctor or go to Urgent Care immediately. *Do not wait.*

continues

continued

PROTECT YOUR FEET FROM HEAT AND COLD

Hot water or hot surfaces are a danger to your feet. Before bathing, test the water with a bath thermometer (90°–95° F is safe) or with your elbow. Wear shoes and socks when you walk on hot surfaces, such as beaches or the pavement around swimming pools. In summer, be sure to use a sunscreen on the tops of your feet.

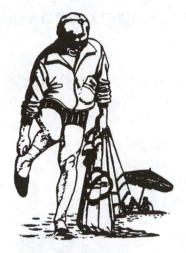

Wear shoes to protect your feet from hot surfaces.

You also need to protect your feet from the cold. In winter, wear socks and footwear, such as fleece-lined boots, to protect your feet. If your feet are cold at night, wear socks. Don't use hot water bottles or heating pads—they can burn your feet.

SHOES AND SOCKS

Wear shoes that fit well and protect your feet without squeezing your toes together. Don't wear plastic shoes or sandals with thongs between the toes. *Don't walk barefoot, even indoors!*

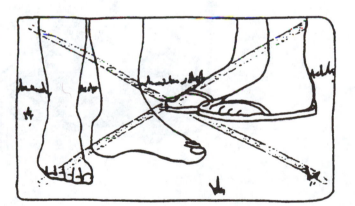

- New shoes should be comfortable at the time you buy them—don't expect them to stretch out. Slowly break in new shoes by wearing them only 1–2 hours a day.
- Always wear socks or stockings with your shoes. Choose socks made of cotton or wool—they help keep your feet dry. Socks should not be tight at the tops!
- Before you put on your shoes each time, look and feel inside them. Check for any loose objects, nail points, torn linings, and rough areas—these can cause injuries. If your shoe isn't smooth inside, wear other shoes.

continues

continued

IMPROVE BLOOD FLOW TO YOUR FEET

- If you smoke, quit.

- If you have high blood pressure or high cholesterol, work with your health care provider to lower it.

- Be physically active, which can help increase the circulation in your feet. Ask about things you can do to safely exercise your feet and legs.

TAKE CHARGE OF YOUR FOOT CARE

Get your health care provider to check your feet and legs every time you visit. As a reminder, take off your shoes and socks when you're in the exam room.

Have your sense of feeling and your pulses checked at least once a year. If you do have foot problems, ask if special shoes would help you.

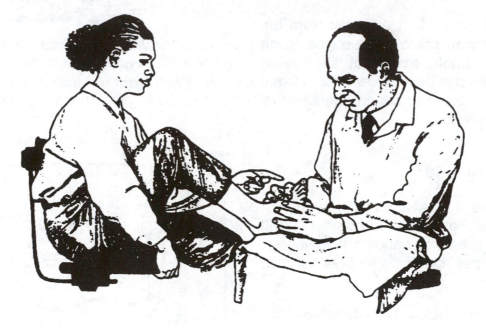

Courtesy of Veterans Administration Medical Center, San Diego, California.

Skin and Mouth Infections

SKIN INFECTIONS

People with diabetes are more likely to develop infections, like boils and ulcers, than the average person.

Women with diabetes may develop vaginal infections more often than other women.

Checking for infections, treating them early, and following a doctor's advice can help ensure that infections are mild and infrequent.

MOUTH INFECTIONS

Infections also can affect the teeth and gums, making people with diabetes more susceptible to periodontal disease, an inflammation of tissue surrounding and supporting the teeth. An important cause of periodontal disease is bacterial growth on the teeth and gums. Treating diabetes and following a dentist's advice on dental care can help prevent periodontal disease.

NOTES:

Source: "Noninsulin-Dependent Diabetes," National Institutes of Health, NIH Publication No. 95–241, September 1992.

Diabetes and Periodontal Disease

DIABETIC CONTROL

People with poor blood sugar control get gum disease more often and more severely, and they lose more teeth than do persons with good control.

BLOOD VESSEL CHANGES

Diabetes causes blood vessels to thicken, which slows the flow of nutrients and the removal of harmful wastes. This can weaken the resistance of gum and bone tissue to infection.

BACTERIA

Many kinds of bacteria (germs) thrive on sugars, including glucose—the sugar linked to diabetes. When diabetes is poorly controlled, high glucose levels in mouth fluids may help germs grow and set the stage for gum disease.

SMOKING

Studies show that smoking also increases the chances of developing gum disease.

THRUSH

Thrush is an infection caused by a fungus that grows in the mouth. People with diabetes are at risk for thrush because the fungus thrives on high glucose levels in saliva. Smoking and wearing dentures (especially when they are worn constantly) can also lead to fungal infection. Medication is available to treat this infection. Good diabetic control, not smoking, and removing and cleaning dentures daily can help prevent thrush.

Source: *Diabetes & Periodontal Disease, A Guide for Patients,* National Institute of Dental Research, National Institutes of Health, Bethesda, Maryland, 1994.

Enfermedad periodontal en los diabéticos

La enfermedad periodontal es una condición causada por bacterias que afectan los tejidos y el hueso que sostienen los dientes y las muelas. Esta enfermedad comienza con la inflamación de las encías. Cuando no se da tratamiento, la inflamación se hace más severa. Eventualmente, la infección destruye el hueso y ligamentos que sostienen los dientes y las muelas. Si no se da el tratamiento adecuado, la enfermedad periodontal hace que los dientes sanos se aflojen y eventualmente se caigan.

Para las personas que padecen de diabetes mellitus, la enfermedad periodontal puede causar problemas serios. La enfermedad periodontal puede hacer difícil controlar el nivel del azúcar en la sangre. Además, si estas personas llegan a perder sus dientes, encontrarán más difícil comer los alimentos adecuados para diabéticos.

¿Qué causa la enfermedad periodontal?

Las bacterias en la boca se adhieren a los dientes formando una capa transparente y pegajosa llamada placa. La placa es una de las principales causas de la enfermedad periodontal porque promueve la inflamación de las encías (o gingivitis).

¿A quiénes afecta la enfermedad periodontal?

La enfermedad periodontal es un problema para muchas personas en los Estados Unidos. De hecho, la mayor parte de las personas de más de 40 años padecen de alguna forma de enfermedad esta, desde una leve inflamación de las encías hasta una infección severa.

Recientemente, estudios científicos han demostrado que los jóvenes y adultos que padecen de diabetes tienen más probabilidad de desarrollar infecciones en las encías y enfermedad periodontal. Esto le sucede especialmente a las personas diabéticas que no controlan bien el nivel del azúcar en su sangre. La diabetes también hace que la enfermedad periodontal sea más frecuente, más severa, y que se presente a una edad más temprana que en las personas no diabéticas.

¿Cómo se desarrolla la enfermedad periodontal?

Gingivitis

La gingivitis, o inflamación de las encías, es la primera etapa de la enfermedad periodontal. Comúnmente, la gingivitis ocurre debido a malos hábitos al cepillar los dientes o al usar el hilo dental. Esto permite que la placa se acumule en los dientes y cerca de las encías. Al principio, ésto causa una inflamación ligera— la encía alrededor de uno o varios dientes se enrojece y se inflama. Después, estos síntomas empeoran, y las encías tienden a sangrar fácilmente. Uno de los primeros síntomas de la enfermedad es cuando las encías sangran al cepillar los dientes. Estos cambios pueden causar que las encías se hagan sensibles al tacto, pero esto no sucede en todos los casos. Debido a que la enfermedad no siempre produce síntomas, en muchas ocasiones el paciente no sabe que la padece.

continúa

continuación

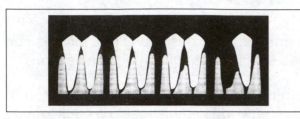

Conforme se acumula la placa alrededor de los dientes, las encías se inflaman y pueden sangrar fácilmente. Se forman depósitos y, con el tiempo, los dientes se aflojan y eventualmente se pueden caer.

Periodontitis

La gingivitis puede controlarse si un dentista limpia regularmente los dientes. También hay que cuidar y limpiar los dientes correctamente en el hogar. Si no se trat la gingivitis, la condición puede progresar hasta convertirse en periodontitis destructiva, que es la etapa más seria de la enfermedad periodontal. Con el tiempo, la placa se endurece formando cálculos (o depósitos de pequeñísimas piedras), y se extiende de la línea entre el diente y las encías hasta la raíz del diente. Gradualmente, las encías se desprenden del diente formando unas bolsas en donde se desarrolla la infección. Estas bolsas tienden a formarse en los espacios entre los dientes a donde no llega el cepillo de dientes.

Pérdida de los dientes

Conforme se extiende la infección, las bolsas se pueden llenar de pus y causar mal aliento. Eventualmente, la infección destruye los ligamentos que sostienen los dientes en el hueso. Esto hace que la mayor parte de la cavidad del diente se desintegre. El diente se afloja y puede llegar a caerse. Es importante mencionar que la persona siente poca o

ninguna molestia mientras que se extiende la infección. Es muy difícil para una persona saber si está desarrollando la enfermedad periodontal.

¿Cuál es el tratamiento para la enfermedad periodontal?

Limpieza de placa

El tratamiento para la periodontitis depende de cuánto ha progresado la infección. En las primeras etapas, el dentista o periodontista (dentista especializado en enfermedad periodontal) saca la placa, los cálculos y el tejido inflamado de debajo de las encías. Esta limpieza profunda, conocida como alisado radicular, elimina la infección. Esto hace posible que las encías vuelvan a pegarse al diente y que se cierren las bolsas de infección.

Para tener éxito en el tratamiento de alisado radicular también es necesario seguir un buen programa de limpieza bucal en el hogar. Prevenir y combatir la enfermedad periodontal en sus etapas tempranas hace posible que el paciente necesite solamente de este tratamiento para curarse totalmente.

Cirugía periodontal

Cuando la periodontitis está muy avanzada, puede ser necesario hacer una cirugía en las encías. Las nuevas técnicas de cirugía le permiten al dentista tener acceso a las áreas con problemas alrededor de las raíces de los dientes. Estas técnicas permiten al dentista o periodontista limpiar cuidadosamente los cálculos y los tejidos infectados. También es

continúa

continuación

necesario alisar las superficies de las raíces del diente que han sido dañadas por la enfermedad. Esta cirugía elimina las bolsas de infección, permitiendo que las encías se vuelvan a adherir a la base de los dientes.

Las encías y el hueso destruidos por la periodontitis avanzada no vuelven a crecer. Sin embargo, hay técnicas especializadas que permiten reemplazar o reconstruir algunas de estas estructuras usando materiales similares al hueso. También se usan transplantes del tejido de las encías sanas para sustituir los tejidos perdidos.

Tratamiento periodontal para las personas diabéticas

Las personas que padecen de diabetes deben consultar a su médico antes de recibir tratamiento para la enfermedad periodontal. El dentista o periodontista también debe hablar con el médico antes de hacer la cirugía periodontal para informarse de la condición física general del paciente. El conocer la salud general del diabético, especialmente si hay problemas de infección o de control del nivel del azúcar en la sangre, le ayuda al dentista y al médico a decidir si se deben dar antibióticos al paciente antes de la cirugía. La decisión de dar antibióticos antes de la cirugía la deben tomar el dentista y el médico, considerando las necesidades especiales y el tipo de tratamiento dental que necesita el paciente.

Las citas para el tratamiento se deben hacer en la mañana, generalmente una hora y media después del desayuno y la inyección de insulina de la mañana. Esto se recomienda para que no se atrasen o se pierdan las comidas regulares del día. Las citas en la mañana también permiten que, durante el resto del día, el dentista pueda observar cualquier efecto de la cirugía de las encías en el nivel de azúcar en la sangre del paciente. Las infecciones agudas, tales como los abscesos, deben ser tratados de inmediato.

Por lo general, los diabéticos que tienen su enfermedad bajo control pueden recibir tratamiento en la oficina del dentista. Las personas con diabetes más severa deben ir al hospital para la cirugía. En el hospital le pueden observar mejor durante y después de la cirugía.

Los pacientes diabéticos toman más tiempo en recuperarse de la cirugía periodontal. Sin embargo, con buen cuidado médico y dental, la posibilidad de complicaciones después de la cirugía es la misma que la de los pacientes no diabéticos. Una vez que se ha tratado la enfermedad periodontal exitosamente, frecuentemente los diabéticos observan que es más sencillo controlar el nivel del azúcar en la sangre.

Mantener sus dientes

Los diabéticos deben entender la importancia de mantener sus dientes naturales. El hueso alrededor de los dientes puede dañarse con la enfermedad periodontal, causando cambios en la forma de los tejidos de las encías. Las encías disparejas pueden hacer más difícil que le adapten dentaduras postizas adecuadamente y cómodamente. Además, los diabéticos toleran menos las dentaduras postizas completas debido a que sus encías son

continúa

continuación

sensibles y duelen al tocarlas. Esto hace necesario que se tengan que readaptar las dentaduras postizas a los cambios de las encías y los tejidos de soporte.

Las enfermedades dentales, especialmente la enfermedad periodontal severa, pueden tener malos efectos en el control de la diabetes porque hacen difícil y doloroso el masticar. Debido a estas molestias, la persona diabética puede decidir comer alimentos que son más fáciles de masticar, pero que pueden no ser apropiados para su dieta. Para evitar estas complicaciones, la persona diabética debe hacer todo lo posible para mantener sus dientes sanos. Con los dientes sanos, los diabéticos pueden controlar su enfermedad comiendo los alimentos correctos, sin tener que sufrir ningún tipo de molestia.

Cómo proteger sus dientes y encías

El mejor consejo, tanto para diabéticos como para no diabéticos, es la prevención. Si se deja que la placa se acumule, las bacterias dañinas atacan constantemente los dientes y las encías. Lo más importante que toda persona puede hacer es evitar la acumulación de la placa. Esto se logra cepillando los dientes y usando el hilo dental cuidadosamente. Si usted hace esto todos los días, puede evitar que se presente la enfermedad.

Los dentistas han notado que los pacientes mejoran una vez que se limpia la placa, incluso en los casos en que la enfermedad ya existe. La inflamación generalmente desaparece en menos de una semana, y las encías se desinflaman y se afirman. Después de algunas semanas los dientes flojos se vuelven firmes. El cuidado dental en el hogar es muy importante para evitar que se presente la enfermedad periodontal otra vez. Normalmente, las personas que limpian la placa correcta y regularmente evitan que se presenten estos problemas.

Cepillar

Cepillarse los dientes es un paso importante en limpiar la placa. Debe hacerlo cuidadosamente y por lo menos dos veces al día. Los siguientes pasos le ayudarán a cepillar mejor sus dientes:

1. Use un cepillo de dientes de nylon blando y con las puntas de las cerdas redondas. También, compre pasta de dientes con fluoruro, ya que esta sustancia le dará mayor protección contra la placa.
2. Cepille sus dientes con el movimiento que le sea más cómodo. Lo que es importante es que no cepille sus dientes demasiado fuerte y que elimine la placa de la superficie de sus dientes.

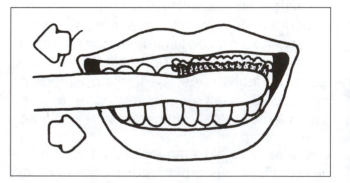

continúa

continuación

3. Se recomienda que trate de usar movimientos circulares, y movimientos cortos de atrás hacia adelante para limpiar las muelas.

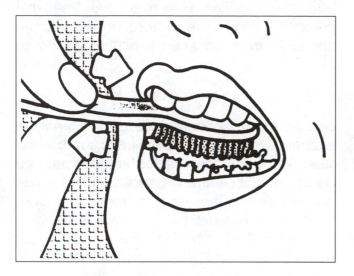

4. Cepille la superficie de la lengua ya que en esta área se acumulan restos de alimentos y bacterias.

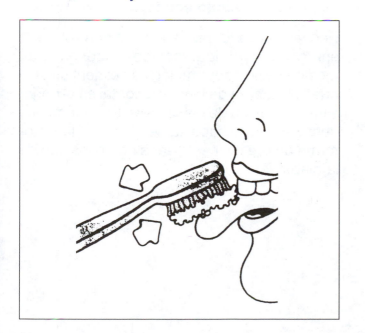

Limpiar con el hilo dental

Use el hilo dental para limpiar la placa entre los dientes y las muelas, que es donde se inician la mayor parte de las bolsas de infección.

1. Manera de sostener el hilo dental para limpiar los dientes de la mandíbula superior.

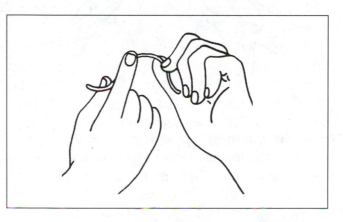

2. Coloque el hilo dental entre los dientes y, moviéndolo cuidadosamente de atrás hacia adelante, súbalo hacia la raíz del diente. Frote suavemente el lado del diente con el hilo desde el interior de la encía hacia la superficie.

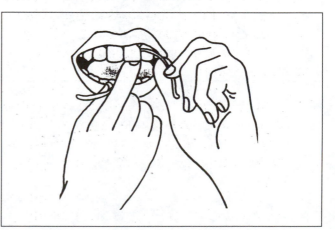

continúa

continuación

3. Manera de sostener el hilo dental para limpiar los dientes de la mandíbula inferior.

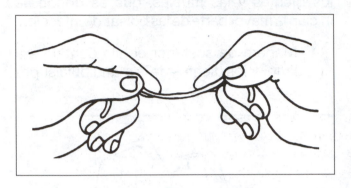

4. Repita este proceso, de uno a uno, con todos los dientes y las muelas. Limpiar cada diente de esta manera rompe las acumulaciones de placa.

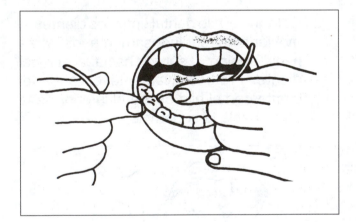

Usar el hilo dental en las muelas y las encías de atrás de la boca es un poco más difícil, así es que probablemente le llevará un poco más de tiempo el aprender a hacerlo. Su dentista le puede enseñar cómo alcanzar estas áreas difíciles. También puede comprar un instrumento especial para sostener el hilo dental y facilitar su uso.

Exámenes dentales

Las personas con diabetes deben tener un examen dental por lo menos cada seis meses. **Asegúrese de decirle al dentista que padece de diabetes.** En estas visitas, el dentista puede quitar cálculos que se pueden haber acumulado. Un examen rápido y simple también ayudará al dentista a encontrar las áreas que pueden necesitar atención especial. El dentista también puede ver si sus encías sangran fácilmente o si los tejidos de las encías se han desprendido del diente.

Trabajo cooperativo

Recuerde que la prevención y control de la enfermedad periodontal depende en gran medida de su cooperación con el dentista. Un buen programa de limpieza dental en el hogar elimina la placa de los dientes. Los exámenes dentales que le hace su dentista son la mejor forma de prevenir esta seria complicación de la diabetes.

Source: "Enfermedad Periodontal en los Diabéticos: Guía para los Pacientes," Office of Communication, National Institute of Dental Research, NIH Publication No. 90–2946-S.

Constipation and Diabetes

DIABETES AND CONSTIPATION

People with diabetes are prone to chronic constipation, for several reasons.

If you have very high blood glucose levels, you'll urinate a lot. To make up for this loss, more water must be absorbed from the large intestine. Your stools will be harder and dryer.

Many people with diabetes have nerve damage. We usually hear about damage to the sensory nerves of the feet. But diabetes can also damage the autonomic nerves—the nerves that control the functions of our internal organs, including the GI tract. When these nerves are damaged, they may lose their ability to coordinate muscle contractions in the intestine. The usual signal from the stomach that triggers the large intestine to move waste into the rectum is gone. Studies have shown that food and waste move far more slowly through the GI tract in people with diabetes.

When severe nerve damage has occurred, home remedies and nonprescription laxatives usually are not effective. People in this situation may need to try other drugs, which are available by prescription, to treat their constipation.

People with diabetes may have other medical problems. Diseases of the heart, kidney, and other organs don't directly cause bowel problems. However, the medications used to treat them may.

What should you do if you think one of your medications is the culprit? Before you stop taking a medication, review all of your medications with your doctor or pharmacist. Ask about their potential side effects. Tell your doctor and pharmacist about the nonprescription drugs, vitamins, and herbal remedies that you regularly take. Some of these products can cause changes in bowel function, and people often forget to mention that they take them.

Most medications don't cause constipation. However, if you discover that one of your medications is known to cause constipation, your doctor can usually prescribe an equally effective drug that is less likely to affect bowel function. Unfortunately, in some cases, you may need to keep taking some constipating medications because they're the only options for a serious medical problem.

FOUR WAYS TO PREVENT CONSTIPATION

- *Take the time to go to the bathroom when you feel the need.*
- *Drink plenty of fluids.* Drink eight 8-ounce glasses of water a day (or, if it sounds better to you, four tall glasses of water a day). Plain water is best: It's cheap, and it doesn't affect your blood

continues

continued

glucose levels. Other drinks, such as fruit juices, regular sodas, alcohol, and drinks with caffeine (coffee, iced tea), can make you urinate more, so you'd be losing ground, and those drinks may affect your blood glucose levels. Try these "tricks" to get your water intake up to eight glassfuls:

—Get in the habit of drinking a whole glass of water when you take a pill, instead of just a sip.

—Keep a glass of water on your desk and sip throughout the day.

—Pour yourself a glass of water at every meal.

- *Eat fiber-rich foods.* You probable won't get constipated if you eat 20 to 35 grams of fiber a day. But if you eat a typical American diet, you eat only half the recommended amount of fiber. Look at how much you get now and then gradually increase the amount. To get more fiber:

—Eat fresh fruits, vegetables, unprocessed grains, and beans. These are nature's best sources of fiber.

—Eat a bran cereal for breakfast. This is a simple way to introduce more roughage into your diet.

—Use a cookbook geared toward healthy eating, so you can plan meals that have plenty of fiber.

Eating fiber-rich foods has other health benefits. Fiber helps you feel full, which may help you control your weight; it may reduce the risk of colon cancer; and large amounts of soluble fiber may lower blood cholesterol levels.

- *Get some physical activity each day.* It may be extremely difficult for some people with diabetes to exercise because of heart disease, a stroke, or a foot amputation. But even simple exercises, like walking and stretching, can help prevent constipation.

A well-balanced meal plan and regular exercise have the added benefit of improving blood glucose control. If you change your diet or level of physical activity, you may need an adjustment in your insulin or oral medication dosage. Monitor your blood glucose levels and let your health care provider know of any changes you see. In the long run, good blood glucose control may prevent or delay the nerve damage that can cause severe constipation.

TREATING CONSTIPATION

If you do get constipated, you may need a laxative. Laxatives, sometimes called purgatives or cathartics, are big business in the United States. The manufacturers extol the benefits of their remedies on television, radio, and in magazines. You can get a fiber, saline, or stimulant laxative, or a stool softener. There are so many that choosing the right product can be difficult.

Even within one product line, there may be different formulations, each containing slightly different ingredients. Many products use a combination of active ingredients. For example,

continues

continued

Haley's M-O contains magnesium hydroxide and mineral oil. Correctol and Peri-Colace each contain a stool softener plus a stimulant laxative.

To arouse consumer interest, some manufacturers make frequent changes in the formulation or the packaging, touting the product as "new" or "improved." Read the label carefully, looking specifically for the active ingredients the product contains. You may find that your good ol' stool softener now has a stimulant laxative, which you may not want.

before making your final selection, it's always wise to ask your pharmacist for advice. Some products are not appropriate for people with diabetes and other medical conditions.

Fiber Laxatives

For many people, a bulk-forming or fiber laxative is the best first step to treat constipation. They're safe, and you'll generally see results within three days.

You need to take fiber laxatives with plenty of fluid for them to work properly. The fiber in bulk-forming laxatives, like fiber-rich foods, encourages water to be retained in the fecal matter, making stools easier to pass. The additional stool bulk helps ensure that there's adequate pressure in the rectum to signal the urge to defecate. While food is the best source of fiber, bulk-forming laxatives are an effective way to increase your fiber intake if eating bran flakes and beans doesn't excite you.

Bulk-forming laxatives do have some drawbacks.

- Many people dislike the gritty feel and unpleasant taste of fiber laxatives. To improve the taste, sweeteners are usually added to these products. Some sweeteners may affect blood glucose levels, so be sure to choose a product that is sugar-free. Fiber tablets have become quite popular because they don't require mixing and are easier to transport.
- Fiber wagers actually taste okay, and some people may be tempted to eat them regularly. Remember that fiber wafers are a baked good similar to cookies and contain calories and fat. They need to be figured into your meal plan.
- Bulk-forming laxatives sometimes cause bloating, abdominal pain, and gas. Over time, these symptoms usually lessen. These are usually less of a problem if you start with a small amount of the laxative and slowly increase the amount you use each day. Try the lowest recommended dose and then, if you need to, increase to the full dose over one to two weeks. If you don't see results after two weeks, see your doctor.
- You may have to use a bulk-forming laxative every day for up to a week to see its full effect.

continues

continued

Choose High-Fiber Foods
(The labels you check may have different amounts of fiber listed.)

Cereal	Serving	Fiber (grams)
All-Bran	½ cup (about 1 oz)	10
Raisin Bran	½ cup (about 1 oz)	4
Total	¾ cup (about 1 oz)	3
Wheat germ	2 Tbsp. (about ½ oz)	2
Oatmeal (cooked)	½ cup	4

Fruits
You'll get about 2 grams of fiber when you eat one of these:
Pear, ½ small, with skin
Apple, 1 small, with skin
Raisins, ¼ cup
Prunes, 2
Orange, 1 small
Banana, 1 small

Vegetables (raw)
You'll get about 1 gram of fiber when you eat:
Spinach, 1 cup
Celery, ½ cup
Tomato, 1 medium
Lettuce, 1 cup

Vegetables (cooked)
You'll get about 3 grams of fiber by eating one of these:
Peas, ½ cup
Canned corn, ½ cup
Potato, 1 large, with skin
Carrots, ¾ cup
Broccoli, ¾ cup
String beans, 1 cup

Legumes
You'll get 6 to 8 grams of fiber when you eat:
Baked beans in tomato sauce, ½ cup
Cooked kidney beans, ½ cup
Cooked navy beans, ½ cup

Bread/Pasta/Rice
Choose a high-fiber food instead of a low-fiber one.

Compare:	Amount of fiber:
Whole wheat spaghetti, 1 cup	4 grams
Regular spaghetti, 1 cup	1 gram
Bran muffin, 1	2½ grams
Wheat bread, 1 slice	1½ grams
Pumpernickel bread, 1 slice	1 gram
White bread, 1 slice	minimal
Brown rice, ½ cup	1 gram
Polished white rice, ½ cup	minimal

continues

continued

- Some bulk-forming laxatives are more expensive than some high-fiber foods. For example, a name-brand fiber wafer costs about 32 cents for one wafer (3.4 grams of fiber). In contrast, if you buy dried kidney beans, you'd pay about 7 cents for a half cup of cooked beans. You'd get about 8 grams of fiber, plus you'd be eating a whole food, with protein, carbohydrate, vitamins, and minerals.

Saline

Saline laxatives draw fluids into the bowel. This increases volume and pressure, which stimulates contractions of the bowel.

Saline laxatives can cause problems, particularly for people with diabetes. Many people with diabetes have kidney problems. Some don't know it. Saline laxative products usually contain magnesium and phosphate. These can be harmful if they build to high levels in the blood. Normally, the kidneys eliminate magnesium and phosphate from the body. However, in a person with kidney damage, magnesium and phosphate may build up in the blood.

Saline laxatives have no role in the long-term management of constipation, for anyone—whether the person has diabetes or not.

No saline laxative should be used for longer than three days in a row or for more than four days a month without your doctor's advice.

Stimulant Laxatives

Stimulant laxatives are thought to work by irritating the lining of the intestines. They may also stimulate nerve activity. When taken at bedtime, these products usually work overnight. They are considered safe for occasional, short-term use.

No stimulant laxative should be used for longer than three days in a row or for more than four days a month without your doctor's advice.

If you can't have a bowel movement without using stimulant laxatives, you may have a serious illness. See your doctor.

If you're thinking of using a stimulant laxative, be aware that:

- Most stimulant laxatives have a special coating, known as enteric coating, which keeps them from being dissolved in the stomach. Don't chew or crush enteric-coated tablets or you'll destroy this special coating, and then you may have severe nausea or vomiting. Furthermore,

continues

continued

> don't take these products within one hour of taking antacids or milk, because these dissolve the enteric coating.
>
> - Ex-Lax and other products containing phenolphthalein may discolor urine, but this shouldn't be a cause of alarm.
> - Stimulant laxatives can cause abdominal cramping and disturbances in fluid balance.
> - Using a stimulant laxative might start a cycle of laxative abuse. You take the laxative. The potent drug completely empties your bowel. You don't have another bowel movement for two or three days because there's nothing left in your bowel. You might mistake this as a sign that you're still constipated. You take more laxatives, and a vicious cycle has started.
> - If you use a stimulant laxative frequently, your bowel may become dependent on the drug.
> - Allergic reactions to stimulant laxatives are rare but can be serious.
> - Castor oil is a very potent stimulant laxative that can cause problems with nutrient absorption and fluid balance. Don't use it!

Emollients and Lubricants

Emollients soften the feces, making them easy to pass. These products, also called stool softeners, are quite safe, and you can use them indefinitely. Some people use them for months or even years. Stool softeners aren't really a treatment for constipation so much as a way to prevent problems. They can be used with a fiber laxative for maximum effect.

If you have had a recent heart attack or abdominal surgery and shouldn't strain to pass stool, your doctor may prescribe a stool softener.

Mineral oil is a lubricant and works like an emollient laxative. It draws water into the feces and softens the stool. But mineral oil has many disadvantages. It can prevent the absorption of the fat soluble vitamins A, D, E, and K. If you use mineral oil for too long, you may develop a vitamin deficiency. Mineral oil, if inhaled (for example, if you gasp when you're trying to swallow it), may cause lipoid pneumonitis, a very serious and potentially life-threatening lung condition. Anal seepage is common with mineral oil use. All in all, mineral oil is not a great choice.

continues

continued

Over-the-Counter Laxatives

If you want to find a store brand that's nearly the same as the name brand (but less expensive), look at the list of ingredients. Find one that has the same active ingredient as the brand name product.

Laxatives	Active Ingredient	Brand Names	Comments
Bulk-Forming (Fiber) Bulk-forming and fiber laxatives work in one to three days. You can use them every day. You need to mix the powders with water. If you take the tablet form, be sure to drink plenty of water.	Psyllium	Metamucil, Konsyl, Perdiem	Must be mixed with fluid.
	Methylcellulose	Citrocel, Cologel	Less gritty. Must be mixed with fluid.
	Polycarbophil	Fiberall, FiberCon, Mitrolan	Available as tablets.
Saline Saline laxatives contain either magnesium or phosphate. If your kidneys aren't working perfectly, as is the case in many people with diabetes, magnesium or phosphase in saline laxatives could build up in your blood. In general, we don't recommend that people with diabetes use these products. Most work in 30 minutes to three hours.	Magnesium citrate	Citroma, various generics	Magnesium may build up to toxic levels in people with kidney problems.
	Magnesium sulfate	Epsom salts, various products	Same as above.
	Magnesium hydroxide	Milk of Magnesia	Same as above.
	Sodium biphosphate	Fleet Enema	Works in 2 to 15 minutes.
	Sodium phosphate	Fleet Phosphas-soda	Phosphate may build up to toxic levels in people with kidney problems.
Stimulant Don't use these products more than three days in a row or for more than four days a month without your doctor's advice. These work in 6 to 10 hours. (Castor oil works more quickly but is not recommended.)	Bisacodyl	Dulcolax, Carter's Little Pills	
	Casanthranol	Lane's Pills	
	Cascara sagrada	various	
	Castor oil	Emulsoil, Purge, various	
	Phenophthalein	Ex-Lax Modane, Laxcaps, Evac-U-Lax	
	Senna	Senokot, Fletcher's Castoria	
Emollient Emollients, also called stool softeners, work in 1 to 3 days. Some people use them every day to prevent problems. If a stool softener alone doesn't do enough for you, you may want to take a fiber laxative as well.	Docusate sodium	Colace, Regutol, D-S-S	
	Docusate calcium	Surfak	
Lubricants	Mineral oil	Agoral Plain, various	Interferes with absorption of vitamins A, D, E, K. NOT recommended.

Source: Elizabeth P. Cowley, PharmD, and Stuart T. Haines, PharmD, "Return to Regular Life," *Diabetes Forecast*, 49(12), American Diabetes Association, © December 1996.

Diabetic Neuropathy: The Nerve Damage of Diabetes

WHAT IS DIABETIC NEUROPATHY?

Diabetic neuropathy is a nerve disorder caused by diabetes. Symptoms of neuropathy include numbness and sometimes pain in the hands, feet, or legs. Nerve damage caused by diabetes can also lead to problems with internal organs such as the digestive tract, heart, and sexual organs causing indigestion, diarrhea or constipation, dizziness, bladder infections, and impotence. In some cases, neuropathy can flare up suddenly, causing weakness and weight loss. Depression may follow. While some treatments are available, a great deal of research is still needed to understand how diabetes affects the nerves and to find more effective treatments for this complication.

HOW COMMON IS DIABETIC NEUROPATHY?

People with diabetes can develop nerve problems at any time. Significant clinical neuropathy can develop within the first 10 years after diagnosis of diabetes and the risk of developing neuropathy increases the longer a person has diabetes. Some recent studies have reported that:

- 60 percent of patients with diabetes have some form of neuropathy, but in most cases (30 to 40 percent), there are no symptoms.
- 30 to 40 percent of patients with diabetes have symptoms suggesting neuropathy, compared with 10 percent of people without diabetes.

DCCT: Can Diabetic Neuropathy Be Prevented?

A 10-year clinical study that involved 1,441 volunteers with insulin-dependent diabetes (IDDM) was recently completed by the National Institute of Diabetes and Digestive and Kidney Diseases. The study proved that keeping blood sugar levels as close to the normal range as possible slows the onset and progression of nerve disease caused by diabetes. The Diabetes Control and Complications Trials (DCCT) studied two groups of volunteers: those who followed a standard diabetes management routine and those who intensively managed their diabetes. Persons in the intensive management group took multiple injections of insulin daily or used an insulin pump and monitored their blood glucose at least four times a day to try to lower their blood glucose levels to the normal range. After 5 years, tests of neurological function showed that the risk of nerve damage was reduced by 60 percent in the intensively managed group. People in the standard treatment group, whose average blood glucose levels were higher, had higher rates of neuropathy. Although the DCCT included only patients with IDDM, researchers believe that people with noninsulin-dependent diabetes would also benefit from maintaining lower levels of blood glucose.

---

continues

continued

Diabetic neuropathy appears to be more common in smokers, people over 40 years of age, and those who have had problems controlling their blood glucose levels.

WHAT CAUSES DIABETIC NEUROPATHY?

Scientists do not know what causes diabetic neuropathy, but several factors are likely to contribute to the disorder. High blood glucose, a condition associated with diabetes, causes chemical changes in nerves. These changes impair the nerves' ability to transmit signals. High blood glucose also damages blood vessels that carry oxygen and nutrients to the nerves. In addition, inherited factors probably unrelated to diabetes may make some people more susceptible to nerve disease than others.

How high blood glucose leads to nerve damage is a subject of intense research. The precise mechanism is not known. Researchers have discovered that high glucose levels affect many metabolic pathways in the nerves, leading to an accumulation of a sugar called sorbitol and depletion of a substance called myoinositol. However, studies in humans have not shown convincingly that these changes are the mechanism that causes nerve damage.

More recently, researchers have focused on the effects of excessive glucose metabolism on the amount of nitrous oxide in nerves. Nitrous oxide dilates blood vessels. In a person with diabetes, low levels of nitrous oxide may lead to constriction of blood vessels supplying the nerve, contributing to nerve damage. Another promising area of research centers on the effect of high glucose attaching to proteins, altering the structure and function of the proteins and affecting vascular function.

Scientists are studying how these changes occur, how they are connected, how they cause nerve damage, and how to prevent and treat damage.

WHAT ARE THE SYMPTOMS OF DIABETIC NEUROPATHY?

The symptoms of diabetic neuropathy vary. Numbness and tingling in feet are often the first sign. Some people notice no symptoms, while others are severely disabled. Neuropathy may cause both pain and insensitivity to pain in the same person. Often, symptoms are slight at first, and since most nerve damage occurs over a period of years, mild cases may go unnoticed for a long time. In some people, mainly those afflicted by focal neuropathy, the onset of pain may be sudden and severe.

WHAT ARE THE MAJOR TYPES OF NEUROPATHY?

The symptoms of neuropathy also depend on which nerves and what part of the body is affected. Neuropathy may be diffuse, affecting many parts of the body, or focal, affecting a single, specific nerve and part of the body.

continues

continued

Diffuse Neuropathy

The two categories of diffuse neuropathy are peripheral neuropathy affecting the feet and hands and autonomic neuropathy affecting the internal organs.

Peripheral Neuropathy

The most common type of peripheral neuropathy damages the nerves of the limbs, especially the feet. Nerves on both sides of the body are affected. Common symptoms of this kind of neuropathy are:

- Numbness or insensitivity to pain or temperature
- Tingling, burning, or prickling
- Sharp pains or cramps
- Extreme sensitivity to touch, even light touch
- Loss of balance and coordination

These symptoms are often worse at night.

The damage to nerves often results in loss of reflexes and muscle weakness. The foot often becomes wider and shorter, the gait changes, and foot ulcers appear as pressure is put on parts of the foot that are less protected. Because of the loss of sensation, injuries may go unnoticed and often become infected. If ulcers or foot injuries are not treated in time, the infection may involve the bone and require amputation. However, problems caused by minor injuries can usually be controlled if they are caught in time. Avoiding foot injury by wearing well-fitted shoes and examining the feet daily can help prevent amputations.

Autonomic Neuropathy
(also called visceral neuropathy)

Autonomic neuropathy is another form of diffuse neuropathy. It affects the nerves that serve the heart and internal organs and produces changes in many processes and systems.

Urination and sexual response. Autonomic neuropathy most often affects the organs that control urination and sexual function. Nerve damage can prevent the bladder from emptying completely, so bacteria grow more easily in the urinary tract (bladder and kidneys). When the nerves of the bladder are damaged, a person may have difficulty knowing when the bladder is full or controlling it, resulting in urinary incontinence.

continues

continued

Diabetic Neuropathy Can Affect Virtually Every Part of the Body

Diffuse (Peripheral) Neuropathy

- Legs
- Feet
- Arms
- Hands

Diffuse (Autonomic) Neuropathy

- Heart
- Digestive system
- Sexual organs
- Urinary tract
- Sweat glands

Focal Neuropathy

- Eyes
- Facial muscles
- Hearing
- Pelvis and lower back
- Thigh
- Abdomen

The nerve damage and circulatory problems of diabetes can also lead to a gradual loss of sexual response in both men and women, although sex drive is unchanged. A man may be unable to have erections or may reach sexual climax without ejaculating normally.

Digestion. Autonomic neuropathy can affect digestion. Nerve damage can cause the stomach to empty too slowly, a disorder called gastric stasis. When the condition is severe (gastroparesis), a person can have persistent nausea and vomiting, bloating, and loss of appetite. Blood glucose levels tend to fluctuate greatly with this condition.

If nerves in the esophagus are involved, swallowing may be difficult. Nerve damage to the bowels can cause constipation or frequent diarrhea, especially at night. Problems with the digestive system often lead to weight loss.

Cardiovascular system. Autonomic neuropathy can affect the cardiovascular system, which controls the circulation of blood throughout the body. Damage to this system interferes with the

continues

continued

nerve impulses from various parts of the body that signal the need for blood and regulate blood pressure and heart rate. As a result, blood pressure may drop sharply after sitting or standing, causing a person to feel dizzy or light-headed, or even to faint (orthostatic hypotension).

Neuropathy that affects the cardiovascular system may also affect the perception of pain from heart disease. People may not experience angina as a warning sign of heart disease or may suffer painless heart attacks. It may also raise the risk of a heart attack during general anesthesia.

Hypoglycemia. Autonomic neuropathy can hinder the body's normal response to low blood sugar or hypoglycemia, which makes it difficult to recognize and treat an insulin reaction.

Sweating. Autonomic neuropathy can affect the nerves that control sweating. Sometimes, nerve damage interferes with the activity of the sweat glands, making it difficult for the body to regulate its temperature. Other times, the result can be produce sweating at night or while eating (gustatory sweating).

Focal Neuropathy
(including multiplex neuropathy)

Occasionally, diabetic neuropathy appears suddenly and affects specific nerves, most often in the torso, leg, or head. Focal neuropathy may cause:

- Pain in the front of a thigh
- Severe pain in the lower back or pelvis
- Pain in the chest, stomach, or flank
- Chest or abdominal pain sometimes mistaken for angina, heart attack, or appendicitis
- Aching behind an eye
- Inability to focus the eye
- Double vision
- Paralysis on one side of the face (Bell's palsy)
- Problems with hearing

This kind of neuropathy is unpredictable and occurs most often in older people who have mild diabetes. Although focal neuropathy can be painful, it tends to improve by itself after a period of weeks or months without causing long-term damage.

People with diabetes are also prone to developing compression neuropathies. The most common form of compression neuropathy is carpal tunnel syndrome. Asymptomatic carpal tunnel syndrome occurs in 20 to 30 percent of people with diabetes, and symptomatic carpal tunnel syndrome occurs in 6 to 11 percent. Numbness and tingling of the hand are the most common symptoms. Muscle weakness may also develop.

continues

continued

HOW DO DOCTORS DIAGNOSE DIABETIC NEUROPATHY?

A doctor diagnoses neuropathy based on symptoms and a physical exam. During the exam, the doctor may check muscle strength, reflexes, and sensitivity to position, vibration, temperature, and light touch. Sometimes special tests are also used to help determine the cause of symptoms and to suggest treatment.

A simple *screening test* to check point sensation in the feet can be done in the doctor's office. The test uses a nylon monofilament mounted on a small holder that has been standardized to deliver a 10-gram force when applied to areas of the feet. Patients who cannot sense pressure from the monofilament have lost protective sensation and are at risk for developing neuropathic foot ulcers. Physicians may order the monofilament (with instructions for use) free from the Gillis W. Long Hansen's Disease Center, Rehabilitation Branch, 5445 Point Clair Road, Carville, Louisiana 70721; telephone (504) 642-4710.

Nerve conduction studies check the flow of electrical current through a nerve. With this test, an image of the nerve impulse is projected on a screen as it transmits an electrical signal. Impulses that seem slower or weaker than usual indicate possible damage to the nerve. This test allows the doctor to assess the condition of all the nerves in the arms and legs.

Electromyography (EMG) is used to see how well muscles respond to electrical impulses transmitted by nearby nerves. The electrical activity of the muscle is displayed on a screen. A response that is slower or weaker than usual suggests damage to the nerve or muscle. This test is often done at the same time as nerve conduction studies.

Ultrasound employs sound waves. The sound waves are too high to hear, but they produce an image showing how well the bladder and other parts of the urinary tract are functioning.

Nerve biopsy involves removing a sample of nerve tissue for examination. This test is most often used in research settings.

If your doctor suspects autonomic neuropathy, you may also be referred to a physician who specializes in digestive disorders (gastroenterologist) for additional tests.

HOW IS DIABETIC NEUROPATHY USUALLY TREATED?

Treatment aims to relieve discomfort and prevent further tissue damage. The first step is to bring blood sugar under control by diet and oral drugs or insulin injections, if needed, and by careful monitoring of blood sugar levels. Although symptoms can sometimes worsen at first as blood sugar is brought under control, maintaining lower blood sugar levels helps reverse the pain or loss of sensation that neuropathy can cause. Good control of blood sugar may also help prevent or delay the onset of further problems.

continues

continued

Another important part of treatment involves special care of the feet, which are prone to problems.

A number of medications and other approaches are used to relieve the symptoms of diabetic neuropathy.

Relief of Pain

For relief of pain, burning, tingling, or numbness, the doctor may suggest an analgesic such as aspirin or acetaminophen or anti-inflammatory drugs containing ibuprofen. Nonsteroidal anti-inflammatory drugs should be used with caution in people with renal disease. Antidepressant medications such as amitriptyline (sometimes used with fluphenazine) or nerve medications such as carbamazepine or phenytoin sodium may be helpful. Codeine is sometimes prescribed for short-term use to relieve severe pain. In addition, a topical cream, capsaicin, is now available to help relieve the pain of neuropathy.

The doctor may also prescribe a therapy known as transcutaneous electronic nerve stimulations (TENS). In this treatment, small amounts of electricity block pain signals as they pass through a patient's skin. Other treatments include hypnosis, relaxation training, biofeedback, and acupuncture. Some people find that walking regularly or using elastic stockings helps relieve leg pain. Warm (not hot) baths, massage, or an analgesic ointment such as Ben Gay® may also help.

Gastrointestinal Problems

Indigestion, belching, nausea or vomiting are symptoms of gastroparesis. For patients with mild symptoms of slow stomach emptying, doctors suggest eating small, frequent meals and avoiding fats. Eating less fiber may also relieve symptoms. For patients with severe gastroparesis, the doctor may prescribe metoclopramide, which speeds digestion and helps relieve nausea. Other drugs that help regulate digestion or reduce stomach acid secretion may also be used or erythromycine may be prescribed. In each case, the potential benefits of these drugs need to be weighed against their side effects.

To relieve diarrhea or other bowel problems, antibiotics or clonidine HCl, a drug used to treat high blood pressure, are sometimes prescribed. The antibiotic tetracycline may be prescribed. A wheat-free diet may also bring relief since the gluten in flour sometimes causes diarrhea.

Neurological problems affecting the urinary tract can result in infections or incontinence. The doctor may prescribe an antibiotic to clear up an infection and suggest drinking more fluids to prevent further infections. If incontinence is a problem, patients may be advised to urinate at regular times (every 3 hours, for example) since they may not be able to tell when the bladder is full.

continues

continued

Dizziness, Weakness

Sitting or standing slowly may help prevent light-headedness, dizziness, or fainting, which are symptoms that may be associated with some forms of autonomic neuropathy. raising the head of the bed and wearing elastic stockings may also help. Increased salt in the diet and treatment with salt-retaining hormones such as fludrocortisone are other possible approaches. In certain patients, drugs used to treat hypertension can instead raise blood pressure, although predicting which patients will have this paradoxical reaction is difficult.

Muscle weakness or loss of coordination caused by diabetic neuropathy can often be helped by physical therapy.

Urinary and Sexual Problems

Nerve and circulatory problems of diabetes can disrupt normal male sexual function, resulting in impotence. After ruling out a hormonal cause of impotence, the doctor can provide information about methods available to treat impotence caused by neuropathy. Short-term solutions involve using a mechanical vacuum device or injecting a drug called a vasodilator into the penis before sex. Both methods raise blood flow to the penis, making it easier to have and maintain an erection. Surgical procedures, in which an inflatable or semirigid device is implanted in the penis, offer a more permanent solution. For some people, counseling may help relieve the stress caused by neuropathy and thereby help restore sexual function.

In women who feel their sexual life is not satisfactory, the role of diabetic neuropathy is less clear. Illness, vaginal or urinary tract infections, and anxiety about pregnancy complicated by diabetes can interfere with a woman's ability to enjoy intimacy. Infections can be reduced by good blood glucose control. Counseling may also help a woman identify and cope with sexual concerns.

WHY IS GOOD FOOT CARE IMPORTANT FOR PEOPLE WITH DIABETIC NEUROPATHY?

People with diabetes need to take special care of their feet. Neuropathy and blood vessel disease both increase the risk of foot ulcers. The nerves to the feet are the longest in the body, and are most often affected by neuropathy. Because of the loss of sensation caused by neuropathy, sores or injuries to the feet may not be noticed and may become ulcerated.

At least 15 percent of all people with diabetes eventually have a foot ulcer, and 6 out of every 1,000 people with diabetes have an amputation. However, doctors estimate that nearly three quarters of all amputations caused by neuropathy and poor circulation could be prevented with careful foot care.

continues

continued

To prevent foot problems from developing, people with diabetes should follow these rules for foot care:

- Check your feet and toes daily for any cuts, sores, bruises, bumps, or infections—using a mirror if necessary.
- Wash your feet daily, using warm (not hot) water and a mild soap. If you have neuropathy, you should test the water temperature with your wrist before putting your feet in the water. Doctors do not advise soaking your feet for long periods, since you may lose protective calluses. Dry your feet carefully with a soft towel, especially between the toes.
- Cover your feet (except for the skin between the toes) with petroleum jelly, a lotion containing lanolin, or cold cream before putting on shoes and socks. In people with diabetes, the feet tend to sweat less than normal. Using a moisturizer helps prevent dry, cracked skin.
- Wear thick, soft socks and avoid wearing slippery stockings, mended stockings, or stockings with seams.
- Wear shoes that fit your feet well and allow your toes to move. Break in new shoes gradually, wearing them for only an hour at a time at first. After years of neuropathy, as reflexes are lost, the feet are likely to become wider and flatter. If you have difficulty finding shoes that fit, ask your doctor to refer you to a specialist, called a pedorthist, who can provide you with corrective shoes or inserts.
- Examine your shoes before putting them on to make sure they have no tears, sharp edges, or objects in them that might injure your feet.
- Never go barefoot, especially on the beach, hot sand, or rocks.
- Cut your toenails straight across, but be careful not to leave any sharp corners that could cut the next toe.
- Use an emery board or pumice stone to file away dead skin, but do not remove calluses, which act as protective padding. Do not try to cuff off any growths yourself, and avoid using harsh chemicals such as wart remover on your feet.
- Test the water temperature with your elbow before stepping in a bath.
- If your feet are cold at night wear socks. (Do not use heating pads or hot water bottles.)
- Avoid sitting with your legs crossed. Crossing your legs can reduce the flow of blood to the feet.
- Ask your doctor to check your feet at every visit, and call your doctor if you notice that a sore is not healing well.
- If you are not able to take care of your own feet, ask your doctor to recommend a podiatrist (specialist in the care and treatment of feet) who can help.

ARE THERE ANY EXPERIMENTAL TREATMENTS FOR DIABETIC NEUROPATHY?

Several new drugs under study may eventually prevent or reverse diabetic neuropathy. However, extensive testing is required by the U.S. Food and Drug Administration to establish the safety and efficacy of drugs before they are approved for widespread use.

continues

continued

Researchers are exploring treatment with a compound called myoinositol. Early findings have shown that nerves in diabetic animals and humans have less than normal amounts of this substance. Myoinositol supplements increase the levels of this substance in tissues of diabetic animals, but research is still needed to show any concrete lasting benefits from this treatment.

Another area of research concerns the drug aminoguanidine. In animals, this drug blocks cross-linking of proteins that occurs more quickly than normal in tissues exposed to high levels of glucose. Early clinical tests are under way to determine the effects of aminoguanidine in humans.

One approach that appeared promising involved the use of aldose reductase inhibitors (ARIs). ARIs are a class of drugs that block the formation of the sugar alcohol sorbitol, which is thought to damage nerves. Scientists hoped these drugs would prevent and might even repair nerve damage. But so far, clinical trials have shown that these drugs have major side effects and, consequently, they are not available for clinical use.

NOTES:

Source: "Diabetic Neuropathy: The Nerve Damage of Diabetes," NIH Publication No. 97-3185, U.S. Department of Health and Human Services, National Institutes of Health, 1995.

Diabetic Ketoacidosis

WHAT IS KETOACIDOSIS?

The body is made of many cells. These cells need glucose from food for energy. When too little insulin is present, the body cannot use glucose for energy. It is then forced to break down fat for energy. The cells cannot use fat completely, and ketones are acids that result. Ketones enter the bloodstream and are toxic (poison) to the body. Ketones are passed out of the body in the urine. When this happens it is a warning sign that diabetes may be out of control. Diabetic ketoacidosis (DKA) is a medical emergency.

WARNING SIGNS OF KETOACIDOSIS

- Nausea, vomiting
- Stomach pains
- Weakness
- Difficulty breathing
- Fruity- or alcohol-smelling breath
- Blood sugar over 240 mg/dL

People who take insulin injections are more likely to experience ketoacidosis.

WHEN TO TEST URINE FOR KETONES

- If you feel sick or ill, test 3–4 times per day.
- When blood sugar is over 240 mg/dL.
- When you have the warning signs of ketoacidosis.

Urine testing strips for ketones may be purchased from the drugstore or diabetes supply center. *Use a fresh sample of urine.* Follow product directions. Examples of ketone testing strips are:

- Chemstrip K
- Ketodiastix
- Ketostix (Foil wrapped)

Call your doctor or nurse if you find moderate to large amounts of ketones in your urine.

Courtesy of Veterans Administration Medical Center, San Diego, California.

Ketoacidosis and Hyperosmolar Nonketotic Coma

KETOACIDOSIS (DIABETIC COMA)	HYPEROSMOLAR NONKETOTIC COMA (HONC)
Usually Type I Diabetes	Usually Type II Diabetes

WHAT IS KETOACIDOSIS?

Ketoacidosis occurs when the body uses fats for energy instead of sugar. This happens when there is:

1. Not enough insulin, *which causes*
2. Blood sugar to get too high, *which causes*
3. The body to use fats for energy, *which causes*
4. Fats to break down and make ketones

WHAT IS HONC?

HONC is a life-threatening emergency. It usually happens to older people with mild type II diabetes. The blood sugar is greater than 400 mg/dL. There is extreme dehydration (lack of fluid) in the body. The person may get confused.

CAUSES

1. Not taking enough **insulin**
2. Illness
3. Too much food
4. Too much stress

CAUSES

1. Dehydration
2. Blood sugar greater than 400 mg/dL
3. Illness
4. Vomiting or diarrhea
5. Operation or injury

SIGNS

1. Fast breathing
2. Fruity smell on breath
3. Pain in stomach
4. Ketones in urine
5. Vomiting
6. Coma

SIGNS

Signs may come on both quickly or slowly.

1. Weakness
2. Tiredness
3. Headache
4. Breathing hard
5. Vomiting
6. Confusion to coma

continues

continued

KETOACIDOSIS (DIABETIC COMA)	HYPEROSMOLAR NONKETOTIC COMA (HONC)
Usually Type I Diabetes	**Usually Type II Diabetes**

TREATMENT

The best treatment is **prevention**. Call the doctor if:

1. Blood sugar is over 250 mg/dL
2. Ketones are in the urine
3. Any of the above signs happen

This cannot be treated alone. If ketoacidosis goes untreated, death may occur.

TREATMENT

Prevention is the best treatment. Drink plenty of water each day. Call the doctor right away if any of the above signs happen. This cannot be treated at home.

Source: St. Joseph Rehabilitation Hospital and Outpatient Center, *Patient Education and Discharge Planning Manual for Rehabilitation,* Aspen Publishers, Inc., © 1995.

Diabetes, Type I, Adult

Patient Pathway

	First Visit after Initial Episode	Second Visit Second Week	Third Visit Third Week	Fourth Visit Fourth Week
Date				
Assessment	Your nurse practitioner or physician will give you a complete physical examination You will be asked what you know about your condition	You will have a physical examination We will go over the results of your blood work, review the results of your fingerstick diary, and discuss any problems you have with taking insulin	You will have a physical examination We will go over the results of your fasting blood sugar test	You will have a physical examination We will discuss the results of your fasting blood sugar test
Testing and Treatments	We will take blood tests and collect a urine sample	You will take a fingerstick test to find out your sugar level	You will take a fingerstick test to obtain blood sugar results	You will take a fingerstick test to find out your sugar level
Teaching and Instructions	You will receive instructions in using the One-Touch machine You will learn how to give yourself insulin properly, the importance of eating the proper foods, and what signs and symptoms to look for to identify elevated or low blood sugar You will learn how to change injection sites and how to dispose of your equipment	You will learn how diabetes, if not controlled, can affect your heart and kidney functioning You will demonstrate your insulin technique and review any other teaching for clarity You will learn the role that diet and exercise play in insulin	You will learn how diabetes can affect your circulation and the importance of foot care You will be shown how and when to calibrate the One-Touch	You will learn how diabetes can affect your nervous system You will learn how diabetes can affect your vision and the importance of a routine eye examination
Medications	You will be taking insulin daily to control the symptoms associated with high sugar in the blood in order to prevent any complications of diabetes	You are to continue with daily insulin The dose is to be adjusted according to your blood sugar levels	You are to continue with your daily insulin regimen	You are to continue insulin

continues

Diabetes, Type I, Adult continued

	First Visit after Initial Episode	Second Visit Second Week	Third Visit Third Week	Fourth Visit Fourth Week
Date				
Consulting Physicians or Services	A nutritionist is available to help you if needed	An exercise instructor is available on request and by appointment	We will make a referral to podiatry to maintain good foot care and prevent complications such as infection	We will refer you to an ophthalmologist for a thorough eye examination
Your Activities	Exercise is very beneficial in controlling glucose Before undertaking strenuous activities, however, an electrocardiogram will need to be taken Eat a well-balanced diet including complex carbohydrates, low cholesterol, and high fiber	After exercise, avoid administering insulin in the exercising limbs to prevent low blood sugar Administer the insulin in the abdomen Supplement three well-balanced meals with three snacks—midmorning, midafternoon, and before bed	You should continue your diet and exercise program, adjusting as required	
Your Questions and Additions	Questions: 1. 2. 3.	Questions: 1. 2. 3.	Questions: 1. 2. 3.	Questions: 1. 2. 3.

Source: Rufus S. Howe, RN, MN, FNP, *Clinical Pathways for Ambulatory Care Case Management*, Aspen Publishers, Inc., © 1998.

Diabetes, Type I, Pediatric—Sample 1

Patient Pathway

	First Visit after Initial Hospitalization	Second Visit 1 Month after Hospitalization	Third Visit Second Month and Every 2 to 3 Months	Annually
Date				
Assessment	Your nurse practitioner or physician will do a complete physical examination We will measure your height and weight on every visit to make sure you continue to grow and develop We will ask you to bring your daily log of your glucose and urine testing, and we will review your log with you We will want to know how you are doing in school and socially—we care about you	We will do a general physical examination with special attention to your injection sites, eyes, thyroid, and feet We will measure your height and weight and make sure you are developing We will review your home monitoring We will ask you how you are doing in school, socially, and how you are coping with your diabetes	We will do a general physical examination with special attention to your injection sites, eyes, thyroid, and feet We will measure your height and weight and make sure you are developing We will review your home monitoring We will ask you how you are doing in school, socially, and how you are coping with your diabetes	Every year we will do a complete physical examination An eye examination will be done by an ophthalmologist We will assess your adaptation and compliance to diabetes
Testing	You may need blood tests if you have not had recent ones during your hospital stay If your blood work is recent, we will ask you to do a fingerstick on your meter so we can check the accuracy of your meter We will test your urine for glucose and ketones	We will test your urine for sugar and ketones We will do a fingerstick for blood glucose level	We will test your urine for sugar and ketones We will do a fingerstick for blood glucose level Hba1c will be done every 2 to 3 months on your visit	Every year we will ask you to collect your urine for 24 hours We will do laboratory work for thyroid tests, chemistry, and cholesterol every year

continues

Diabetes, Type I, Pediatric—Sample 1 continued

	First Visit after Initial Hospitalization	Second Visit 1 Month after Hospitalization	Third Visit Second Month and Every 2 to 3 Months	Annually
Date				
Teaching	By this time you and/or your family should be comfortable with insulin injections, fingersticks, and your meter; we will ask you to demonstrate these techniques. We will continue to review all of your previous inpatient teaching about diabetes including: • Pathophysiology and complications of diabetes • Symptoms and management of hypo/hyperglycemia • Finger testing • Urine testing • Effects of exercise, illness, and stress on glucose levels • Glucagon • Diet • Insulin actions/peaks • Injections • Home monitoring • When to seek medical help Our goal is to make sure you and your family are comfortable dealing with your diabetes	We will continue to review all of your previous teaching. We will help you and your family with the management of your diabetes. We will ask and answer questions about your diabetes. We will review your diary at every visit and make adjustments, so be sure to bring it each time you come. By this time you and/or your family should be proficient at insulin injections and fingersticks; let us know if you are experiencing difficulty	We will continue to review all previous teaching, helping you and your family identify areas of needed education. We will continue to teach you and your family management of diabetes and how to adjust insulin requirements. By this time, you should be eating a well-balanced diet. Insulin injections and fingersticks have become part of your daily routine—done easily	We will review and modify your treatment based on your diary and physical examination. By this time, you and your family are managing most of your own care
Medications	We will review your insulin dosages and your sliding scale and make adjustments. We will train your family on how to use glucagon in case of an emergency	We will review your insulin dosages and sliding scale and make adjustments as needed	We will continue to review your insulin dosages and make adjustments. If you are experiencing a lot of high and low blood sugars, we will talk to you about an insulin pump	We will readjust insulin as needed if you have grown and gained weight

continues

Diabetes, Type I, Pediatric—Sample 1 continued

	First Visit after Initial Hospitalization	**Second Visit 1 Month after Hospitalization**	**Third Visit Second Month and Every 2 to 3 Months**	**Annually**
Date				
Consulting Physicians/ Referrals	You will have a nutritionist to help you plan your diet If you and your family are experiencing difficulty coping with your diabetes, we will arrange for you to talk to a psychologist to help you	We will give you a list of support groups to attend for children/families with diabetes We will tell you about special camps for children with diabetes that you may want to attend We will encourage you to see the dietitian if you are having difficulty with the diet We will ask your family to inform your school nurse and teachers about your condition	We will provide you a list of names and phone numbers of other children/families with diabetes with whom you may want to talk	Every year, we will ask you to see an ophthalmologist to examine your eyes Every year, we will arrange for you to see your nutritionist to make needed calorie adjustments in your diet
Activity	We want you to have a normal life with diabetes You can continue with sports We will ask you to check your blood sugar before and after exercising You may need to take a snack to boost blood sugar prior to activity You should stop if you feel weak, sweaty, or nauseous Always wear an identification bracelet and carry a snack Drink plenty of water to prevent dehydration	We may need to change your insulin dosages/snacks during exercise/sports It is important you continue to test your blood sugar before and after activity and report to us any symptoms of hypoglycemia so we can figure out what treatment is best for you Wear comfortable shoes/ sneakers to protect your feet Do not exercise alone	Your activity level may change daily so continue to keep track of your blood sugar before and after We want to make adjustments so you can be as active as you want without complications	By this time, you should see a pattern between exercise and blood sugar You will have a better idea of the snack you need and insulin coverage during exercise to prevent hypoglycemia
Your Questions and Additions	Questions: 1. 2. 3.	Questions: 1. 2. 3.	Questions: 1. 2. 3.	Questions: 1. 2. 3.

Source: Rufus S. Howe, RN, MN, FNP, *Clinical Pathways for Ambulatory Care Case Management,* Aspen Publishers, Inc., © 1998.

Diabetes, Type I, Pediatric—Sample 2

Patient Pathway

	First Visit 1 to 5 Days after Release from Hospital	Second Visit 6 to 14 Days after Last Visit or Sooner	Third Visit 2 Weeks after Last Visit or Sooner	Fourth Visit 2 to 3 Weeks after Last Visit or Sooner	Monthly Visit for 3 Months
Date					
Assessment	Your nurse practitioner or physician will perform a complete physical examination Special attention will be given to your heart, chest, stomach, eyes, and kidneys Your finger will be pricked so that we may determine the level of sugar in your blood A urine sample will also be obtained	A physical examination will be performed but it will be much quicker than the previous examination Your finger will be pricked to get blood to test for sugar The diary that you are keeping for blood sugar will be reviewed We will discuss your diet and exercise	Your finger will be pricked so that your blood can be tested for sugar The diary that you are keeping for blood sugar will be reviewed We will discuss your diet and exercise	A physical examination will be performed Your blood will be tested for sugar The diary that you are keeping for blood sugar will be reviewed We will discuss your diet and exercise	A physical examination will be performed Your blood will be tested for sugar We will review the diary you are keeping on your blood sugar We will discuss your diet and exercise
Testing and Treatments	You may need to give us blood and urine if recent results are not available Your weight will be taken	A urine sample will be needed You will be weighed	A urine sample will be needed You will be weighed	A urine sample will be needed You will be weighed	A urine sample will be needed Your height and weight will be measured A special blood test will be collected

continues

Diabetes, Type I, Pediatric—**Sample 2** continued

	First Visit 1 to 5 Days after Release from Hospital	Second Visit 6 to 14 Days after Last Visit or Sooner	Third Visit 2 Weeks after Last Visit or Sooner	Fourth Visit 2 to 3 Weeks after Last Visit or Sooner	Monthly Visit for 3 Months
Date					
Teaching and Instructions	We will teach you the proper way to store and get insulin ready We will show you how to fill a syringe with insulin and how to inject the insulin You will be told the warning signs when your blood sugar may be too high or too low We will show you how to measure the sugar in your blood and how to keep a diary on the readings that you get The diet that you should be eating will be discussed	You and your provider will discuss a plan so that your blood sugar will remain under control The warning signs of low or high blood sugar will again be discussed You will be shown how to rotate the place where you inject the insulin An exercise plan will be constructed and the preparations for exercise will be discussed You and your family will learn about a special medicine that may have to be injected when your blood sugar is too low	We will review and modify your treatment plan with special emphasis on how you are dealing with insulin injections, your diet, and exercise	We will review and modify your treatment plan based on your diary and physical examination	We will review and modify your treatment plan based on your diary and physical examination
Medications	You will be using two very different types of insulin One is regular insulin, which is very short acting and will reduce your blood sugar in a short time The other insulin is NPH, which will lower your blood sugar later in the day It is important that you give yourself the right amount of each type of insulin	You will give yourself the right amount of insulin at the right time as determined by you and your provider You will also learn about another medicine that you or your family can give you if your blood sugar is too low	You will take your insulin according to the treatment plan you and your provider created in regard to your diet and exercise	You will continue to use the correct amount of insulin that your body requires for the diet and exercise that you have maintained	By now you will have balanced your insulin needs with your diet and exercise

continues

Diabetes, Type I, Pediatric—Sample 2 continued

	First Visit 1 to 5 Days after Release from Hospital	Second Visit 6 to 14 Days after Last Visit or Sooner	Third Visit 2 Weeks after Last Visit or Sooner	Fourth Visit 2 to 3 Weeks after Last Visit or Sooner	Monthly Visit for 3 Months
Date					
Consulting Services	You will meet with a dietitian who will plan your diet with you. The dietitian will explain the foods that you need to avoid and the foods that you can eat				Once a year a physician will examine your eyes to make sure that they are okay. You should see your dentist twice a year to make sure that there are no problems with your teeth
Your Activities	You are going to have to avoid simple sugars that are found in candy, cakes, ice cream, juices, and so forth. On special occasions (e.g., your birthday) you can enjoy these things as long as your provider is aware. It is very important that you stay on the diet that is provided	It is important that you learn when your blood sugar may be high or low by the way you feel	You and your provider will try to balance your insulin, diet, and exercise with your activities	You and your provider will try to balance your insulin, diet, and exercise with your activities	By this time you and your provider will have balanced your insulin, diet, and exercise so that your activities will not be limited
Your Questions and Additions	Questions: 1. 2. 3.	Questions: 1. 2. 3.	Questions: 1. 2. 3.	Questions: 1. 2. 3.	Questions: 1. 2. 3.

Source: Rufus S. Howe, RN, MN, FNP, *Clinical Pathways for Ambulatory Care Case Management*, Aspen Publishers, Inc., © 1998.

Diabetes, Type II—Sample 1

Patient Pathway

	First Visit	Second Visit 2 to 3 Days after Visit	Third Visit 1 Week after Second Visit	Fourth Visit 2 Weeks after Last Visit	Every Month
Date					
Assessment	Your nurse practitioner will perform a physical examination on you			Today your nurse practitioner will listen to your heart and lungs and check your pulses and your feet	Today and each month, you will have a complete physical examination
Testing and Treatment	We will need to take blood and urine tests today These tests will determine if you have any sugar in your blood or urine As you were instructed on the phone, we need to take these tests *before* you eat anything	Please do not eat before your visit today We will need to take a sample of blood from your finger to check your blood sugar before you eat breakfast We will also need to do an electrocardiogram to see how well your heart is functioning	Please do not eat before your visit UNLESS you are taking medication for diabetes If you are taking medication, eat and take your medication as instructed We will again be taking a sample of blood from your finger This test will see how well you are doing with your treatment regimen and will help your nurse practitioner to adjust your medication properly	Same as last visit	Each month we will take a blood sample from your finger Please remember to take your medications as instructed Every 3 months we will do a special blood test to see how your blood sugar has been during that time period Once a year we will test your blood and urine and do an electrocardiogram to see how well your heart is doing
Teaching and Instructions	Today we will discuss the symptoms of diabetes and how family history and obesity play a role in who gets the disease	Your nurse practitioner will discuss the results of your laboratory tests with you today If your blood sugar is high today, you will receive a card to carry stating that you are a diabetic	Today your nurse practitioner will discuss with you what you learned from the nutritionist Also discussed will be why exercise is important for you and how to safely start an exercise program	Today your nurse practitioner will discuss with you why it is important to monitor your blood sugar at home and tell you how to obtain a machine to do this	Your blood glucose log will be reviewed Your nurse practitioner will discuss sick day routine with you today

continues

Diabetes, Type II—Sample 1 continued

	First Visit	Second Visit 2 to 3 Days after Visit	Third Visit 1 Week after Second Visit	Fourth Visit 2 Weeks after Last Visit	Every Month
Date					
Medications	Depending on the amount of sugar in your blood today and at the next visit, you may be started on an oral medication to help lower it	If your blood sugar is high today, you will receive a prescription for a pill to help lower it You will also be told the possible side effects of this medication	We will continue to monitor whether or not to keep you on medication (or to raise the dosage if necessary)	We will continue to adjust your medications according to what your blood sugar values are	Same as last visit
Consulting Physicians or Services		You will be referred to a nutritionist to help you understand what types of food are best for you	Because diabetes can affect your eyes and your feet, your nurse practitioner will refer you to an ophthalmologist and a podiatrist	Diabetics tend to have problems with their teeth and gums If you do not have a dentist, your nurse practitioner will refer you to one Today you will receive the telephone number of the American Diabetes Association Please call to find out about support groups for diabetics in your area	
Your Questions and Additions	Questions: 1. 2. 3.	Questions: 1. 2. 3.	Questions: 1. 2. 3.	Questions: 1. 2. 3.	Questions: 1. 2. 3.

Source: Rufus S. Howe, RN, MN, FNP, *Clinical Pathways for Ambulatory Care Case Management*, Aspen Publishers, Inc., © 1998.

Diabetes, Type II—Sample 2

Patient Pathway

	First Visit after Diagnosis	Second Visit 1 Month after Initial Visit	Third Visit 2 Months after Second Visit	Fourth Visit 3 Months after Third Visit	Fifth Visit 3 Months after Fourth Visit	Sixth Visit 3 Months after Fifth Visit
Date						
Assessment	Your nurse practitioner will obtain a complete history and will physically examine you with special attention to your skin, eyes, thyroid, heart, lungs, pulses, feet Your height, weight, blood pressure, pulse, respiratory rate will be taken We will measure your glucose level	You will have an interim physical examination of your heart, lungs, thyroid, pulses, feet, weight, and vital signs (pulse, respiratory rate) We will measure your blood glucose level	You will have an interim physical examination We will review your home monitoring diary We will evaluate glycemic control We will measure your blood glucose level We will assess the signs and symptoms of hyper/hypoglyce-mia	You will have an interim physical examination We will review your home monitoring diary We will evaluate glycemic control We will measure your blood glucose level We will assess the signs and symptoms of hyper/hypoglyce-mia	You will have an interim physical examination We will review your home monitoring diary We will evaluate glycemic control We will assess the signs and symptoms of hyper/hypoglyce-mia We will measure your blood sugar level	You will have a complete physical examination once a year
Testing and Treatments	You will need a few blood and urine tests to obtain a baseline to help guide your treatment	You will need your blood sugar tested	You will need your blood sugar tested and have a blood test to determine your blood sugar over the past 3 months	You will need your blood sugar tested	You will need your blood sugar tested and have a blood test to determine your blood sugar over the past 3 months	Once a year you will have all your initial blood and urine tests repeated

continues

Diabetes, Type II—Sample 2 continued

	First Visit after Diagnosis	Second Visit 1 Month after Initial Visit	Third Visit 2 Months after Second Visit	Fourth Visit 3 Months after Third Visit	Fifth Visit 3 Months after Fourth Visit	Sixth Visit 3 Months after Fifth Visit
Date						
Teaching and Instructions	You will meet with a dietitian to guide your meal planning You will receive instructions about your medicines and diet/exercise control of your diabetes You will learn to recognize and treat low blood sugar and the signs and symptoms of high blood sugar You will learn about diabetes mellitus and its complications	You will receive instructions and demonstration of how to use your home glucose monitor and how to keep a diary of blood sugar You will take your medication according to your treatment plan, which you and your provider will develop We will discuss ways to control your blood sugar	We will discuss obstacles to glycemic control and how to manage them We will review and modify your treatment plan based on your physical examination, blood glucose, and home glucose diary You will know when to seek medical care	We will review and modify your treatment plan based on your home glucose diary and physical examination	We will review and modify your treatment plan based on your home glucose diary and physical examination	We will review and modify your treatment plan based on your home glucose diary and physical examination
Medications			Individuals with type 2 diabetes mellitus produce some insulin Oral medications work with the insulin your body produces or on the production or utilization of sugar	You will take your medication according to your treatment plan	You will take your medication according to your treatment plan	You will take your medication according to your treatment plan

continues

Diabetes, Type II—Sample 2 continued

	First Visit after Diagnosis	Second Visit 1 Month after Initial Visit	Third Visit 2 Months after Second Visit	Fourth Visit 3 Months after Third Visit	Fifth Visit 3 Months after Fourth Visit	Sixth Visit 3 Months after Fifth Visit
Date						
Consulting Physicians or Services	You will meet with a dietitian to help plan an acceptable daily menu to manage your diabetes. Diabetes mellitus can affect your eyes; you will see an ophthalmologist who will dilate and examine your eyes	If you are a smoker we will talk to you about a program to stop. If you develop complications of diabetes mellitus you may need to see a physician who specializes in treatment of that complication	You may want to speak with others who are experiencing similar feelings and are adjusting to diabetes. You may want to join a support group		You may meet with the dietitian if you have questions or want to review your diet	Once a year you will have your eyes examined by an ophthalmologist who will dilate your eyes
Your Activities	Exercise/walking daily or at least three times a week for 30 minutes can help to control your blood sugar and improve your circulation	You may need to limit some activity if you develop pain in your extremities. You may want to adjust your diet according to amount of exercise	You should continue to exercise. You should wear supportive sneakers and thick cotton socks. Exercise/walking increase to five times a week for 30 minutes	You should continue your exercise and meal plan	You should continue your exercise and meal plan	You should continue your exercise and meal plan
Your Questions and Additions	Questions: 1. 2. 3.	Questions: 1. 2. 3.	Questions: 1. 2. 3.	Questions: 1. 2. 3.	Questions: 1. 2. 3.	Questions: 1. 2. 3.

Source: Rufus S. Howe, RN, MN, FNP, *Clinical Pathways for Ambulatory Care Case Management*, Aspen Publishers, Inc., © 1998.

Diabetes, Type II—Sample 2 continued

This is an explanation of the visits you will make to _____ to learn about your diabetes.

The telephone number is _____.

The name of your health care provider is _____.

In managing your diabetes you may experience times of high or low blood sugar, or be unable to control your blood sugar because of an illness. If you need help managing your diabetes at any time call us.

Your next appointment is _____.

_____

Questions I want answered at my next appointment:

1. _____
_____

2. _____
_____

3. _____
_____

4. _____
_____

5. _____
_____

Source: Rufus S. Howe, RN, MN, FNP, *Clinical Pathways for Ambulatory Care Case Management,* Aspen Publishers, Inc., © 1998.

Diabetes, Type II—Sample 3

Patient Pathway

Date	Follow-up Week 1	Follow-up Weeks 2 to 3	Follow-up Weeks 5 to 6	Follow-up 3 Months
Assessment	Your nurse practitioner will do a thorough physical examination, check your weight, pulses, blood pressure, heart, lungs, and skin Your personal support system will be discussed	Same as first visit We will review entries in your diary over the last 2 weeks such as diet, activity, symptoms of frequent thirst, hunger, urination, and feelings of weakness or low blood sugar	Same as first two visits	Same as first two visits
Testing and Treatments	A urine specimen and a fingerstick blood test will be performed to check your sugar	Same as first visit	Same as first visit	Same as first visit A venous blood test called Hba1c will be done to monitor your blood glucose pattern over the last 3 months
Teaching and Counseling	Your nurse practitioner will discuss with you the importance of understanding and accepting the diagnosis of diabetes You will be shown how to keep a diary of events, activities, and symptoms We will discuss five important topics: diabetic diet, daily exercise, medication that you may need to take every day, how to check your blood and urine at home, and how to recognize and take action when hypoglycemia occurs	We will review the first visit We will review diet planning, foods to avoid, meal selection, and preparation of foods Diabetes management literature will be made available to you	We will briefly review the first visit We will discuss exercise planning and foot care	We will stress the need for regular eye examinations We will discuss the need to avoid alcohol and tobacco We will address the use of Medic-Alert tags

continues

Diabetes, Type II—Sample 3 continued

	Follow-up Week 1	Follow-up Weeks 2 to 3	Follow-up Weeks 5 to 6	Follow-up 3 Months
Date				
Medications	The nurse practitioner will discuss with you the medications (if any) that you need to take and how to take them. The nurse practitioner will also discuss over-the-counter drugs and drugs that interfere with your new medication	Same as first visit	Same as first visit	Same as first visit
Consulting Physicians or Services	At any time you may be asked to see a specialist to recheck your eyes, feet, and heart. You may be asked to see another practitioner who is an expert in diabetes	If you wish to attend seminars for diabetics, or you wish to get additional help with losing weight or meal planning, you can be referred to a dietitian	The American Diabetes Association and the public library are sources of helpful information for you	Remember, too, that you can consult your practitioner when you have questions or problems or a change in symptoms
Your Activities and Outcomes	You can probably continue your routine activities as long as you do not have severe symptoms of hypoglycemia and/or as long as you can incorporate your new diabetic regimen of diet, exercise, medications, and glucose monitoring as instructed	You will need to plan for proper snacks and plan for emergency care for low blood sugar by keeping a simple sugar (like candy) in your car, at work or school, and always nearby or in your pocket. You will need to check with your insurance company for payment for the home glucose monitoring kit and supplies	You will have to take extra good care of your feet by wearing proper shoes, preventing calluses, and reporting any foot or skin infection (even if it seems minor) to your practitioner promptly	Always report that you are diabetic to any practitioner that you are treated by
Your Questions and Comments about Diabetes	Questions: 1. 2. 3.	Questions: 1. 2. 3.	Questions: 1. 2. 3.	Questions: 1. 2. 3.

Source: Rufus S. Howe, RN, MN, FNP, *Clinical Pathways for Ambulatory Care Case Management*, Aspen Publishers, Inc., © 1998.

Index

Social Security income, disability income, 239
Socks, 255
Sodium consumption, 64
Stimulant laxatives, 269–270
Stress, 154
Stroke, 7
Sucrose consumption, 63
Sulfonylureas, 34–35, 161
Surgery, 149
Sweating, 276
Sweets, concentrated, 193
Symptoms, 112
Syringes, caring for, 179
Systolic Hypertension in the Elderly Program, 52

T

Teaching plan, NIDDM, 67–69
Teaching sheet, 70–71
Therapy
  algorithm, type II diabetes, 11
  nonpharmacological, 34
  pharmacological, 34–35
Thrush, 258
Toddler feeding guidelines, 197
Toenails, 253
Tolinase, 170
Tonometry, 244
Tooth brushing, Spanish version, 262–263
Tours, 163
Transcutaneous electronic nerve stimulations, 278
Transplantation, 214
Traveler's diarrhea, 160
Traveling, 156–163
Treatment, 6
  of cardiovascular disease, 44–45
  of constipation, 266–271
  of diabetes, 117
  of diabetic ketoacidosis, 18

of diabetic neuropathy, 48, 277–279, 280–281
of eye disease, 40
of foot problems, 50–51
of gestational diabetes, 23–24
of hyperglycemic hypersomolar nonketotic coma, 283–284
of hypoglycemia, 20, 45
of kidney disease, 41–42, 220–221
patient involvement in, 16
of periodontal disease, 37
of pregestational diabetes, 22–23

U

Ultrasound, 277
Urea reduction ratio, 229, 230
Urinary problems, 217, 279
Urination, 274–275
Urine test, 28, 115, 127, 282

V

Vanadium, 181
Vegetarian exchange lists, 198–202
Veterans Administration benefits, 239
Visceral neuropathy, 274–276
Vision
  altered, 32
  blurred, 240
  loss, 210, 213
  problems, 240
Visual abnormalities, 31. *See also* Diabetic retinopathy
Visual acuity test, 244
Vitrectomy, 241, 246

W

Weakness, 279
Weight, 43
Women, heart disease and, 216